D0029779

Please turn the page for more reviews. . . .

THE NATURE OF
ANIMAL HEALING

The Path to Your Pet's Health,

Happiness, and Longevity

MARTIN GOLDSTEIN, D.V.M.

BALLANTINE BOOKS · NEW YORK

A Ballantine Book
Published by The Random House Publishing Group

Published in the United States by Ballantine Books, an imprint of The Random
House Publishing Group, a division of Random House, Inc., New York, and
simultaneously in Canada by Random House of Canada Limited, Toronto.
Originally published in a slightly different form
by Alfred A. Knopf, a division of Random House, Inc., in 1999.

www.ballantinebooks.com

This book is intended to reach readers about therapies and supplements used by
Dr. Martin Goldstein in his veterinary practice, and to serve as a guide for them in
seeking treatment for their pets. However, this book is *not* intended as a substitute
for proper veterinary care. Readers whose pets may be experiencing medical
problems or symptoms should consult a veterinarian.

Grateful acknowledgment is made to The Random House Publishing Group, a
division of Random House, Inc., and the Denise Marcil Literary Agency, Inc., for
permission to reprint the "Shiki" anecdote from *Keep Your Dog Healthy the
Natural Way* by Pat Lazarus, copyright © 1999 by Pat Lazarus. Reprinted by
permission of The Random House Publishing Group, a division of Random House,
Inc., and the Denise Marcil Literary Agency, Inc.

Library of Congress Catalog Card Number: 00-190159

ISBN 0-345-43919-8

This edition published by arrangement with Alfred A. Knopf, a division of
Random House, Inc.

Manufactured in the United States of America

Cover photo by Leo Sorel

First Trade Paperback Edition: June 2000

16 18 19 17

CONTENTS

ACKNOWLEDGMENTS

Whenever I read a book, I start with the acknowledgments and try to picture the network of people who have supported the writer, enabling him to complete his work. I realize that, like Academy Award speeches, these tributes should be kept short. But I also think it is vital to acknowledge those who have loaned that extra hand, since no one can really do it alone.

To brother Bob and sister Susan for playing this game with me;
To the very special people who were there during those times when extra support was needed: Karen Miller, Suzen Ellis, Cathy Soukup, Barbara Lazaroff, Milly Duncan, Barbara Newington, Rosemarie Frigerio, Andrea Eastman, Colleen Camp-Goldwyn, Carol Marangoni, Marty Leaf, and Cindy Meehl;
To Dave Worthen for being in a class by yourself;
To Dr. Martin DeAngelis, whose ethics and guidance have helped construct my walls of responsibility, and whose rigorous criticisms of this book in manuscript were so extraordinarily helpful;
To my cowriter Michael Shnayerson for your relentless support and intuitive communication, and for helping me convert my thoughts and work into this book;
To my editor, Peter Gethers, and my agent, Meredith Bernstein, for your faith in my work;
To all my staff at Smith Ridge, both past and especially present, for your incredible support and effort. Special thanks to Julie, Michael, Linda, Meg, and Nancy;
To Dr. Lawrence Burton, for your genius and dedication to the fight against cancer;
To L. Ron Hubbard, whose works have enlightened me on my path;
To Mom and Dad, may you already be back to read this;
To Roscoe, a golden retriever who introduced me to Helen, Paul, and Lena, and who serves as a fitting example of all the animals through whom I have made some of my dearest acquaintances;
To the rest of my family and friends, too numerous to list, for all your love and support.

And two very special acknowledgments:
To the healing force of Nature for always being there. And to the Animals— your presence in my life has made it all worthwhile, and your absence would make it all so empty.

THE NATURE OF
ANIMAL HEALING

Saving the Kingdom

If animals could talk, here's what they'd say.

For starters, *about that food.* Why, they'd ask, do you give me the same boring pet chow day after day? *You* don't have that kind of diet. You have different foods for every meal—and the foods you eat are *real*! Why wouldn't we want real food, too? Don't we have the same bodily needs? As it is, the dry kibble is boring, the canned food is gross, and neither kind seems to impart much nutrition. How, they'd ask, can a pet expect to feel peppy—never mind healthy—on that?

Perhaps, they'd add, having thought long and hard on the subject, there's some connection between poor food and poor health. Certainly you take us to the veterinarian more than ever before. Yet why, they'd ask, do visits to the clinic often leave us feeling worse in the long run? We come in with a skin inflammation, we're given a steroid; for a while we feel better, but then the effect fades. We go back with a fever, get an antibiotic; the fever goes down, but something else comes up. We get vaccines—five, six, seven ingredients at a time—meant to protect us against disease, yet days or even months later we feel sluggish and sick. Just as we're finally shaking off the ill effects, back we go to the veterinarian for more.

And if all that conventional medicine is supposed to keep us well, they'd ask, why are so many animals getting seriously sick? Why, in particular, is there so much cancer? Why are so many dying before their time?

Pets don't talk to me either, but they don't need to. I see the results of bad diet and misguided conventional medicine every day. Admittedly, my clinic is somewhat different from the standard veterinary hospital. Like the doctors on *ER*, we take more than our share of desperate cases—basket cases, as some of my colleagues in the field put it. Though I certainly see healthy pets, many of the animals I treat have been given less than a month to live. They have some form of severe, premature degeneration: arthritis, kidney or liver failure, hyperthyroidism, or, most frequently, some form of cancer.

If I were just seeing a small, steady trickle of extreme cases, year in, year out, you could stop reading right now. What, you could say, are the chances of your pet becoming one of those statistics? And if he did, that would just be fate, right? Bad luck out of the blue?

Unfortunately, it's not that simple.

Twenty-five years ago when I started out in practice, the pets I saw with these diseases were old. Their conditions seemed to be age-related, and slow-growing enough to be accepted. Of the cases I see now, many are young and don't live past the age of five. It's no longer unusual to see a three-year-old cat with kidney failure. Or an eighteen-month-old dog with part of its jaw eaten away by cancer.

If the age of these patients is troubling, so too is the rate at which their diseases now grow. Not that long ago—in April 1997—I treated a seven-year-old Rottweiler named Wrinkles who had a huge, mushroom-shaped tumor next to her rectum; the tumor, a spindle cell sarcoma, had already grown back after being removed by a board-certified surgeon. I dug in, with my hands and instruments, *four inches* to grasp the extent of it and cut it out. Then I froze the remaining diseased cells with liquid nitrogen, destroying nearly 100 percent of her clinical cancer. Two weeks later, Wrinkles' owner called to report that the tumor had begun growing back, and was already the size of a walnut. That was on a Thursday. I asked the owner to bring her in on Monday to prepare her for another surgery. By then, the tumor was the size of a grapefruit. It was a case that even I, who rarely gives up on any pet, conceded was hopeless; I put her to sleep.

Fortunately, we're able to save many of the pets we treat—to restore them to health, or at least to give them an extended period of happy life which they weren't expected to have. But the challenge grows as the conditions we see get more aggressive, more unpredictable, and more bizarre.

The fact that we're now treating up to thirty-five new cases of cancer a *week*, far more than just a few years ago, is in a sense misrepresentative: cancer-stricken pets from all over the country are flown or driven in to us now, through clinic referrals or, increasingly, the Internet. But ask your local veterinarian if he's seen more cancer in recent years. Of course he has. A 1998 survey of disease-related death among pets by the nonprofit Morris Animal Foundation bears this out. Of 720 canine deaths reported, 479 were cancer-caused. The next highest category was heart-related problems (12 percent), followed by kidney (7 percent) and epilepsy (4 percent). Among 468 feline deaths, cancer also ranked highest (32 percent), followed by kidney and urinary disease (23 percent) and heart problems (9 percent). This raises the obvious questions: Why? And can anything be done about it?

As a holistic veterinarian, I don't view cancer as a mysterious disease that attacks the body. *It's the ultimate manifestation of ill health.* It's what happens when the body's immune system, under siege for too long, at last surrenders, letting cell growth go awry. To me, it's clear that more and more pets are getting cancer and other degenerative diseases because they're being hit with more and more toxins that eventually mutate their genes, weakening successive generations.

The assault begins with those processed and packaged foods that most of us give our pets. Mediocre at best, they often contain toxins in their chemical additives and preservatives, or in reprocessed "meat" unfit for human consumption. Other toxins are absorbed from tap water or ground chemicals. A great number of cancer-producing toxins in pets come, I believe, from certain conventional drugs meant to *improve* their health. All this is accelerated, of course, by animals' relatively short life spans. Just in the time most of us have been alive, many generations of pets have come and gone. With each generation, the incidence of genetic diseases, including cancer, has increased.

Cancer is the far marker, the defining outer limit of how toxic our world has become, and of what those toxins can do to animals. But almost every lesser manifestation of ill health is also aggravated by toxins that inhibit the immune system and keep an animal from healing itself. And all too often, when an animal desperately needs its toxins reduced, conventional medicine responds by adding *more*.

Some years ago, a white terrier named Blake was brought into our clinic. At twenty-eight months of age, he had skin that was darkened, flaky, smelly, highly inflamed, and so itchy that he'd scratched off half his fur. He was truly suffering. We see a lot of patients with skin problems, by the way, and we see more of them now, in worse shape, than we did a decade ago. A conventional veterinarian had initially concluded—correctly—that Blake had severe allergies to such items as grasses, wool, fleas, and molds. Also, he had a secondary bacterial infection of the skin. The veterinarian had deduced that the rugs in the house contained the most immediate allergens tormenting Blake, and so the rugs had been removed. At the same time, Blake had been put on a series of different hypoallergenic diets. He'd also been subjected to a battery of desensitization injections after undergoing allergy testing, treatments with cortisone, antibiotics, and medicated shampoos, and finally even chemotherapy. When nothing worked, the veterinarian recommended having Blake put to sleep.

First, we put Blake on dietary supplements, most of which were based on his individual deficiencies, determined by blood analysis. We administered homeopathic remedies, initially by injection, then orally. We also gave him naturally derived injectable cortisone. As we did, we weaned him off all the prescription drugs he was on. Nine months later, Blake had perfect skin, his fluffy white coat had grown in fully, and he was a happy, healthy dog. My silent partner in Blake's revival? Blake. The dietary supplements gave him new strength, then Blake simply healed himself.

The rugs, by the way, eventually went back into the house. They did contain allergens, but with Blake's immune system back in top shape, they didn't bother him at all.

This is where holistic medicine begins: with the belief that *the best way to cure an ill patient is to help him cure himself.*

"Cure" is a risky word to use—in our society, it implies a promise of eradication of symptoms for life. However, a *reasonable* state of cure, more appropriately known as remission, in which the patient's pain diminishes and his sense of well-being improves, is definitely and readily attainable when the patient is able to martial his own immune system to combat ill health. The body's immune system is the best defense, far better than man-made drugs. Keep it strong, restore it if it's weak, and the body, which is one amazing creation, will do almost whatever needs to be done to heal what's ailing it. When health has been restored, it *can* be maintained—if the immune system is sustained.

Once, those words would have seemed naïve, if not blasphemous, to me. I didn't start out as a holistic veterinarian. I graduated in 1973 from Cornell University's College of Veterinary Medicine, considered by most in the field to be among the top-rated in the United States, and began my practice with as conservative an outlook on medicine as any of my colleagues. Little by little, out of curiosity, I began opening up, trying "new" alternatives that predated conventional medicine, from acupuncture to homeopathy, and finding, to my surprise and delight, that they worked. Today at the Smith Ridge Center I oversee in South Salem, New York, we still apply conventional medicine when needed: from setting broken legs to administering the occasional direly needed antibiotic. But we find that 95 percent of the cases we take on can be treated alternatively. That includes healthy pets, whom we put on our special regimen of good food and dietary supplements to *prevent* their health from deteriorating. And it applies almost without exception to pets with common irritations—fleas, flaky skin, allergies, colitis—who are conventionally treated with drugs and chemicals that can do more harm than good. As for pets with extreme conditions whom we treat holistically, it's important to realize that we're not miracle workers: we don't save every one we treat. *However, of the pets we do save, most have been deemed hopeless by veterinarians using conventional medicine.*

In the twenty-five years I've been in practice, a growing number of veterinarians have come to call themselves holistic. The American Holistic Veterinary Medical Association has seven hundred members, all veterinarians trained at conventional veterinary schools for the four years it takes to be licensed (after four years of undergraduate work). Just as it's becoming more and more accepted in the medical treatment of humans, so too has holistic treatment gained at least some credibility in helping animals. But it still isn't as commonplace as it could and should be.

At Tufts, considered one of the most liberal veterinary schools, a group of some thirty holistically minded students had to lobby hard and long last year before being allowed to arrange a two-day, unaccredited seminar in acupuncture. At other schools, acupuncture simply doesn't exist as a course of treatment, much less one deserving of academic status. The result: Many graduating veterinarians remain ignorant of such holistic approaches, and of the actual harm they're doing to animals by perpetuating certain conventional methods. Only by seeking out alternatives on their own can they begin to change the way they practice. But how many have the curiosity—let alone the time—to do that? And of those few who do, how many are willing to implement what they've learned?

In the pages that follow, I'll explain how I approach different medical problems, and go into some detail on administering complementary products and preparations for disease and health states. I believe that this approach, and all it entails, will keep your pet healthier and happier, and prolong his life. But I don't mean for this to be a how-to book of holistic medicine that tells you, as a pet owner, all you need to know to be a do-it-yourself veterinarian. Those books exist for any who wish to find them; in my experience, as illuminating as they may be, they also lead to frustration. More times than I can count, an owner has brought in his obviously sick pet and rattled off a list of vitamins he's tried. His pet, however, is still sick. Our pets, like us, are all individuals, all with different requirements. So what works for one may not work for another. A young pet, for example, will often have an immune system far more capable of repelling a serious illness than that of an older pet. But sometimes a young pet is so genetically predisposed to immune deficiency that he will not respond as well as an older patient who has slowly built up his immune deficiency. Treatment for each should vary accordingly.

My aim with this book is a more immediate one: to demonstrate the ways in which our pets are being ill served by us, by their environments, and, yes, by some aspects of conventional veterinary medicine. I hope to be, in effect, a voice for these pets, because they cannot talk. I want to show that with the right care, they can still lead healthy lives. And I intend to make clear that we are not the true healers of our pets; *they* are. The best we can do is to help them grow as strong as they can, both physically and emotionally, so that they can best tackle the hard work they must do to regain and maintain their own health.

The fact is, with the right *diet*, a healthy kitten, puppy, or other young animal may not need any sort of veterinary care beyond annual checkups. I have three dogs of my own: Nina, a five-and-a-half-year-old Pomeranian; eighteen-month-old Kooper, also a Pomeranian; and Clayton, a six-year-old poodle. They have a proper, balanced diet of real food, nutritional supplements, and pure water. Aside from receiving an initial round of minimal vaccines, none of them has had to make the short trip to my office for professional care. The same holds true for my cats: Jasmine, a fifteen-year-old Siamese, The Geeter, a Maine coon, age twenty-three, and my new kitten, Squeeki. My pets almost never get treated, and their health is maintained exclusively through proper nutrition.

For pets less fortunate than mine, who do have weakened immune systems that render them more vulnerable to disease, holistic veterinary medicine offers a rich, almost overwhelming array of treatments and possibilities. Underlying all, I've realized after practicing them for so long, is a series of fundamental principles that are the root of all we know and practice in holistic medicine. Read them now, and keep them in mind as you read this book.

THE PRINCIPLES OF NATURAL HEALING

1. Disease is an absence of health, and vice versa: health is an absence of disease. But health was here first!
2. Disease is a process used by nature in an attempt to get itself healthy.
3. Degenerative disease is not *caused* by nature. It is an aberration of nature (caused mostly by—in my opinion—man).
4. Cancer is nothing more than a *severe* aberration of nature manifested in and by the body.
5. Sickness is an excuse to get healthy.
6. Don't mess with Mother Nature!
7. The mechanism for healing is already built into all individuals. Healing therefore occurs most rapidly when we realign with the natural laws governing that mechanism.
8. Pure health is spontaneous healing.
9. The immune system functions maximally and at peak efficiency in its totally unaltered state.
10. The degree to which we have to work toward health is directly proportional to the amount we have messed it up in the first place. Health is simple; disease brings in complexity.
11. Generally, it's not what you put into the body that restores health; rather it's what you let the body eliminate.
12. Physically, health isn't everything, but without it, everything is nothing.
13. Food, including the necessary vitamins and minerals, was intended not to improve, but rather to maintain, the body. Therefore, the need for treatment reflects the degree to which the individual has strayed from nature.
14. The body does not have to degenerate or age nearly as quickly as we presume. Each body cell has the ability to replicate itself 100 percent, and the process should continue for longer than we currently expect if we minimize deleterious effects on the cellular structure. It is only what we choose to do to the body, both consciously and unconsciously, that leads to the premature aging we experience.

15. Genetic predispositions to disease are only predispositions, and do not have to manifest if health is maintained. Once a genetically predisposed disease condition appears clinically, it *can* be reversed, although with more difficulty, as a course toward health is taken.

16. Nature and the being itself are the true healers. The practitioner, in the guise of being the healer, is truly the guide. Or: Physician, heal thyself!

17. Nature uses disease to establish balance. Only when our bodies are out of balance are we subject to disease, and if we can just endure the natural healing process, the disease will soon abate, having restored us to the balance that is optimal health!

18. In the holistic perspective, there is no such thing as coincidence.

One final thought before we begin. This is a book about animal care, but the guidelines of holistic veterinary medicine are, of course, based on those originally devised to help human beings. If we're going to give animals purified water because we realize what a silent killer ordinary tap water can be, why not drink purified water ourselves? If good foods and dietary supplements boost our pets' health, why not start applying the same nutritional lessons to improve our own? If acupuncture and homeopathic medicines work on animals, why not incorporate them into our own lives? We've done so much for our pets—perhaps saving them from being put to sleep at the shelter, taking them into our lives, caring for them, and showering them with love. If by chance you come to apply this book's principles of holistic health and diet to your own life, then your pet will have done, I believe, the best single thing he can to pay you back.

PART ONE

UNDERSTANDING DISEASE

CHAPTER ONE

Unraveling the Mystery of Disease

We live in a society that's riddled with disease. Looking for cures, our doctors diagnose us, give what ails us a name, and put us on drugs to make the problems go away. Unfortunately, all too often, that's like dealing with a car that has black smoke spewing from its exhaust system by trying to fix the tailpipe. Not until you examine the car's inner workings can you hope to figure out what's causing the exhaust problem and go on from there to solve it. More often than not, a basic tune-up is what's needed.

With pets, the distance between symptoms and true causes is often harder to trace than with cars—or with people. Pets can't answer questions that might produce clues. Often with a pet, all you *have* are signs. Perhaps your pet is lethargic. Or his coat is dull and matted, or his skin is scaly, or reddened and sore, or itchy. His eyes may be cloudy or reddened, his nose running, or his breath foul-smelling. Maybe he's stopped eating, or has intestinal gas. Perhaps he has diarrhea or a discolored stool; perhaps he's started urinating more often or in the house for the first time. These are the signs leading owners to conclude that their pets must "have something wrong." Pets can't tell you they have headaches or stomachaches; they can't say they're feeling feverish or generally punk, or that they remember eating something suspiciously odd-tasting yesterday in the woods.

An animal's inability to say what he's feeling exacerbates the tendency of modern medicine to focus on the immediate problem and treat *that*, as fast as possible, typically with drugs, or surgery, or both. A human patient with a flu may report he's nauseous, he has a fever and chills, perhaps diarrhea, and he looks pale. Chances are, he'll be given the oldest advice in the book: rest easy, drink plenty of fluids, maybe take some vitamin C, and, if need be, call back in a couple of days. Unless he feels worse, he'll recover without drugs. An animal presented to a veterinarian with those symptoms will be considered a more serious case, perhaps even an emergency. Given a choice, the animal would go off to recover on his own in isolation. In a conventional veterinary clinic, he'll be given antibiotics for his fever. For the nausea, he may well be subjected to a series of X rays, even sometimes in conjunction with having barium or some other contrast medium "forced" down his mouth to see why he's vomiting. If there's a skin irritation involved, he'll be given some form of cortisone, too. For a pet, prescribing drugs suggests a certainty of diagnosis and response reassuring to veterinarian and owner alike. But if drugs are the easiest answer, promising direct and immediate action, they may not be the correct answer. They may fail to address the underlying cause of the problem.

Let's look more carefully at those telltale signs that most commonly bring a pet in for medical attention. All seem to suggest specific ailments. Generally, trouble with a pet's coat or skin means allergies or skin infections. Cloudy eyes could suggest hardening of the lenses, which may indicate cataracts; a nasal discharge, cough, or foul breath indicates a viral or bacterial infection. Urinary problems suggest bladder infections or stones; stool irregularity might mean anything from intestinal problems that developed because a pet ate something he shouldn't have, to parasites or colitis. Underlying all of these symptoms or signs is the dark, lurking possibility of cancer.

Generally, a conventional veterinarian first prescribes antibiotics and/or some form of cortisone. The drugs treat the symptoms directly, and the ailments usually go away—antibiotics aren't used the world over for nothing. The problem *may* not return. More likely, however, it will, either in the exact way it did before, or in another, more insidious, form.

This is because drugs are essentially suppressive mechanisms. Typically, they suppress the symptoms of ill health that make you feel sick, rather than grapple with whatever might have provoked those symptoms in the first place. (Hence the enduring affection for aspirin for aches and pains, itself just a suppressive mechanism.) If the symptoms go away, you feel better. And, in fact, the body may be able to correct the underlying cause of your illness while the drug is at work on the outward signs, and restore itself to health—especially if you've chosen to rest easy, take lots of vitamin C, and drink lots of fluids, and so helped the body help itself. But don't credit the drug (or the vitamin C).

A pet put on antibiotics for some unexplained illness may not be so lucky. Suppressing symptoms will make him feel better for a while, but if the underlying cause of his ill health remains untended, it will reassert itself—somehow, somewhere. Why? Because the problem isn't an isolated one. The body's immune system works in an integrated way to protect our health, supply us with energy, give us our strength. The system should be able to fix itself, sending help to repair damaged or diseased cells at various points. If it can't, the problem is going to reappear elsewhere.

This is not to suggest that as a holistic veterinarian I stand back when a sick dog is brought in and do nothing, letting the body heal itself—or not. But instead of just treating the external sign—changing the tailpipe, in effect—I work to improve the dog's whole immune system so that it can better, and perhaps more quickly, expel the toxins that made it sick in the first place. I do this with nutritional supplements; I also use homeopathic remedies, good diet, acupuncture, chiropractic adjustments, herbs, and several other approaches that all come under the broad umbrella of holistic, complementary, or alternative therapy. In Chapters Five and Seven, I'll explain in detail which remedies I use with many different diseases. Here, let me just say that I've seen these practices work, consistently and completely, in thousands of cases during the years I've been in veterinary practice. And because they're not toxic, and are noninvasive, they have virtually no adverse side effects. Indeed, many modern drugs either use or replicate some natural herb or plant as their core ingredient. It's the synthetic chemicals that are substituted or mixed in to produce more immediate (if short-term) results which begin to cause problems.

Appreciating how central the immune system is to health—and ill health—is fundamental to alternative therapy. *All healing has to do essentially with the body's immune system.** Disease begins when the

---

*Medically, the internal immune system is like an army composed of many ranks of soldiers, many of them found in the bloodstream. Within the blood are antibodies, including B lymphocytes and the four immunoglobulins (IgA, IgE, IgG, and IgM), as well as helper cells, K cells, phagocytic cells, and catalysts such as complement and properdin. We also have the cell-mediated immune system, comprised of T lymphocytes, macrophages, and the "offspring" of these cells, lymphokines, monokines, and cytokines. But the whole immune system consists of much more than these blood components. It actually starts with the skin and the respiratory and alimentary systems, and includes the nervous and endocrine systems.

body is either not absorbing the nutrients it needs to maintain the immune system, or is failing to expel excess toxins and/or diseased cells which then keep the immune system from doing its job. Whatever the name or symptoms of the disease, it will last until the immune system, through its various channels, has finished purging. Physical healing is about what the body can get rid of—its ability to expel, or purge, toxicity.

Conventional doctors accept the notion that the body recognizes toxins and works to purge them: every day of our lives, toxins are processed by the liver and then expelled from the body via urine or feces. It's also understood that when those systems get overwhelmed, they may not work as they should. It seems an easy enough leap to see that other channels must then be employed, and that different diseases are nothing more or less than varied efforts by the body to remove toxicity and restore itself to health. Why do so many veterinarians resist this idea? Perhaps because they weren't taught it in school.

In fact, toxins are expelled within mucus from the nose or mouth, within tears or gummy matter from the eyes, or within wax from the ears. There's a basic logic here: the body has orifices through which the immune system can do its work. If the toxins are too far from one of those routes, they come up through the skin, as inflammations of one kind or another. What is a pimple? Nothing more than an example of detoxification. The process may not be pretty, but it's entirely natural and healthful. In many cases, if left alone, the body will finish the task of detoxifying itself, then heal the discomfitted site through which the toxins were expelled. With more severe cases, internal support will be needed to assist the process. That, in essence, is what holistic medicine does.

If, on the other hand, toxicity is suppressed, it will fester and reappear elsewhere in the body as some other disease or medical condition, likely more toxic than before, with a new name bestowed upon it to make it seem distinct. Not until the immune system succeeds in purging it will health return.

In the introduction, I said that cancer is the ultimate manifestation of ill health. Another way to put it is that many cancers are typically an extreme result of toxicity trapped within the body. Unable to purge that toxicity by any of the usual means, the body's immune system finally surrenders: the rebels take the garrison and begin to loot and plunder the cells with a violence the body cannot control.

When a pet is diagnosed with cancer, typically no cause will be given for how this chaos of the cells evolved, or why. No link will be made between the cancer and a pet's history of ill health—let alone its treatment. In pets, as in people, cancer is regarded as a random, inexplicable curse, coming out of nowhere. In Chapter Eight, I'll discuss at length my experience in treating cancer in pets, and my view that cancer arises in part from lesser stages of ill health; what's important to understand here are the fundamentals of how conventional and alternative medicine perceive—and treat—the disease.

When it appears in pets, cancer is usually treated by surgery, chemotherapy, and/or radiation. I make these choices sometimes, too, but only when they're needed to save a patient's life. To me, a treatment as toxic as chemotherapy is like taking a shotgun to the kidnapper who's making off with your child. You may kill the kidnapper, but you may also hurt or even kill the child. Certainly, chemotherapy rocks the immune system as it zaps disease cells. Too often, as a result, it brings short-term improvement at the expense of long-term health. Sometimes the improvement justifies the assault. Against a ravaged immune system, however, the cancer often strikes back—and wins.

Treating cancer with alternative therapies doesn't always work. Sometimes the cancer is too aggressive or pervasive; sometimes the pet is just too far gone. But I've seen alternative therapies succeed far more often than conventional ones.

The idea that toxins cause the conditions we call disease, and that health comes from letting the toxins *out* of the body, not treating them with drugs and pushing them further in, may seem radical to a practitioner of modern veterinary medicine. In fact, it is anything but new.

"Disease is an effort of the body to eliminate waste, mucus and toxemias," wrote Professor Arnold Ehret nearly a hundred years ago, "and this system assists Nature in the most perfect and natural way. Not the disease but the body is to be healed; it must be cleansed, freed from waste and foreign matter, from mucus and toxemias accumulated since childhood. You cannot buy health in a bottle, you cannot heal your body, that is, cleanse your system in a few days, you must make 'compensation' for the wrong you have done your body all during your life."

Still all but unknown to conventional doctors, Ehret (1866–1922) was a German-born writer and lecturer whose conclusions about health, toxicity, and fasting are central to the practice of holistic medicine today, both for people and pets. His seminal works, *Rational Fasting* and *The Mucusless Diet Healing System*, might have benefited from catchier titles, but their message—that the body can be purged of its toxins and achieve a mucusless state of perfect health—seems all the more urgent in a society pervaded by toxins . . . and drugs. "The diet of civilization is never entirely digested and the resultant waste eliminated," Ehret wrote. "In addition to mucus and its toxemias in the system, there are other foreign matters such as uric acid, toxins, etc., and especially drugs if ever used. . . . Drugs are NEVER eliminated as is the waste from foods, but are stored up in the body for decades. . . . Th[e] entire pipe system [of the body] is slowly constipated, especially at the place of the symptom and the digestive tract. This is the foundation of every disease!" And guess what? It applies to animals, too.

Ehret's father was actually a veterinarian who instilled in him a keen medical curiosity. That stood him in good stead when his health began to suffer for no apparent reason. By the age of thirty-one, burdened by kidney trouble among other ailments, Ehret set off on the first of five rest cures, then consulted twenty-four doctors, only to be told that his case was hopeless and that he would soon die. Nearly bankrupt and deeply depressed, he decided to seek his own answers based on a succinct, if unproven, assumption: "that wrong eating was the *cause* and right eating might be the *cure*."

First, Ehret tried vegetarianism, though with indifferent results. As he points out in his book, vegetarianism was all the rage in Berlin at that point (the mid-1890s), but vegetarians with their sallow complexions and lack of energy seemed no healthier than meat eaters. Then he tried a diet of nothing but fruit, initially supplemented by a pint of milk a day—fasting, in effect, for days at a time. When his health improved dramatically, he became an exuberant convert to the theory that the grape sugar in the fruit was the "essential material of human food, giving the highest efficiency and endurance, and at the same time was the best eliminator of debris and the most efficient healing agent known for the human body." (The grape sugar wasn't as important as he thought; it was the water, of which grapes are mostly comprised, that was so beneficial. Essentially, he was fasting.) This, in turn, led Ehret to his theory that mucus and the toxins which provoke it are the cause of all the forms of ill health which doctors call disease—the theory I've come to adopt in both my life and my practice as the best way to understand ill health in pets.

In the first two decades of the twentieth century, Ehret developed an international following of "Ehretists" dedicated to his regimen of intermittent fasting on a fruit-and-nut milk diet to cleanse the body of toxins. His own complexion glowed with brilliant health, and he radiated energy, so much so that he embarked on marathon bicycle trips and hikes, stopping only to lecture along the way. At the same time, his own fasts grew longer and longer—one lasted forty-nine days. Unfortunately, on October 9, 1922, while "enjoying a superior state of health known but to few men of present-day civilization," as a sympathetic biographer noted, Ehret slipped on an oil-slick street in Los Angeles, fell backward, and hit his head on a curb with enough force to cause instant death. Which just goes to prove one of the key principles stated in the introduction: health isn't everything!

Though without it, of course, everything is nothing.

In his own way, Ehret was rebelling against the essential presumption of modern science: that all things in the natural world can be rationally understood. Diseases can be analyzed, named, and codified; and drugs can be concocted sooner or later to cure them. (Science would cure his illness eventually, too, his doctors at the sanitariums had told him, just not soon enough to save *him*.) Ehret intuited that the body could cure itself if allowed to do so. He had no idea exactly how the body did so, but he didn't care! About the body and its workings, in other words, he could tolerate a certain mystery, as long as he saw some results.

In holistic medicine, that sense of mystery is ingrained. I can't tell you why an almost infinitesimal amount of a few minerals in a homeopathic remedy, when administered to a cat radically crippled with arthritis for months, can result in the cat walking almost normally in two hours when conventional medicine failed to have any beneficial effect after three months of continuous therapy. For all my conventional and alternative medical education and experience, I can surmise, but *I really don't know*. What I know is that these homeopathic remedies, as well as so many other forms of complementary or alternative therapy, work. That's enough for me—and it's usually enough for the owners whose pets I treat. With results, they come to feel as I do: that if a society obsessed with naming and treating symptoms is getting sicker, perhaps a new perspective is in order.

A few years ago, I found a passage that touched on this point in a most unlikely place: Michael Crichton's *Jurassic Park*. Crichton, of course, is a medical doctor by education and former practice, and very literate, too; one reason his books are so popular is that a reader gets fascinating science and history lessons as those thrilling plots unfold. In *Jurassic Park*, Crichton, in the person of Malcolm, also a doctor, observes that modern science, with all its empirical force, is only five hundred years old. It arose in part, he observes, because it seemed better than what preceded it, but also because what preceded it had failed. And now its own logic is outmoded, too.

> The basic idea of science—that there was a new way to look at reality, that it was objective, that it did not depend on your beliefs or your nationality, that it was *rational*—that idea was fresh and exciting back then, it offered hope and promise for the future, and it swept away the old medieval system which was hundreds of years old. The medieval world of feudal politics and religious dogma and hateful superstitions fell before science. But, in truth, this was because the medieval world didn't really work anymore. It didn't work economically, it didn't work intellectually, and it didn't fit the new world that was emerging.
>
> But now, science is the belief system that is hundreds of years old. And, like the medieval system before it, science is starting not to fit the world anymore. Science has attained so much power that its practical limitations begin to be apparent. Largely through science, billions of us live in one small world, densely packed and intercommunicating. But science cannot help us decide what to do with that world, or how to live. Science can make a nuclear reactor, but it cannot tell us not to build it. Science can make a pesticide, but cannot tell us not to use it. And our world starts to seem polluted in fundamental ways—air and water and land—because of ungovernable science. . . . This much is obvious to everyone.
>
> . . . And so the grand vision of science, hundreds of years old—the dream of total control—has died, in our century. . . . Science has always said that it may not know everything now but it will know, eventually. But now we see that isn't true. It is an idle boast. As foolish, and as misguided, as a child who jumps off a building because he believes he can fly.

As a doctor, I deal every day with mysteries I'm sure I'll never understand. Why did your cat get a bladder infection? When will your dog be better? How long will its recovery last? Yes, experience helps you make a better estimation. But really, *who knows?* No doctor knows these things. The difference is that as a holistic doctor, I *cele-brate* the mystery, which is why I can also embrace improvements I don't understand but which are natural and benign—and which work.

I'd love to tell you that I came to holistic medicine from some deep intellectual yearning for truths I hadn't found in conventional medicine. In fact, I was just trying to keep from losing my hair.

Barely in my mid-twenties, I was losing it fast to classic male-pattern baldness. My health wasn't so great either—I had degenerative bursitis and arthritis of my left shoulder—but I was less worried about that. I loved my hair! So much so that I'd worn it shoulder-length all through vet school, which *nobody* else did at Cornell, even in the late 1960s. When I happened upon a book called *You Are All Sanpaku*, left behind in my house by a friend, I picked it up with curiosity but skepticism. The author, Sakurazawa Nyoiti, also known as George Oshawa, addressed, among many other issues, the problem of hair loss and disease in general.

As I began to read, I was riveted by the concept Oshawa called "sanpaku," which means "three-sided." When people die, he related, their eyeballs roll up somewhat, so that the whites of their eyeballs are not merely on either side of the iris but below it as well. In some people, however, this condition appears while they're in ostensibly good health. This sanpaku condition is a sign of impending ill health, a foreshadowing, really, of death. When I looked in the mirror after reading about sanpaku, I was shocked: I had the condition myself.

At first, I just figured I was tired and needed more sleep. But after several days of rest, I was still sanpaku, and my arthritis pains kept getting worse despite ultrasonic therapy. The reason my doctor gave me for why I had arthritis in one shoulder was that I was getting "old." But what sense did that make? After all, my other shoulder was also twenty-seven years old and doing fine! That was when I decided to give Oshawa's dietary recommendations a try.

To cleanse the body and restore it to health, Oshawa recommended a macrobiotic diet consisting in large part of grains, specifically brown rice. I'd always loved eating, and as a schoolchild had earned the nickname "Porky." As a grown-up, I was still somewhat overweight. Nervously, I embarked on the diet, looking in the mirror every time I felt my resolve start to flag. On the third day, I had a major headache—just as the book predicted. The next morning, I felt looser and healthier than I had in years. My arthritis felt better. I went to the mirror: the sanpaku was gone.

When I'd lost twenty pounds in eight days, my brother became curious about the diet. He's a veterinarian, too—my mother liked doctors—and, also like me, tended to be overweight. The diet helped him as dramatically as it did me. One day, as we sat talking about it, we came to the simultaneous decision that we should try the diet on pets and see if it improved their health, too. "For starters," my brother said, "why not try it with Leigh?"

Certainly we had nothing to lose. A seven-year-old golden retriever, my brother's dog Leigh was a woeful compendium of medical disasters. He had hip dysplasia—degeneration of the hip joints—that had led to arthritis so painful he was crippled. He had allergies so severe that we had to bandage his legs to prevent him from chewing them. Plus, as he was getting old—or what we thought was old for him—his red muzzle had turned white. As conventional veterinarians, my brother and I had given Leigh regular injections of cortisone to control his symptoms; soon, we thought we'd have to put poor Leigh to sleep.

In truth, we hadn't thought about Leigh's diet at all. Diet wasn't a subject that came up often in veterinary school, and when it did, it was more associated with the quantity, not the quality, of food for animals. Leigh, as a result, had been raised almost solely on Top Choice and Gaines Burgers, the semimoist burger patties that seemed so carefully prepared in their clear plastic wrapping, and felt so fresh when pulled out and put in Leigh's bowl. Now, instead, my brother put Leigh on a diet of brown rice, spinach, and hamburger.

In days, Leigh began to walk better. Soon the bandages came off his allergy-ridden legs. Most astounding to us, Leigh's muzzle began to grow in red again. We kept him on the brown rice diet, of course, and eventually threw out our year's supply of Top Choice and Gaines Burgers. Leigh continued to have hip dysplasia, considered an irreversible condition. But he was no longer in pain, he walked without effort, and plainly he was infused with an energy—nothing less than a life force—that we'd never have imagined we'd see in him again.

So disease might be combated more effectively with the right diet than with the right drugs! For my brother and me, this was a turning point in our practice. Along with it came the recognition that while Leigh was still diseased, he wasn't dis-*eased*.

A recent *Webster's* defines "disease" as any process that serves to "interrupt or impair any or all of the natural and regular functions of an organ in the body; to afflict with pain or sickness." At the same time, the dictionary includes an obsolete definition of disease as "uneasiness; distress." What a fascinating evolution in meaning! The modern definition embodies the attitude of conventional medicine that all sickness is disease, and contains the implication that all disease must be wiped out before a person can be deemed healthy. The old definition is underscored by the word's root meaning: a disease is anything that dis*eases* the body. So if a condition like hip dysplasia can be kept from producing painful symptoms by the right diet, and an animal can go on to live a relatively long, *easeful* life, is it diseased? We thought not, and Leigh's subsequent experience confirmed our new view. Rambunctious enough to wander off for days at a time to neighboring towns, alert enough to return, Leigh remained relatively dis*ease*-free until the day he died.

At seventeen and a half.

For myself, I stayed with the brown rice, adding some vegetables to it and sometimes a bit of meat—it's hard to change your diet so quickly. As I persisted with it over several months, I realized that my hairline was no longer receding. By now I'd begun exploring other books of Eastern thought, taking lessons from them for my own life, but also for the pets I was treating. Acupuncture was particularly fascinating to me, as it quickly eliminated the last twinges of pain from my bursitis. By 1976, I'd incorporated it into my practice, with amazing results.

At that time, the medical establishment still regarded acupuncture with wariness as a pain reliever for people. As an approach to veterinary care, the very mention of it stirred horror in my colleagues—particularly the seven with whom my brother and I had just begun a collective practice in the New York suburb of Mount Kisco.

Early into that ill-fated venture, one of my new partners was treating a weimaraner who had had a seizure in the middle of the night. The dog was given a lot of Valium and then slipped into a coma. In the Veterinary Hospital for Special Services, but still in the coma one week later, the dog was about to be put to sleep. By now I had earned my certification in veterinary acupuncture, so I suggested trying acupuncture on the dog as a last resort. The idea was met with scornful laughter. "Anyway," I was told, "you're not the attending doctor, you'd have to get permission." As much out of irritation as anything else, I called the hospital and spoke to the attending veterinarian, who, as it happened, had had acupuncture himself and was bullish about it. The veterinarian called the owners, who gave their permission reluctantly, having no expectation that it would work but understanding that their pet's case appeared to be hopeless. And so I went over with my needles to give it a try.

Most of us now know that acupuncture, which predates modern science by thousands of years, is the Chinese practice of gently inserting fine needles into the body to relieve pain or certain disease conditions. Less known is the idea behind it: that the body is a network of linked energy channels, like interconnected waterways, and that the needles, serving as conductors, effectively loosen the dam that constricts the flow. To treat the weimaraner, I chose six points along its energy-flow network indicated for neurological problems. I put the first five needles into their respective points and got no response. The sixth was at a point just above the dog's paw. I inserted it, turned it—and the dog woke up! I was stunned. So were the attending veterinary technicians, who backed off as if they'd just witnessed witchcraft. The next day, when I got to the sixth point, the dog sat up and started barking.

Over the next three weeks, I put the dog on a basic macrobiotic diet that I had learned about while studying acupuncture from Dr. Norman Ralston, considered by many to be the grandfather of holistic veterinary medicine. Sure enough, the dog started to detoxify. I witnessed for the first time what I would later recognize as a healing crisis: a seeming turn for the worse that conventional veterinarians would identify as disease and try to suppress, but which was actually a purging of toxins as the body worked to recover its health. The dog's coat turned from gray to tan, then started to fall out in clumps. Whoever touched the dog broke out in a rash, including me. Soon enough, however, the dog's chronic ear problems vanished and he began to grow a beautiful new coat of soft gray puppy hair. The healing crisis was over, the toxins expelled, and the dog was rejuvenated.

No one has demonstrated in a scientific way exactly how and why acupuncture works. Nor did I know how to analyze the weimaraner's healing crisis; indeed, I didn't know while it was occurring how it would end. But the fact that what I'd witnessed was, in the eyes of modern medical science, a mystery, didn't bother me at all. It worked. Indeed, the mystery of it fascinated and awed me: the body, I realized, knows far more about how to take care of itself than modern science can hope to know. Back at our Veterinary Hospital for Special Services weeks later, though, the head of medicine took a cynical view of how things had turned out. The dog, he declared, had undergone "spontaneous remission" of a stroke. Clearly, the veterinarian added, the dog would have experienced this same remission without treatment.

"If that's true," I asked him, "then why did you recommend euthanasia?"

Along with an appreciation of mystery, the weimaraner case taught me the importance of patience. Drugs are expected to work fast; if they don't, others are quickly tried. Then, if there's no response, a case is declared "hopeless" and out comes the call for euthanasia. Patients aren't given enough of a chance to heal, and a worsening condition may not be recognized as the purging that leads to health. That's why, whenever I get a "hopeless" case, the first thing I do is to try to take a pet off drugs as I put him on alternative therapies. And then I *wait*— for the pet to start healing himself. This is not to say that drugs are bad. They do have their role in society and, used at a minimum, in my practice. But our goal should be to wean our patients from them as soon as possible, and let true health be our best protection against disease.

Viewing health and illness as a function of toxicity, appreciating the importance of diet, and opening oneself to the good that holistic medicine can do, mysterious as it may be—these are the first steps toward a whole new way of caring for your pet.

CHAPTER TWO

The Struggle for Health

Now, when your pet gets sick, you'll understand that his symptoms are the result of the immune system's effort to purge, or failure to purge, toxins and unhealthy cells. How does that help you treat illness or, better yet, prevent it? It doesn't. Until, that is, you begin to appreciate where disease comes from, and what you can do to help fend it off.

How often, when you bring your pet to the veterinarian, is anything said about what may have *caused* the symptoms he's experiencing? To be sure, some problems do have obvious origins. Lyme disease is contracted from a deer tick. Heartworm is carried by infected mosquitoes. And fleas are fleas. Most illnesses, however, seem to grow without such explanations, especially when they appear internally, as flus or fevers, accompanied by symptoms that range from lack of appetite to diarrhea. Instead, as your veterinarian writes up the prescription for antibiotics, he usually mentions one of those two catch-all causes: virus or bacteria. Where have they come from? Why have they targeted your pet now?

I'm the first to admit that nature works in mysterious ways. But to me, the biggest mystery about viruses and bacteria is why they're still so universally assumed to be the causative agents of so many diseases.

Consider how viruses are defined: as submicroscopic germ organisms, smaller even than a single cell, that travel through air or water from person to person, animal to animal, infecting us with various diseases. Without exception, a flu victim will have been exposed to a flu virus. But did the virus cause the disease? Or did the disease bring on and support the virus? *The fact is that viruses infrequently appear outside diseased tissue.* So again: Which comes first, the virus or the diseased tissue? I think the latter; otherwise, the virus would have to evolve out of thin air. The diseased tissue somehow engenders the virus—not the other way around. At which point the virus "sets up home" in the diseased environment, concentrates, and then *appears* to cause the disease and "spread" to others.

Granted, feline leukemia, a major killer of cats, appears to be virus-borne. So does feline infectious peritonitis, a horrible disease that swells the abdomen appallingly; and feline immunodeficiency virus, the so-called feline AIDS, among others. But these are relatively new diseases, brought on, I believe, not by new viruses appearing out of nowhere, but rather from our unfortunate success in affecting nature—and ourselves. The result, in the broadest sense, is that we've disrupted the balance between the two, allowing viruses to take opportunistic hold. Even so, I don't believe they initially cause these diseases on their own.

My first inkling that something other than viruses might be involved in causing disease came in the course of my attempts to improve my own health. Before I changed my diet, I used to get bad flus half a dozen times a year. High fevers, achiness—I'd be down for the count. Since then, over more than two decades, I've probably been exposed to thousands of viral flu bugs and have not caught one. Just luck? I don't think so.

One of the first veterinary cases that served to confirm my suspicions concerning illness actually involved feline leukemia. A woman came to the clinic in the early 1980s with a cat diagnosed as having feline leukemia virus (FeLV) of the spinal cord. The cat, it turned out, was one of six the woman owned. Within a three-month period, two more of her cats incurred the disease, one also in the spinal cord, one in the chest. There was nothing I could do for any of them; all three cats died. Yet the other three cats remained healthy. That mystified me. If feline leukemia was a virus and the survivors lived in close quarters with the cats who died, why didn't they contract it, too? In fact, the three cats who died were related to each other; the three who survived were not. Something more than the virus had to be involved. Something in the infected cats' immune systems had allowed the virus to take over. Something, perhaps, that had been instilled in an earlier generation and passed on genetically.

My practice has kept me too busy to address the mysteries of feline viral diseases in a systematic way, but Dr. Deva Khalsa, a holistic veterinarian in Pennsylvania, has confounded the conventional wisdom that feline infectious peritonitis is a 100 percent fatal virus. She hasn't tried to knock out the virus or rather, she's focused on building her feline patients' immune systems by using certain homeopathic remedies: apis mellifica, made from honeybees; pulsatilla, made from anemone; and hydrastis, made from goldenseal. "It turns out from studying their genomes that most cats carry FeLV and FIP, even wild ones," she explains. "But in many cats it remains dormant. Why does it manifest itself more in some breeds than others? Inbreeding seems to be one reason: in Persians and Bermans, both very inbred, the virus tends to get a foothold and develop as disease." It seems no coincidence, Dr. Khalsa adds, that inbred cats tend to have shoddy immune systems.

Parvovirus, a potential killer that's earned its own vaccine in the standard annual lineup of canine inoculations, offers more evidence that viruses aren't independent causal agents. Parvo is spread when dogs ingest the feces of infected animals (often just by stepping in the excretions, then licking their paws clean later). Diarrhea, often bloody and watery, ensues, usually along with vomiting, lack of appetite, and a fever. Yet the parvovirus, which might seem as established as rabies, distemper, and the other scourges combated by annual vaccines, was only discovered in 1978! At some point not long before that, the parvovirus either appeared out of nowhere—unlikely—or existed as a benign organism. What caused that benign organism to become a viral scourge? One of two things. Either we as a society changed the organism's makeup by introducing some chemical into the environment, or, more likely, we changed our pets, inhibiting their immune systems by various means intended to help them. Either way, a natural balance between dogs and parvo was upset, and so the virus took hold.

Most veterinarians still say that parvo is a viral disease, and that the way to prevent it is with the parvo vaccine. I'll have more to say—a lot more—on the subject of vaccines in Chapter Four. For now, let me just note that in my experience, boosting pets' immune systems with nutritional supplements—and without annual vaccinations—has produced a tremendous success rate: not one incidence of parvo among the thousands of dogs I've seen in the last half dozen years. And this is despite the reported appearance of new strains of the viral disease.

Here's one more indication why viruses no longer seem to me to be the sole cause of the diseases to which they have been linked. In recent years, as we have come to treat patients on a national basis at Smith Ridge, reports of similar viral illness have come in, often almost simultaneously, from different parts of the country. It seems kind of odd to me that viruses could be *that* simultaneously contagious, or would coincidentally "pop up" everywhere.

Unless, of course, other factors are at work, precipitating the disease—and the virus.

Bacteria are a similar story, with the same conclusion. All of us, people and pets, have millions of friendly bacteria, or single-celled germs, in our bodies. They help us maintain good health by facilitating digestion, producing certain vitamins, and keeping a proper ecological balance in the body. Yet when a dog starts coughing or sneezing and its nose begins to run, the first thing a veterinarian will likely do is put the dog on antibiotics as a matter of course to kill the bacteria causing it. After all, if the doctor takes a culture from the dog's throat, it will probably show an abnormally high level of bacteria. And strictly speaking, the bacteria *have* caused the dog's condition. So the culture will appear to confirm the wisdom of prescribing antibiotics. Within a short period, hopefully, the cough will abate, along with the dog's other symptoms.

The dog may stay well. Just as likely, however, his cough will return weeks or months later, more racking than before. What's to explain it?

In short, the bacteria aren't necessarily the problem. They're part of the body's natural solution of eliminating acquired toxins through the respiratory system. Already, the body has generated mucus as part of the process of transporting toxins out through the dog's mouth and nose. As that happens, the dog's normal flora of throat bacteria have multiplied and become more virulent, producing toxins themselves, but for a very healthy reason: to help destroy excess mucus. (The bacteria actually live on the toxin-rich mucus, absorbing it as food.) The cough is the sound of a healthy battle: of the bacteria destroying the mucus and thus finishing the elimination.

What happens when the bacteria succeed? Now that they've multiplied, won't they hang around the throat and keep causing the dog to cough even after the toxins are gone? Not at all: our bodies are too clever for that. If left alone—not wiped out by antibiotics—the bacteria will then be reduced to normal levels by white blood cells brought to the scene by the body's immune system. You know they've arrived because the blood that brings them wells up as an inflammation, or sore throat. (Simply put, an inflammation is the reddening caused by surplus blood bringing immunity to an afflicted area.) So an associated sore throat, too, is a sign of health being restored—naturally, by the body—not of sickness to be knocked out by drugs.

If antibiotics are used at this juncture, they kill the bacteria, so the cough goes away, along with the runny nose and sore throat, and your dog feels better relatively quickly. But the mucus that the bacteria would have ingested remains, to linger in the throat or trickle back into the lungs or cellular structure. At the least, it will return in another attempt to be discharged. At worst, it will become a foundation of chronic illness, such as chronic bronchitis or even cancer. Many of the cancer cases I see, particularly nasal and bladder cancers, have a history of repetitive antibiotic therapy with partial or repetitive response. The connection is unproven but worrisome.

A traditionally trained doctor will observe, to be sure, that bacteria do cause many diseases in pets and people alike: medical science proves it every day. And antibiotics do kill the bacteria, which enables the immune system to strengthen itself. To which I say: That's holding the telescope the wrong way. Strengthen the immune system first, keep it free of toxicity, and bacteria, like viruses, will remain benign. Use antibiotics instead, and the result will be an immune system that soon either loses the capacity to repel bacteria on its own or, in growing lax, allows other benign conditions to become virulent, precipitating more disease.*

To question whether bacteria cause disease may seem as foolish and unscientific as arguing that the world may not be round. In fact, bacteria's role as an agent of infectious disease was defined but a moment ago in world history: by Louis Pasteur, who in the 1880s proved that bacteria could cause anthrax in sheep. Pasteur was at least half right: bacteria did cause anthrax in the sheep he tested. But a holistic practitioner would ask about bacteria, as with viruses: Were they the only cause? Or did something make them more virulent?

Even as Pasteur was conducting his most famous experiments, a contemporary French physician and pharmacist named Antoine Beauchamp reached an opposite conclusion. Beauchamp, as authors John

---

*That said, I don't rule out the use of antibiotics altogether. Nor should any responsible doctor. Why? Because almost every day we see pets with conditions so severe that their immune systems are overwhelmed. Without antibiotics, those pets could die. You can believe absolutely in alternative therapy, as I do, but you can't practice it on a dead pet. As a result, I'll employ antibiotics or other forms of conventional medicine. Reluctantly. Sparingly. And for as brief a duration as possible. When the pet is out of danger or his immune system starts to kick in, I'll withdraw or ease him off the antibiotics or other drugs as judiciously and rapidly as I can.

Diamond and Burton Goldberg recount in *An Alternative Medicine Definitive Guide to Cancer*, believed that bacteria alone could not cause disease in a healthy body. Indeed, he theorized, bacteria readily invade a body and take up residence within its cells, but if the cell "terrain" is balanced, they cause no harm. When the cell terrain becomes unbalanced, however—perhaps from poor diet, stress, or toxins, especially carcinogens—the bacteria can then change shape, or "morph," into increasingly pathogenic forms that do bring on disease. Beauchamp called his theory "pleomorphism" (*pleo* means shape, and to *morph* is to change), as opposed to Pasteur's "monomorphism," which held that bacteria or any other microbe have one unchanging shape and cause damage by invading from outside the body. By the time Beauchamp published his findings, the germ theory had gained universal acceptance, and he was ridiculed. But according to authors Diamond and Goldberg, Pasteur on his deathbed repudiated his own concept and endorsed Beauchamp's, declaring, "The microbe is nothing; the terrain is everything."

Remember: Before disease, there is health. The world in its natural state, which is to say before man began subverting nature to his own ends, probably had little in the way of what we would identify today as degenerative disease. Animals relied on nature for food, and the strongest survived. They fought for turf, and those forced to move on may have starved or been killed as a result. Granted, our medical advances have increased life expectancy, but look at how disease-ridden and compromised those extended years so often are. The more diseases man has conquered, the more that have arisen to plague him. What's wrong with this picture?

I believe that the myriad diseases that afflict pets today are attributable directly or indirectly to modern man's activities on the planet. These vary in kind and degree, from the global results of the claimed greenhouse effect to the emotional impact of a hypertense person on the physical well-being of his pet. In essence, however, I place the causes of disease in four categories:

1. dietary
2. environmental
3. emotional/spiritual
4. genetic

Inevitably, the causes become commingled. And the more serious the disease, the more likely it is that all four are involved.

In clarifying the role of diet in disease, I always use this analogy: If you put Sterno in your gas tank, your car won't run very well. If you give your dog or cat a standard brand of mass-market pet food, the results will be more subtle but, over time, just as real and unfortunate. We really *are* what we eat, and when what our pets eat is at best devoid of the nutrition they need, and at worst actually dangerous to their health, then diet will lead to disease as surely as Sterno will ruin the internal workings of your car.

Diet is so important to a pet's health—and a contributory if not fundamental cause of so much ill health—that the whole of Chapter Three in this book is devoted to it. If you have time to read only one more chapter, make it that one—please. Simply by reconsidering what you feed your pet, you can do more to improve his physical health, and more to prevent future disease, than a veterinarian can with most Western medicine. Plus, the effects will be longer-lasting!

The body, after all, is literally made from food. Proteins from food are the building blocks of cellular structure—and the body is composed mostly of cells. That's how an embryo is formed; it's also how a body sustains itself out of utero. Over a period of seven years, it is said, every cell in the human body is replaced: you are literally not the person you were seven years ago. Because dogs and cats have shorter life spans than humans, I've always felt that their total cellular structure is replaced every two to three years. A poor diet, as a result, may affect their health sooner, and more profoundly, than it does human health.

How? Basically, the body does three things: absorb, assimilate, and eliminate. All require energy. The worse a diet is, the more toxins it contains. Toxins need to be eliminated, because they're of no use and because they're harmful; that's what the processes of urination and excretion are all about. Normally, a body does much of this work during sleep, when it needn't expend its energy in other ways; excretion often occurs right after waking because of this nocturnal process. The more energy a body has to expend passing toxins, the less it has for using nutrients and maintaining its immune system. Energy is also used up for the assimilation of food; that's why a pet (or person) sometimes feels sleepy after a big meal, and indeed sleeps longer than another creature that eats lightly. Over time, then, a poor diet weakens the body, including the immune system. Incoming toxins from more bad food may not be eliminated, but instead reside in the eliminative organs and in the blood, festering. A stressed-out immune system is also more vulnerable to viruses and bacteria from outside. Strictly speaking, a poor diet may not cause disease. What it does is create conditions that *lead* to disease.

I remember a painful incident in my own life that helped me appreciate the true nature of disease. I know exactly when it happened: on a late-fall Sunday afternoon in 1986, at exactly two minutes before one o'clock. Every Sunday, I would rise at four o'clock in the morning and try to get all my casework and errands done in time to be sitting in front of the television, with my lunch on my lap, at the kickoff of the weekly pro-football game. Usually, as hard as I worked, I still slid into my seat a few minutes late.

This day was different. This day, I was on time. At two minutes before one o'clock, my lunch fully prepared, I slipped around my kitchen counter toward the TV room. Just as I did, the little toe on my right foot encountered one of the legs of a wood-burning stove. That hurt. I hobbled to the TV room anyway, and watched the game, but noticed that the toe was askew and assumed I'd dislocated it. Later that night an X ray confirmed that I'd broken it.

The next morning, I described the incident by phone to my chiropractor, and decided to do nothing more than wear loose-fitting sneakers and let it heal itself. Within a few days, I was able to jog without undue pain, and the toe, though a little red at the fracture site, appeared to be on the mend. Then, that Saturday night, I was invited to a party where all kinds of tempting, rich foods and drinks were served. Having stuck for weeks to a rigorous diet of all-healthy, all-natural meals, I splurged on every snack in sight. Two hours later at the party, my toe began to throb. When I took my sneaker off at home later that night, I saw that the toe had swelled to twice its size. Sunday morning, it was black and blue for the first time—a week after the injury. This incident got me to see what really causes disease.

There's no better first step for your pet than recognizing just how toxic his diet probably is. Even a pet who eats nothing but healthy food, however, is subject to a broad range of threats from his immediate environment. Not all are visible; not all can be dispelled. Still, a pet's environment is the next crucial factor to consider in maintaining his health.

In the course of a year, many pounds of dirt and dust are blown in or tracked into your house or apartment. Much of it may be benign; some of it, however, may include pesticides dangerous to your pet's health. Lead particles from auto exhaust, flaking paint, or even the ink from color-print newspapers may, if ingested in quantity over time, lead to vomiting, diarrhea, and various internal problems. At the same time, synthetic fibers from certain factory-made rugs may cause respiratory problems. Far worse, of course, is asbestos, which while no longer in use can occasionally be found as insulation in older houses. Though no house can be completely pollutant-free, some obvious measures can be taken: keep your house as clean as possible; avoid deep-pile synthetic rugs; and check to see that you have neither lead-based paint nor asbestos insulation (both of which, to be sure, pose health hazards to the rest of your family as well). One other step: install an air filtration or purification system that removes dust motes (and mites), environmental toxins, and fumes. I'm partial to a brand called Alpine, which has the added advantage of an ion and ozone generator. I've got an Alpine system at the clinic and at my house (Smith Ridge is a distributor). When I walk into my home from outside, it's like walking into a rain forest.

If you live in a house with a yard, your pet is probably fenced in from passing cars. But what about the yard itself? You may have a gardener who uses weed killers like Roundup that a pet might lick off the patio—or his own paws. As well-known holistic veterinarian Richard Pitcairn and his wife, Susan, report in their *Complete Guide to Natural Health for Dogs and Cats*: "The National Cancer Institute found in 1991 that dogs whose owners used 2, 4-D, a common broadleaf weed killer, had twice the rate of lymphoma (a cancer of the lymph system) as dogs whose owners did not use it." Your gardener might also use a poison for moles and voles, or you yourself may put out rat or ant poison.

Those toxins, at least, you can control. Beyond your property, alas, other potential hazards lurk. If you live near cultivated fields, pesticides will almost certainly be used to protect the crops, and a breeze may blow them your way. A pet may ingest other toxins in the neighborhood which his owner wouldn't because the pet spends so much of his life with his nose to the ground and tends to lick whatever he smells. Antifreeze, which tastes deceptively sweet, is one of the most common and destructive dangers; motor oil is another. The chemical-saturated runoff water from a nearby golf course can be terribly toxic. In the city, toxins are leaked by passing traffic. You can't hope to eliminate them altogether, either in the city or in the country: the fact is that your pet (and you!) lives in a world infinitely more toxic—and disease-ridden—than it was a century ago.

Many of these toxins come to us as pollutants in water and air. But all of us who inhabit this planet—on two legs or four—are now subjected to low- and high-frequency radiation, invisible to us but almost certainly a contributory factor to the steep rise in many cancers. Human beings, who created the dangers, absorb the most direct of them: X rays and radiation, long-term proximity to power lines, microwaves, computer screens, and more. As man-made pollution erodes the ozone layer, more ultraviolet rays than our skin can safely withstand beam down on us, adding to the increased incidences of skin cancer. Whether or not pollution at the same time creates the so-called greenhouse effect, or whether El Niño is to blame, the fact is that aberrant weather conditions of recent years favor certain species at the expense of others, and may even lead to rising water levels that imperil entire landmasses and the life-forms on them.

All this may seem remote from the present condition of your pet, and in a sense it is. There isn't any yardstick by which to measure how much a decreased ozone layer has contributed to the melanoma I might have to excise on a Tuesday morning from a worried-looking golden retriever. Nor is it easy to tell if the antifreeze your dog lapped up is what's given him kidney failure—unless your veterinarian suspects it and does a screening test for it. But certain climactic changes do affect the health of our pets in obvious and quite dramatic ways.

Take violent storms, of which there've been so many more in recent years—either as a result of imbalances created by global warming, or coincidence, take your pick. The old farmer who says he can predict a storm by feeling it as pain in his bones is right. The falling barometric pressure of an impending storm packs the air with positive ions. The calcium in the farmer's bones and joints also carries a positive charge. The positives repel each other, like two positive magnets. That stirs the calcium in the farmer's bones, and causes his arthritis to flare up. Some measure of calcium will actually be displaced into the blood as the storm arrives; as a result, the farmer's urine during and after a storm will change in hue as the calcium is excreted.

Animals with arthritis—or bursitis, or hip dysplasia—are irritated by oncoming storms, too. Last summer, during a string of summer storms, the phones at the clinic began to ring off the hook. Pets who'd been doing fine, their arthritis tamed by acupuncture, homeopathic remedies, and nutritional supplements, were experiencing discomfort, some even to the point of near paralysis. Increased acupuncture and homeopathic treatments helped—but so did a change in weather.

Back in the mid-1970s, I started noticing that electrical storms also appeared to provoke urinary problems in both dogs and cats. When a breeder I knew complained that cats in her cattery were experiencing bladder infections, especially during seasonal changes, I informed her of my suspicions about positive ionic charges. Intrigued, the breeder bought two negative ion generators to neutralize these effects on her animals, and during seasonal changes ran them twenty-four hours a day. From then on, the incidence of bladder infections diminished substantially.

Barometric pressure and the positive ions it produces may also be what causes many domesticated dogs to react fearfully to approaching electrical storms. Well before the first thunderclap, many dogs are under a bed or chair, literally trembling with fright. I think the barometric pressure is affecting the fluids in their brains, exerting a pressure that gets communicated as a signal of change that may be dangerous. If that seems crazy, consider the proven effect of a full moon on all the water on our planet, from the ocean's tides, which can rise several feet during a lunar cycle, to the fluids in our brains, which lunar pressure affects, too—provoking, if we set store by the root meanings of words, lunatics and fits of lunacy. More traffic accidents occur during full moons; hospital emergency rooms report increased bleeding from patients, whatever the direct cause may be. In my own practice, I've noticed that epileptic dogs have more seizures when the moon is full, too. Just last week I treated Bud, a dachshund, for chronic lower back pain. "My nickname for Bud is Budrometer," his owner told me, "because his back always gives out with severe shifts in barometric pressure."

You can argue, if you like, that the ozone layer is fine and that UV light is the same as it ever was; you can shrug off global warming and say that the heat waves and hurricanes of the last decade are merely a historical blip. But no one can dispute the fact that the pollen count is reported in certain areas to be higher than ever before—aggravating allergies in pets and people alike—and that a changed environment of warmer weather is the cause.

Almost every year now, in most of the United States, winter shrinks and the growing seasons expand. Goldenrod and the many other plants that pollinate have more time in which to do so; sufferers from hay fever and other allergies struggle that much more to cope. In dogs, for example, a common allergy called atopy is a hereditary predisposition to react to certain allergens: molds, trees, ragweed, wool, flea saliva, and house dust chief among them. In recent years, I've seen far more pets with allergies than ever before, enduring the four standard symptoms: sneezing, itching, tearing, and paw licking. (We rub our eyes; dogs lick their paws.) Both dogs and cats can be helped with homeopathic remedies, herbs, and nutritional support, and these, like other holistic treatments, boost the immune system first rather than suppressing the symptom chemically.

Simply put, an allergy is the reaction of an antibody to an antigen. The flea saliva, to take one of those provocations, is the antigen; the immune system's antibodies react to it. A healthy body is strong enough not to be thrown out of balance by the antigen. In other words, it's *insensitive* to the allergen, which is good. In an unhealthy body, toxins overwork the antibodies of the immune system and so *sensitize* them to this antigen, causing the allergic reaction.

Why, to put it another way, do we know that pollen doesn't itself cause hay fever and other allergies? Because if it did, all of us would have these diseases. That most of us don't is an indication, to some doctors, of the role of hereditary traits. I see it as yet another issue relating to immunity, which is affected by the environment but also, with proper care, easily helped. And again, what persuaded me was personal experience.

As a child, I had more allergies than anyone I knew. Every week, I had to go to Dr. Gould, a stern allergist who, after 177 skin-testing injections, determined that I was allergic to dozens of agents, some of which I'd never eaten, seen, or been affected by in any way. I refused to go in after that for regular allergy shots, and fortunately, my mother backed me up. The allergies persisted into my early teens. Almost overnight, as I went through a maturation process and grew six inches taller within several months, they disappeared. From then on, the only allergen that caused a reaction was fleas, but the swellings from their bites diminished to pinpricks after I changed my diet and got healthier in my thirties—until one memorable Sunday.

After a week away at a health retreat, during which my pets stayed with a friend, I walked into my house to meet a cloud of fleas that had taken up residence in our absence and grown voraciously hungry. I was their meal for the few minutes it took me to stash my gear and change clothes for a Sunday picnic with friends. But in my state of optimal health, I barely noticed the tiny red dots the flea bites provoked. At the picnic, all manner of tempting foods was served: sugary, nonnutritious foods. Forgetting my new diet, I ate and drank everything in sight. Within two hours, the flea bites, which had almost vanished, swelled to huge red welts. The lesson was inescapable: what had provoked my allergic reactions were the toxins I'd ingested, which then stimulated my white blood cells to "remember" how they used to react to the allergen—what's known as an anamnestic response.

If you've owned a dog or cat in the last five years, you hardly need me to point out two other unfortunate consequences of warmer weather on animal health. But think of them now within the larger picture of global change and disease.

Not so long ago, fleas were a manageable nuisance during summer and fall, peaking during Indian summer but gone with the second or third frost. About a decade ago, however, I began to see flea cases well past autumn. During the warmer winters, they persisted right on until spring, when the insect population traditionally reappears. Powerful new products are currently on the market, as a result, to try to keep the fleas at bay: pills, collars, chemical baths, sprays and liquids, even concentrated, flea-deterring chemical drops that are applied to the skin between a pet's shoulder blades, along with the ever-stronger battery of toxic insecticides sprayed throughout the home by professional exterminators. I'll consider those products specifically in Chapter Seven, along with holistic alternatives. Suffice it to say here that they're not part of the solution. They're part of the problem.

In the last five years, too, much of the Eastern Seaboard has become overrun by white-tailed deer infested with deer ticks that carry Lyme disease. An earlier change in the environment brought about by humans produced the burgeoning herds in the first place: the development of rural areas chased away or simply wiped out the deer's biological predators. But now warmer weather has extended their calving seasons, and seemingly fostered additional tick hatchings. And so a disease that appeared only yesterday—its first case recorded in 1975 in Old Lyme, Connecticut—is now a widespread health threat to people and pets alike. I'll consider Lyme at length in Chapter Seven, but let me say this for now: for pets, the Lyme vaccine does much more harm than good.

Most of the environmental causes of disease discussed so far have to do with the environment around us: how the changes we've worked upon it have worked changes upon our health. But here and there are glints of a different kind of environmental factor: the drugs given to people and pets that all too often do less to cure disease than cause it.

For pets, probably the most commonly prescribed drug—the number one drug of choice the veterinary world over—is cortisone. Over the years, it has acquired a reputation as "the reliever of all and curer of none." It's a steroid that brings quick but short-term results. And it comes in many forms. It's used topically, for inflammation of the skin. It's in eye ointments and ear preparations. It's also given orally, or injected, for everything from allergies and asthma to colitis and joint disease. Although I use it, I do so in doses small enough to avoid provoking the side effects so commonly seen at prescription-dose levels. Then I back up its effects with natural products that either have the same effect as the drug itself or enhance those effects at a much lower dose until the pet can be successfully weaned from it.

Nearly as ubiquitous are antibiotics. Penicillin, the first and best-known, isn't used much anymore. It derives from a fungus and is, in that sense, more natural than its successors, but the new synthetic antibiotics are more effective, especially against bacterial infections that have grown penicillin-resistant. Amoxicillin is a common choice. So is tetracycline, which comes in a black-and-yellow capsule, and Baytril, which comes as a pretty purple tablet. All affect the immune system in the long run. But that's not all they do.

The fact is that antibiotics don't merely subvert the body's natural process of expelling toxins. They add toxins—from the drugs themselves, from the chemicals used to bind their components together, from the synthetic agents used to color their casings. Those toxins fester in the body, straining and eventually nullifying the immune system's power to heal. At the same time, the drugs lose their capacity to suppress disease symptoms. In China, the use of antibiotics is so pervasive that many diseases are no longer affected by them at all. In the U.S., too, there's growing concern among doctors that antibiotics are losing their efficacy in cases where people and pets have ingested too many of them. More alarming, certain bacteria appear to be growing impervious to antibiotics altogether by mutating to new strains. In the U.S., staphylococcal infections were once easily thwarted by penicillin. When penicillin began to lose its effectiveness against staph, other drugs were used. Gradually, some strains of staph have become impervious to all of them; doctors now acknowledge that unless some new, even more potent antibiotic can be devised, they'll have nothing left in their medical arsenal. And so staph will be, in a word, unstoppable.

Even antibiotics that do appear to work effectively—if treating symptoms, rather than curing disease, can be said to be effective work—are often used excessively to a patient's detriment, especially if that patient is a pet.

Take a dog at six months old that begins to exhibit itchiness, inflammation, and pustules containing staphylococcal bacteria (a condition called staph or juvenile pyoderma). A conventional veterinarian will assume that this is a bacterial infection of the skin, and administer antibiotics. A holistic veterinarian, mindful that the skin is a powerful eliminator of toxins, will first consider that any inflammation is part of a healthful process. As in throat infections, toxins that are being eliminated promote bacterial growth, which white blood cells then "clean up." What do I do about it? Nothing more than support the overall health of the patient—and perhaps add a homeopathic remedy or herbal preparation to help relieve symptoms—because this elimination, and the bacteria that appear with it, is part of a pet's maturation, just as acne is associated with puberty in humans. If the bacteria are killed by antibiotics, the symptoms will subside, but the overall effect will be one of retained toxicity, especially if cortisone is used in conjunction with the antibiotics. Then the dog's dermatitis—*itis* means inflammation—will reappear as another inflammation, perhaps of the ear (otitis) or the throat (tracheobronchitis), the intestines (enteritis) or the anal sacs (anal sacculitis).

Externally and internally, a pet's body, like a human body, heals via inflammation. Sprain an ankle, and it swells. Get a cut, and the skin around the cut inflames. Ingest poisons, and the liver will swell. As the poisons get eliminated, the lining of the colon will inflame (i.e, colitis). A body whose inflammations are repeatedly suppressed by drugs will exhibit increasingly serious symptoms, or "diseases," until they grow powerful enough to be potentially lethal.

The first two causes of disease we've considered are tangible, at least. They can be analyzed and measured, and many of the instances of either can be changed. But what are we to make of emotion? How a pet feels might seem, at best, an indirect cause of disease. Indeed, to most conventional veterinarians, it still does. It shouldn't, however. Two decades ago, the emotions of a human patient with cancer were given minimal consideration. Today, cancer doctors take for granted that the degree to which a patient "fights" his illness with a positive attitude is integral to his chances of recovery. More cautiously, many doctors allow that some cancers may, in some patients, be precipitated at least partly by emotions as well. A pet, as we know, is not capable of intellectual thought. He does, however, feel strong emotions which, I believe, affect both his likelihood of incurring a chronic, degenerative disease and his chances of beating it back.

This too is a factor so important for pets that much of Chapter Nine addresses it in one way or another. Here, let me raise just a few questions that point toward the role of emotions in disease.

- Does your pet love you?
- Does he care about you?
- If you became incapacitated, how might he feel?
- If you began to act brusquely toward your pet for some reason—perhaps because you were sick, or distracted—how would he feel?
- If he couldn't win your approval and love, which he craves, how might he react?
- If he incurred a debilitating disease and you conveyed only anxiety and fear, how do you think he would feel? And might those feelings affect his condition?

Of the four causes of disease, three, at least, are within our power to influence today. The fourth, sadly, will only change with time.

When I began my practice, I would have said that environment was the principal cause of disease among pets. As my perspective broadened, I began to appreciate the role that diet played. Eventually, I came to see how important the emotions are, too. I discovered, from my training, that some diseases do get passed genetically from one generation to the next. But I would not have said, until very recently, that mutant genes do more to cause disease in pets than any of the other three causes. I say it now partly because I've treated more pets and the evidence has grown. Partly, it's because there's more genetic disease—much, much more—than there was a quarter century ago.

At first glance, that might seem a curious supposition to make. If a pet inherits a mutated gene that makes him likely to get a certain kind of cancer, then surely a parent, or a grandparent before him, had the same genetic predilection, right? Wrong. Most genetic traits, it's true, tend to appear in every generation, or every other generation, in a pet's line, stretching back as far as we can document it. So are genetic predilections among humans: that's why we can look at a sepia-toned photograph of a long-dead great-great-grandfather and see strong hints of our own physical features. Unfortunately, a genetic tendency toward disease can be introduced into a current generation and then become ingrained in a pet's genetic code. In fact, the mutation can worsen in successive generations.

What introduces those mutations? Any of the environmental factors mentioned above. Principal among them, I feel, are the myriad chemicals brought into the world within the last thirty or forty years—chemicals whose genetic effects on living creatures we don't yet fully understand. Since pets' life spans are so much shorter than ours, and since so many generations have come and gone just in the course of my own human life, those effects have grown more evident, more various, and more imbedded. So quickly is medical science advancing the frontiers of genetics—by the time this book appears, the whole human genome may be identified and catalogued, an unbelievable prospect even ten years ago—that in our lifetimes, science may manage to undo some of the genetic damage it has caused. Meantime, all we can do with genetically passed diseases is to treat them on an individual basis, strengthening the immune system and, sometimes, enabling a pet to heal himself.

This I know: that the more we change the environment, the more any animal's body will be changed. The more we prop up the body with chemicals instead of encouraging it to protect itself from those changes, the weaker it will be in the long run. We perceive that weakness as disease, because the body isn't what it used to be. In fact, the body is simply creating a new balance with nature, one that takes such changes into account. It may die, as a result, but that's of no concern to nature, only to us. Or it may reacquire the balance it used to have, the one we call health, if we help it to help itself.

PART TWO

TAKING ACTION

CHAPTER THREE

It All Starts with Food

Beside my computer right now is a 13.2-ounce can of Ken-L Ration Grand Recipe dog food with "homestyle chunks in sauce." I chose it at random this morning at the local supermarket, along with a few other kinds of dog and cat food that we'll get to in a minute. Have you ever stopped to read the ingredients on the food you give your pet? Let's give it a whirl with Ken-L Ration, as common a brand as you can find.

The first ingredient listed for any food, as you may know, is the weightiest one. The first ingredient in Grand Recipe is "water sufficient for processing." Just how much water are we talking about here? The answer appears on another part of the label called "guaranteed analysis": moisture is listed as constituting 82.0 percent of the contents. So a good part of this can will simply be passed by your dog as urine or will serve to dilute the potency of his stomach's acids needed to help digest the meat. Hearty chunks indeed!

The second ingredient is "poultry by-products." Uh-oh. "Poultry by-products" are not simply the parts of the chicken you'd rather leave on the platter as it goes around the family dinner table. According to the Association of American Feed Control Officials (AAFCO), an independent group that issues guidelines approved by the Food and Drug Administration, poultry by-products "must consist of non-rendered clean parts of carcasses of slaughtered poultry such as heads, feet, viscera, free from fecal content and foreign matter except in such trace amounts as might occur unavoidably in good factory practice." So this product may include chicken heads and feet, and viscera—an inclusive term that refers not only to intestines but to any internal organs, such as the heart and lungs, thorax and abdomen. I don't know whether any of those parts might be in this or any other can of Grand Recipe; the can label does not specify the nature of the poultry by-products included, nor is it required to do so. But the term is hardly cause for celebration. The reference to fecal matter in the AAFCO guidelines sounds more reassuring until I start to wonder how even a slaughter-house determined to observe "good factory practices" could remove all or even any of the fecal matter from each of the thousands of chickens being slaughtered and processed at its plant each day. (Now *there* would be a job!) And what about that other assurance, that the by-products must consist of "non-rendered clean parts of the carcass." Just what is rendering anyway?

More on that below.

Next on the ingredient list of Grand Recipe we come to soybean meal. Sounds vaguely healthy, doesn't it? Sort of . . . vegetarian? Not remotely. Soybeans are not easily digestible by dogs, so much of their protein is wasted, especially when they're exposed to high heat and processing, as nearly all pet foods are. Worse, certain breeds tend to be allergic to soy protein, including Akitas, Dobermans, German shepherds and Labrador retrievers. "Soybean meal," however, isn't even straight soybeans. After most of the oil—the part that's somewhat beneficial for people, if not for pets—is removed from soybeans, the husks that remain are ground up as "soybean meal."

Wheat flour, the third ingredient in Grand Recipe, might seem less disconcerting than soybean meal. In itself it's not a problem. Unfortunately, AAFCO allows wheat flour to include "the tail of the mill," a quaint phrase that means anything swept up from the wheat mill floor at the end of the week.

Finally, with the fourth ingredient, we get substance: *meat*. Here at last are those hearty chunks, in whatever modest percentage of Grand Recipe that remains after water, by-products, and meal. Though about that word "meat": What does it mean? According to AAFCO, meat can be derived from any skeletal muscle of any slaughtered animal. It can come from the tongue, diaphragm, heart, or esophagus, and it can include fat or skin. "If it bears a name descriptive of its kind," AAFCO's guideline goes on to say of meat, "it must correspond thereto."

Since the Ken-L Ration label does not specify which kind of meat is contained in Grand Recipe, your guess is as good as mine. For that matter, your guess is as good as AAFCO's, because this group's only job is to declare what *should* be stated on pet food labels.* Each state has an agricultural department or office of state chemist that may enforce AAFCO guidelines—or not. The FDA helps AAFCO draft its guidelines, but does nothing to enforce them. Indeed, the FDA takes no action on pet food matters unless a claim is made on a label that may be fraudulent, such as that a cat food may help feline lower urinary tract disease (formerly known as feline urological syndrome) when it does no such thing. There is, in other words, no federal agency that polices the pet food industry at all, and at best a patchwork of state regulators who may, from time to time, make inquiries. Unfortunately for your dog or cat, the pet food industry pretty much regulates itself.

In 1983, the Hills company, a large pet food producer, waged an advertising campaign to show how much better its brand was than the competition. To help make its point, it created an ad that showed how you could produce a blend of shoe soles, coal, and crankcase oil that would meet AAFCO's minimum requirements for protein, fiber, fat, and other nutrients. We tend to assume that pet foods have improved in quality over time: after all, the packaging on most brands is better than it used to be, with reassuring buzz phrases like "complete nutritional diet" and "scientifically proven." Unfortunately, no one who's made an effort to analyze pet food in recent years from outside the industry and government has been able to determine that the products *are* any better than they ever were. An investigative report by the Animal Protection Institute of America, a national nonprofit animal advocacy organization, is both impressive in its scholarship and utterly depressing in its conclusions. A book by Ann Martin titled *Food Pets Die For* is even more damning.

For starters, let's consider the basic appeal of almost any pet food: meat or fish. We like to think that commercial brands contain at least some decent cuts of one or the other. The truth is they contain none. Any cuts fit for human consumption are consumed by humans: they're too valuable not to be. Only the heads, feet, and various organs are set

*Though AAFCO is independent in this pursuit, much of its funding comes from the sale of publications that contain its guidelines and other information—publications bought, largely, by the pet food industry, according to an AAFCO representative.

aside for pet food. And that's the *best* of what's in commercial pet food.

Fish parts, at least, are free of hormones, drugs, and disease—though they may contain high levels of mercury or some other toxin that makes them unfit for human consumption. More troubling, however, is the livestock fated to end up as pet food.

The poisoning of pet food meat begins with the hormones fed to livestock to make them grow faster, so they can be slaughtered that much sooner. People who eat hormone-fattened meat are, in my opinion, taking a certain health risk. But at least they're eating choice cuts, and their diets are varied. Pets who eat hormone-injected, ground-up and processed meat by-products every day are definitely at greater risk. As Richard and Susan Pitcairn observe in *Dr. Pitcairn's Complete Guide to Natural Health for Dogs and Cats*, laboratory animals have developed cancers when fed proportionately as many hormones as livestock is.

The daily feed of livestock is also laced with "maintenance doses" of antibiotics intended to prevent disease. As likely, these drugs instill toxicity that increases cancer risks, both in the livestock and the pets that feed on processed meat. Industry guidelines direct farmers to wean their livestock from antibiotics thirty days before slaughter; ostensibly, that's enough time for the antibiotics to work their way out of the animals' systems. But is it? My own sense is that it's unlikely a powerful antibiotic will be flushed out entirely in that time. And again, a pet fed the same diet of antibiotic-laced substandard meat every day is at far greater risk of cancer than a person eating choice cuts on an occasional basis.

These guidelines, such as they are, ignore a whole other category of livestock: the direly sick animals who collapse from one disease or another and, as a result, never reach the slaughterhouse. These animals are deemed unfit for human consumption, killed, and sent off to "rendering" plants which supply meat protein used in pet food.

Nine years ago, as a result of her own dogs' illness, Ann Martin found herself thrust into an investigation she'd never considered pursuing: determining the role that rendering plants play in the composition of pet food. Her book *Food Pets Die For* is to the pet food industry what Rachel Carson's *Silent Spring* is to the petrochemical industry. (In fact, that comparison is made in the book's introduction by Dr. Michael Fox, a vice president of the Humane Society of the

United States; I just heartily echo his view.) In her native Ontario, Martin discovered that rendering—at its best, the boiling of any animal substances discarded by slaughterhouses as unfit for human consumption—is an established, if little-publicized industry, and that "rendered" animal substances go directly into livestock and pet feed. These substances may include "4-D" meat: meat from dead animals, dying animals, and diseased and disabled animals. (To that I add a fifth D for "drugged.") These 4-D carcasses may have cancerous tumors, worm-infested organs, and the like—basically, anything and everything goes in the pot. Worse, Martin found, rendering plants happily accept roadkill, dead zoo animals, and, most appallingly, euthanized pets from animal shelters and veterinary clinics.

Shocked by the standards she found in Canada, Martin sent a questionnaire to the state governments of all fifty of the United States, asking, among other things, if state laws allow euthanized pets to be rendered, and if rendered material is freely used for livestock and pet feed. Twenty states replied blithely that no laws forbid the rendering of euthanized pets or their use in pet food. The remaining thirty states did not reply, suggesting their standards are just as lax. "Finding companion pets eating dead cats and dogs objectionable is more than just aesthetics," Martin writes. "Safety is at stake."

Indeed it is, since most pets are euthanized with sodium pentobarbital, which medical authorities acknowledge may be dangerous or deadly, even absorbed indirectly after some days or weeks, by healthy cats and dogs. Just how significant is this unpublicized aspect of the commercial pet food chain? Martin found that the main rendering plant in Quebec was rendering *11 tons of dogs and cats per week*. On March 11, 1997, the *New York Times* reported that the city of Los Angeles sends two hundred tons of euthanized cats and dogs to a company called West Coast Rendering every month. Most veterinarians Martin spoke with had no idea that the pets they euthanized were ending up at rendering plants; they assumed that the services they paid to remove the animals were cremating them. When Martin explained the situation, all switched to a reputable cremater. In other parts of Canada, however, and throughout the United States, the rendering continues, apparently without the awareness of nearly any veterinarians.

A couple of years ago, the *Los Angeles Times* ran a story about the sad fate of two circus elephants so maltreated that they died of tuberculosis during the circus's run. The story was tragic, but so, too, was the following detail mentioned in passing about one of the elephants: "Workers used a forklift to put the animal's body on a truck for transport to the San Bernardino State Diagnostic Lab. A necropsy showed that 80 percent of Joyce's lung tissue was infected either with cancer or tuberculosis. The body was taken to a rendering factory to be processed into animal food."

As bad or worse than the "meat" in many pet foods are the chemicals used to make the "meat" look and taste fresh. Not until after my brother and I had stopped feeding Leigh Gaines Burgers did we learn that of all the dog foods, the "semi-moist" kinds may be the worst in this regard. To keep them looking fresh and moist, manufacturers use chemicals called humectants and emulsifiers. The most common—and most notorious—in this class is propylene glycol, a compound whose molecular structure is nearly identical to that of ethylene glycol, which is antifreeze. Though propylene glycol is harder to find on ingredient labels than it used to be, all "semi-moist" foods are loaded with sugar and various preservatives to keep them moist in their plastic wrapping for literally years.

Take Purina's Moist & Meaty, another brand I picked up this morning at the supermarket. Dogs love the "chopped burgers," declares the package, because "real beef is our #1 ingredient." Beef *is* listed first—whatever "beef" means to Purina—so that it is, ostensibly, the heaviest ingredient in the recipe. But look at what's second: high-fructose corn syrup.* Corn syrup is not only useless to pets, it's actually harmful, overstimulating the production of insulin and potentially causing diabetes or other diseases. The "burgers" loaded with it are sickeningly sweet, and have nothing to do with the ground chuck we associate with the words "burgers." Perhaps Purina should advertise these "chopped burgers" as Moist & Meaty Sugar Burgers!

Let's look at one other dog food I bought this morning: Ken-L Ration's Gravy Train. Dry "kibbles" are reputed to have more protein than either semi-moist "burgers" or canned "wet" food. The

---

*The makers of Gaines Burgers used to list two forms of corn syrup separately—"high-fructose corn syrup" and "corn syrup." Yet the two types of corn syrup are basically the same. If the two had been combined, "corn syrup" would have been the first—i.e., greatest in volume—ingredient in that product, a disconcerting discovery for any owner who thought he was feeding his pet real "burgers."

moisture content of Gravy Train, for starters, is "not more than 10 percent," which sounds impressive: the remaining 90 percent, one would guess, must contain protein. In fact, we can determine exactly how much protein this remaining "dry weight" contains by a simple equation. All we have to do is divide the dry weight into the "crude protein" figure listed in the same place on the label. When we do that, it turns out that our can of Grand Recipe, despite its high water content, actually has more "crude protein" than Gravy Train. So the canned food actually beats the kibble! But remember, "crude protein" may contain such ingredients as chicken feathers and beaks. The "crude protein" constitutes some, if not most, of the protein. So all you're getting is more of what you didn't want in the first place. Lose-lose.

Cat food, too, appears as kibble or "wet" food (also as clear-packaged semi-moist chow, in the case of Tender Vittles, though the word "burgers" is omitted because, presumably, it sounds unfeline) and contains many of the same dubious ingredients: digests, by-products, and meals. On a can of Friskies "mixed grill formula" I bought this morning along with those other tasty provisions is the especially unimpressive mention of *bonemeal*. What bones? What meal? Who knows? AAFCO's guidelines define "meat and bonemeal" as "the rendered product from mammal tissues, including bone, exclusive of any added blood, hair, hoof, horn, hide trimmings, manure, stomach and rumen contents, except in such amounts as may occur unavoidably in good processing practices." As Ann Martin observes, however, even this modest requirement seems unlikely to be met at the rendering plant. How easy is it for a renderer, after all, to remove those offending parts from every animal he throws into the pot? In fact, Martin's investigation led her to believe not only that whole pets are rendered but that some of their collars and tags are thrown in, too!

For cats, all this rendered and highly processed meat, even if not of dreadful or dangerous quality, poses a special concern. Cats need a certain amount of taurine, an amino acid, to avoid retinal atrophy and a heart disease called cardiomyopathy; they can only absorb it from meat. In recent years, many pet food manufacturers have begun adding taurine after a disturbing incidence of these diseases in cats. Of course, if there was enough unadulterated healthy meat in their products to begin with, adding taurine would be unnecessary. Cats, as Ann Martin observes, also tend to suffer from excess levels of iodine from the commercial foods they're given. Too much iodine can lead to hyper-thyroidism (an overactive thyroid) in cats.* (It can also lead to hypothyroidism—an underactive thyroid—in dogs.) And lower feline urinary tract disease has also been linked to the high levels of ash, phosphorous, and magnesium in commercial pet food.

Pet owners who do read ingredient labels will probably find some reassurance from the many vitamins listed after the main ingredients on nearly any pet food label. Ken-L Ration's Grand Recipe, for example, includes "vitamin E supplement, niacin supplement, vitamin A supplement, riboflavin supplement, vitamin B_{12} supplement, and vitamin D_3 supplement." The other brands on my desk contain the same or similar ingredients. Why "supplements"? Because Grand Recipe's "hearty chunks" of dubious no-name meat, once cooked at high temperatures, have such little nutritional value that vitamins must be added to provide the overall minimum level of nutrition requested by AAFCO. A premix of these vitamins adds up to 130 percent of the established minimum daily requirements to compensate for the loss incurred by the heating process. But while a food analysis will show an ample or excess amount on the label as a result, these vitamins are then cooked at high temperatures, so their quality is, to say the least, diminished.

The roll call of ingredients of all mainstream pet foods ends in a jumble of nearly unpronounceable chemicals used as preservatives, and a smattering of colors with numbers. Packaged food for people has preservations too, of course, but not, for example, propyl gallate, which some doctors believe causes liver damage. Sodium carboxy-methyl-cellulose is an edible plastic filler that used to be put in thick shakes at some fast-food franchises to make them thicker, until the FDA outlawed it—for human consumption. It's still in some pet foods, along with ingredients like cellulose gum and guar gum—all used to bind beak bits, ground bones, and other ingredients into chunks, "burgers," or kibble. BHA and BHT are still almost universally used; both are suspected carcinogens. (Foods for people contain BHA and BHT too, but in minute quantities; and again, people don't eat the

---

*Research being done at the University of Georgia's College of Veterinary Medicine suggests that various other substances in cat food called goitrogens may also contribute to hyperthyroidism. Identifying and eliminating these goitrogens may help produce a decline in hyperthyroidism from its current epidemic levels.

same food at every meal.) One of my favorites is potassium sorbate, a preservative used to preserve the things that weren't preserved before they went in! And then, on my package of Purina Moist & Meaty, is ethoxyquin, currently the most notorious preservative of the bunch.

Ethoxyquin, also used in many "better brand" foods, was concocted in the 1950s by Monsanto, originally as a rubber stabilizer. It is, in fact, the major preservative in tires, keeping the rubber in them from oxidizing. As a synthetic antioxidant, it works the same magic in food, too, keeping fats from turning rancid so that the food is more or less edible forever. It's used in most farm feeds, especially for poultry, which is to say that people, not just pets, absorb it. But only in pet foods is it used directly. And as the Animal Protection Institute of America (APIA) observes in a recent investigative report on pet foods, ethoxyquin has been associated with a staggering array of medical complications, including infertility, neonatal illness and death, skin and hair coat problems, immune disorders, thyroid, pancreas, and liver dysfunction, and behavioral disorders. I know of three academic studies—by researchers in Australia, Norway, and Mexico—that found strong links between ethoxyquin and various ill effects in laboratory rats or chickens, including significant degradation of livers and kidneys. *Bad stuff.* Moreover, as the APIA observes, ethoxyquin need only be listed on a label if the pet food manufacturer was the one who put it in the product. When it enters the pet food chain at the slaughterhouse or rendering plant, it need not be listed. And over the years, its use has increased.

"The FDA kept allowing more usage in pet foods because it was more concerned about the animals that were part of the human food chain," the report states. Now neither the FDA nor the consumer has the means to measure whether even those lower standards are being met. "There is absolutely no way of knowing if the pet food companies are complying with the law or not."

Also near the bottom of most pet food ingredient lists are a number of colors, usually accompanied by numbers. These, of course, are artificial dyes. Ken-L Ration's Grand Recipe has Red 3, Purina's Moist & Meaty has Red 40, while Ken-L Ration's Gravy Train sweeps the derby with Yellow 5, Yellow 6, Red 40, and Blue 2—what a beautiful pageant! Unfortunately, all are inorganic and toxic. Since neither dogs nor cats perceive color nearly as well as we do, why do the pet food makers bother? To impress you! After all, you wouldn't buy Moist & Meaty if it looked naturally gray rather than sirloin-fresh red.

Synthetic flavorings, on the other hand, are only for pets. Phosphoric acid, for one, tingles animals' tongues and so acts as an artificial appetite stimulator, especially in cats. Beef digest, poultry digest, salt, and sugar are all also used to perk up tasteless food. Barely a nutrient among them.

Imagine waking up in the morning and coming down to the kitchen to make yourself breakfast. You take some soybean grits, mix them with some tainted cattle-meat meal, throw in a few beaks and feathers, smother your concoction with processed sugar syrup and chemicals, then sprinkle on a few preservatives and dyes. Pressure-cook the hell out of it, let it cool—and dig in!

What if you were told that this is exactly what you'd eat at every meal for the rest of your life? Is it any wonder our pets have degenerative diseases? That so many get cancer? That so many die before their time?

Even if these foods were as hearty as advertised, even if the meat was real meat, the vitamins not destroyed when added back in, the color and taste untampered with, would it seem beneficial for a pet to eat the same meal day after day, year after year? Due to our own laziness as owners, we've bought the idea that a bowl of "complete and balanced nutrition" is best for a pet, so we can feel we're filling his dietary needs simply by filling the bowl with the same food every day. In fact, no animal in the wild typically eats meals of "complete and balanced nutrition" every day. And so, over the course of history, surviving species have developed internal systems that work best when *not* fed ingredients considered to be "complete and balanced" at every meal. Cats and dogs, in order to adapt to domestication as they have, likely no longer have such internal systems. But that's not to say they're the healthier for it.

Because the food most pets eat is so *un*healthy, the toll it takes is that much worse. Every day, a pet living on most commercial-brand foods absorbs not the "complete and balanced nutrition" intended for him but a host of toxins that his body must struggle to expel. The more toxins he absorbs, the more his body needs real nutrition to help his immune system do its job. Then comes the catch-22. His body can't use these inorganic substances, so it tries to void them. If it succeeds, they take a variety of forms that seem symptomatic of disease: as mucus, flaky skin, diarrhea, and the rest. On come the drugs, to tamp them back down: the cough suppressants to stop that route of expulsion, the antiseborrheic shampoos to stop the flaky skin discharges, the

Imodium to stop the mucous-laden stool. When the immune system gives up, blocked by drugs or simply exhausted by the shortage of enzymes and vitamins it needs, the toxins begin to reside in bodily tissues, precipitating more severe disease.

You can boost your pet's health profoundly by making one simple decision. All you have to do is to change his diet from unhealthy, commercial-brand fare to something you may never have imagined giving him: *real food!*

Think about that a minute, and then gauge your reaction. Chances are, the notion of feeding a pet "real food" seems peculiar to you, or foolish, or just plain wrong. *Chicken stew for your Afghan, madam? A T-bone steak for that hungry-looking Lab? The vegetarian plate for Miss Fifi today?* Yes, it does sound odd. And yet what could be more natural than an animal eating . . . food?

There's a lack of logic here, and it isn't accidental. Over the decades, the pet food industry has grown to be a powerful force in America's economy. We've been taught by it to believe that pet food comes out of a can or package—period. Advertising leads us to believe that the only question before us is which well-known commercial brand to choose over the others. Supermarkets reinforce the perception by offering the major brands—all highly processed, low-quality fare—and nothing else. Even the few newer brands of relatively good-quality prepackaged pet food are almost never found at mainstream markets. Partly that's because major brands monopolize shelf space. Partly it's because small manufacturers can't afford to supply the chain stores: pet food is too heavy in bulk, and has too narrow a profit margin, to be transported in anything less than huge volumes, thanks to the way the majors have defined the business (low-quality food at low cost). As for finding *fresh* pet food at the market—forget it. There is no such thing. Though in one sense, none need be added: the fresh food you buy at the market for yourself is the food you should give your pet, too.

The pet food industry appears to be a cynical one, focused mainly on the corporate profits its prepackaged product lines bring. The very idea of animals eating fresh food is, to put it mildly, not one it seems to encourage. But it's not the only culprit in the Great Pet Food Conspiracy. Another is AAFCO, with its standard that all of a pet's dietary needs—proteins, fats, carbohydrates, vitamins, and minerals—be present in every meal. AAFCO means, of course, to aid pets by assuring they get the nutrients they need. Unfortunately, it has the opposite effect. The quality of nutrients isn't there in prepackaged foods to begin with, since oversight is nill. The food that isn't nutritious but appears to be thus becomes a pet's *in*complete meal day after day after day. And the pet food industry gets to sell the greatest possible volume, can by can and box by box, with the least real variety.

AAFCO's guidelines are misleading us when they suggest that standard pet food can fill a pet's dietary needs, but also its fundamental premise is wrong. There *is* no such thing as a meal providing "complete and balanced nutrition," either for pets or for people, because the nutritional needs counteract one another. Mix proteins and fats in the same meal, for example, and the oils from the fats coat the walls of the stomach, keeping the stomach's acids from breaking down the proteins so that they can be used by the body. The way a pet *should* eat is the way we too should eat, ingesting different food types from meal to meal. If the foods are healthy in their own different ways, they supply complete nutrition in the aggregate, with the nutrition of one food not blocking out that of another.

In their own way, that's how dogs in the wild ate, too, a long, long time ago. Like wolves, wild dogs would hunt down their prey in packs. But unless they were starving, they wouldn't eat the dead animal in its entirety at once. Instead, they'd open its belly and eat the contents, along with the internal organs, then bury the carcass. A few days later, when they grew hungry again, they'd dig up those parts and have another full meal: leg of lamb, loin of pork, or whatever other savory haunches they'd hunted. The time between courses enabled the dogs to digest these very different kinds of nutrition without having them block each other out. (The meat of their prey contained fat, but in a raw, natural form that did not get processed in the stomach and thus did not block the digestion of protein.) And because the carcass had been buried in warm earth, it would have fermented by the time they dug it up, which would have increased its enzyme content and thus made it more nutritious. Today, the only vestige of that behavior—and diet—is a dog's instinct to bury a bone.

If dogs survived well enough in the wild, they also seemed to cope as pets in more recent centuries, before prepackaged pet food. So, for that matter, did cats. And yet the conventional wisdom among most veterinarians remains that pets should never eat table food. Pets in nature ate table food; they just didn't have tables!

The foolishness about table food underscores a larger point: that veterinary schools are the third culprit in the Great Pet Food Conspiracy. When I was in veterinary school, the whole issue of animal food was addressed only as one of percentages: what percentage of a pet's (unvarying) meal should be protein, carbohydrates, fats, and so forth. Quantities were stressed; quality was all but ignored. Switching my brother's dog Leigh from Gaines Burgers to a macrobiotic diet was the first step we took toward questioning our teachers' approach.* Soon enough, I realized that the *ideal* diet for a pet was the polar opposite of what he gets in a can or box. It's what he ate in the wild! After centuries of domestication, of course, dogs and cats have evolved into tamer creatures incapable of hunting as they once did, much less eating their prey, and their systems have changed accordingly. But with a little experimentation, I found I could give my pets a diet ideally suited to their present-day constitution. And it sure didn't come out of a can.

When I tell an owner that a change of diet can affect her pet's health in a matter of days, the first reaction is usually delight, sometimes even exhilaration. Toss out the prepackaged food, I say. Soon, symptoms you've grown all too accustomed to—or tried in vain to dispel with antibiotics—may improve dramatically. Everything from skin irritations and dull, matted fur to bad breath and digestive problems to lethargy and lack of appetite can be alleviated. All you have to do, I add, is to start preparing your pet's meals yourself.

At that, the owner swallows nervously. A guilty look comes over her face. I know what she's thinking. *Cook for my pet? When I (a) don't even have time to cook for myself, or (b) already cook dinner for my spouse and children as it is, or (c) don't know how to cook at all?* Let's face it: the fourth culprit in the Great Pet Food Conspiracy is probably you.

Feeding your pet from a can or box is easy, quick, and seemingly cheap: the reasons the pet food industry rose up in the first place. And cooking or preparing for your pet may seem like one extra burden you don't need in your life. But it can be easier than you think, certainly easier than it appears from the few available holistic pet care books that list dozens of complex recipes and all but order you to become your pet's *haut chef de cuisine*. Consider what I do for my pets every Sunday morning.

---

*Although this new diet did contain various combinations of food, its quality and wholesomeness were such a step in the right direction toward proper nutrition.

First, I take a raw free-range chicken and put it in a pot of good water (i.e., purified water!). I throw in a little sliced garlic and a pinch of salt, boil the water, then let it simmer for perhaps fifty minutes. (That's for a bird of about two and a half to three pounds.) Then I take the chicken out and put in about a pound of organic brown rice, cooking it on low heat for an hour or so, or millet for about half that time. (For both brown rice and millet, figure two and a half cups of water to one cup of grain.) Just before the grains are done, I put in a 12-ounce bag of frozen vegetables. Suffused with the taste of chicken, the cooked grains and vegetables will be especially appealing to my crew. Meanwhile, I will have removed the chicken meat from the carcass and added it back into the mixture. Refrigerated in plastic containers, the grain-and-vegetable mix and the rest of the chicken will last my (mostly small) pets several days if interspersed with two or three other home-cooked meals. When I use an especially big turkey that yields more containers than I can use in a week or so, I'll just freeze the rest.

Simple as that recipe is, it raises complex issues. Not forgetting that the recipe *is* simple, let's consider them one by one.

First of all, the food is cooked, not raw. But if we're trying to put our pets on a more natural diet, how does cooked food square with that scene of wild dogs of yore, eating freshly killed prey? Strangely enough, it does. The animals brought down by wild dogs were herbivores—deer, for example—who ate grains and berries. When a wild dog tore open a deer's belly, the food he found inside was already chewed, further decomposed by saliva, stomach acids, and enzymes, then heated to about 102 degrees Fahrenheit by the stomach's natural warmth. It was, as a result, processed enough to be considered cooked.

Ah, you say, but when the wild dogs finished what was in the deer's belly and moved on to the deer itself, the deer was *raw* meat. So why cook the chicken?

The issue of raw-meat feedings to pets is a contentious one among holistic veterinarians. It's true that raw meats do accord with pets' natural diets and supply, among other nutrients, the amino acid taurine, found only in flesh-based protein. My hesitation is that I don't trust the meat. The *E. coli* outbreak that led to a huge federal recall of frozen hamburger patties in 1997, the widespread incidences before that of salmonella in chicken—these were, I feel, only the latest indications that our meat is unsafe. So I cook my pets' meat as a rule. Then, to compensate for what has been destroyed by cooking, I add specific supplements and enzymes. If you have a source you trust, though, you might give organic raw meat a try—as I did, sort of by accident.

I kept my own pets away from raw chicken when I first began cooking for them, even though I used only free-range chicken. Then one evening I had to rush out on an emergency call and left a nearly defrosted raw chicken on the kitchen counter. I came back to find parts of a picked-clean carcass on the floor, with five very self-satisfied dogs and cats munching on chicken bones in the living room. I was sure that if the meat didn't poison them, they'd choke on the bones. Guess what? They were fine.

For a while I continued to play it safe, cooking the chicken and putting the carcasses in garbage bins with locking lids. When my crew figured out how to unlock the bins and had several more bone fests without incident, I began to relax. And the day my golden retriever Daniel dragged a dead wild boar out of the Westchester woods (I *swear* it was a boar; it was big, black and white, and hairy) and polished it off, bones and all, without getting sick, I officially changed my position.

Though not, I have to say, without regrets. The fact is that I'm a vegetarian myself, and have been for more than twenty years, for all the obvious reasons. I hate the inhumane ways animals are raised for slaughter. I'm sickened that they're slaughtered at all when we have so much other food to eat. It depresses me to think of how much river water is diverted, at great expense, to irrigate grazing lands for cattle and cows (not to mention the very real environmental hazard of methane gas being emitted as a waste product from millions of cows). And as a doctor, I understand the ways in which red meat especially can constrict human blood vessels with fat and cholesterol, in bodies likely never intended to consume meat at all.

That's the vegetarian view. As a veterinarian, however, I know that both dogs and cats were meant to eat meat in the wild, and that as modified as their systems are by the modern world, they do still need meat, raw or cooked. They aren't merely drawn to it by their biological instincts as a fun food choice. Specifically, they need more protein and calcium than a vegetarian diet can provide—which is also to say more protein and calcium than humans need. Because dogs and cats *are* carnivores.

If I'd had any doubts that pets should eat meat, they were dispelled some time ago by a visit from several vegans. Vegetarians in the extreme, vegans will not touch any products connected in any way with living creatures. So no dairy products for them, not even yogurt; no soups or sauces made with chicken or beef bouillon; and no fish (or caviar!). The vegans arrived at my clinic one day with their eight-and-a-half-year-old shepherd mix, named—guess what?—Vegan. And of course Vegan had been raised on a strict vegan diet. Unfortunately, she was dying of mammary cancer. I asked the vegans exactly what they were feeding Vegan, and to me it sounded great. But in addition to her cancer, Vegan the dog was acting so aggressively—lunging at me with intent to kill, or at least bite—that the diet appeared to have damaged her emotional state as well as her physical being. "Your diet sounds great," I said, "but something's wrong here, because if it was properly balanced for Vegan, I don't think she'd be dying or trying to kill me."

I tested Vegan's blood for its immune protein content, and was shocked by how high it was. You might think, when a disease like cancer takes hold, that protein levels in the blood would drop, but that's not the case. The protein level goes up because the body's immune system, working improperly, doesn't efficiently use these immune proteins. Since the body isn't using protein as it should, the immune system begins to drain protein from the muscles instead. Diseases like cancer and AIDS are typically "wasting diseases" because as the body saps the muscles of protein, the muscles waste away. It helps, at least, to give a wasting-disease patient red meat, because it contains protein that the body can recognize and use, thus allaying the wasting process. "If this dog doesn't get some meat as soon as possible," I told the vegans, "she will die."

But the vegans wouldn't permit that. Their only concession was to allow injections of specifically isolated, naturally occurring immunological protein from healthy donor dogs. Vegan wouldn't actually be eating the protein, they rationalized, and another animal was not being killed to produce them. They left as a group by car for Florida, and called me a day or two later from Virginia: Vegan had gotten really weak. "Come on, guys," I pleaded with them. "Give this dog some protein." At last, they bought her a can of red-meat dog food—and Vegan roused herself to attack it. Still, the protein came too late. Within another day, Vegan was dead.

. . .

On the issue of raw food for pets, I've recently gone from wary endorsement to real enthusiasm. I've been inspired by its benefits as shown in the work of animal health advocate (and former Miss Rheingold!) Celeste Yarnall (author of *Natural Cat Care* and *Natural Dog Care*). And seeing the effects that an increase in raw food has on animals has led me to increase the amount of it for my pets as well as in my own diet. One day, I fully expect all the members of my household to be living *exclusively* on raw foods.

My cats will go for raw food as much as the dogs do, by the way—and even organic red meat (though they still prefer cooked food). I also let them have the bones, which they adore. I know this violates a cardinal rule of conventional pet care, and I realize that some pets have gotten bones stuck in their throats or stomachs, so I won't promise you that bones are safe for *your* pet. The fact is, though, that over many years, neither my dogs nor my cats have ever had a problem with poultry bones, raw or cooked. (Many veterinarians caution that cooked bones are more dangerous than raw ones because the heating process has made them more likely to splinter; it hasn't happened at my house but to be safe, I advise owners to stick to raw bones.) I do see animals who have gastroenteritis as a result of bone eating—intestinal inflammations that brought on vomiting and diarrhea. But in my house, my small dogs get bones, mostly cooked, from organic chicken, lamb chops, and even huge turkeys, at least twice weekly, and I can't recall a single bone-swallowing incident. And think about it: Have animals in the wild, including poultry predators like wolves and wild dogs, ever seemed troubled by bones? Nature just wouldn't be designed that way. To be sure, wild dogs had stronger jaws than domesticated dogs do, and more muscular stomachs, and more powerful hydrochloric acid to help in the digestion of troublesome bones. But especially as pets become healthier on good diets, they seem to grow more capable of handling bones, too.

Raw fish poses another dilemma that gets judged either way. Many holistic veterinarians now recommend raw fish as well as meat, both to provide nutrition and to serve as a measure of prevention against degenerative diseases like cancer. I don't believe that a raw-food diet is nearly as effective against cancer as certain colleagues of mine do, though I occasionally recommend it in addition to other measures when a sick animal might benefit from the quick jolt its protein can provide. With my own pets, I steer clear of raw fish out of fear that it may contain toxins. But I do serve cooked fish on occasion, and as it happens, my dogs like it as much as my cats do. I'm actually more surprised that cats like fish than that dogs do, given how much they fear being immersed in water. Did cats in Egypt hang out by the shores of the Nile, waiting for fishermen to go through their nets? Or did their fish craving come later, when they hung out as alleycats by nineteenth-century fish markets? Or do they just embody Oriental souls who as human beings liked sushi? Whatever the reason, they adore any fish I give them.

I feed my pets a wide variety of raw vegetables, which contain important enzymes lost during the cooking process. These range from alfalfa sprouts to zucchini, and include asparagus, carrots, and even lettuce (though tomatoes aren't usually a hit). I feed them fruits, too, including grapes, peaches, plums, and bananas. I once had a cat named Sparsely Populated who loved cantaloupe and had an absolutely uncanny affinity for it. I have a house with a long front lawn, and Sparsely would be in the woods at the end of it. I'd take a cantaloupe out of the refrigerator and start slicing it—with the windows closed. As I looked out the window, Sparsely's head would instantly go up. He couldn't smell it, he couldn't see it, but still he'd zoom home to get some! This cat would kill for cantaloupe; cooked winter squash, too.

In fact, both my dogs and cats happily dine on a far wider range of real food than I ever imagined when I threw out the Gaines Burgers those many years ago. Yesterday, I took two organic potatoes, diced them up, and simmered them in a skillet with some olive oil and water. Then I put in a lamb burger and some broccoli, and just before they were done, I added a few pieces of organic cheese. Admittedly, that took twenty minutes. But it was a one-pan dish that required no more than a bit of slicing and stirring, and both my dogs and my cats loved it. Other nights I'll cook some yellow squash and mushrooms, or scrambled eggs with leftover chicken and rice. Or pasta! Pasta in a pesto sauce with broccoli rabe is their new fixation. Tonight, as I was working on this chapter, I gave my dog Clayton my leftover sautéed garlic veggies over chopped lettuce salad and watched him lick the bowl clean. Is that sort of cooking such a sacrifice, really, for the joy and good health it brings?

Dairy products I serve somewhat sparingly to my pets because they're mucus-forming (as they are in people), but my pets love them, so I include them in moderation. Almost any hard or semisoft cheese will be happily received; just stay with the blander choices (no Stilton, even for English breeds!) and avoid soft cheeses like Brie, which have too much cream in them. For that matter, stay away from cream or half-and-half altogether. But you might try a little cottage cheese, an easily digestible source of good nutrition, and also yogurt. The fruit-laced yogurts usually find takers, but if not, you can almost always get a dog or cat to eat plain yogurt. Just as it helps us by providing friendly bacteria for our digestive tracts, so it helps pets, especially those with gas or diarrhea, and should definitely be given in conjunction with—and especially after giving—antibiotics for digestive support. (Acidophilus, available in pill, powder, and liquid form at your local health food store, also helps digestive problems; administer just one pill or its equivalent each week. See Chapter Seven for more on diarrhea.)

Eggs, by the way, are fine, too, once or twice a week. (I'd strongly suggest you only use organic eggs.) Some health food advocates suggest pets be fed raw yolks. (The white must be cooked, as it contains a substance called avidin, which destroys the B vitamin biotin.) But I prefer to give my own animals cooked eggs. They all love omelettes. Sunday morning, I'll sauté some vegetables and tuck them in, along with a helping of the brown-rice-and-chicken combo, add a couple of pieces of organic cheese, and voilà. With pets, as with people, just avoid having eggs on too regular a basis.

Some of these foods, admittedly, are less than ideally healthy, and purists may grumble. But they're also the foods my pets happen to like! And to me, one of the fundamentals of life is to enjoy what one eats. For that matter, my old dog Danny was just wild about pizza. Once in a while—not often enough to bring on the food police, I promise!—I would stop off as we were driving to get a couple of slices, one for me, one for Danny. Pizza certainly seemed to have no ill effects on him: he lived nineteen years, a remarkable life span for a golden retriever.

To almost any sautéed dish, garlic is a healthy and tasty addition. Plus, it makes the kitchen smell great! I try to add some, minced, to any cooked meal I make for my crew, figuring roughly a half clove for each ten pounds of pet. Most dogs and cats like garlic as much as people do, so it's hardly a tough sell. But garlic is also useful, along with yogurt containing lactobacillus acidophilus, in addressing digestive tract problems. And it's a very effective natural antidote to fleas. Just as we exude garlic through our skin the morning after a garlicky meal, so do pets. Fleas, fortunately, appear to hate the smell and taste of garlic, and tend to stay away from a pet who's been eating garlic on a daily basis as summer unfolds. (See Chapter Seven for a fuller discussion of garlic as a flea fighter.) And, of course, a garlic-rich pet is great for repelling vampires.

The real-food choices for your pet are nearly as wide-ranging as they are for you, assuming you're the sort of person who makes a habit of eating healthy foods. Indeed, they may seem too wide-ranging. So here's a simple equation to help in the menu writing. Generally (which is to say, don't feel you have to abide by this every day), I recommend that a dog's meals be approximately one-quarter meat, two-quarters grain, and one-quarter vegetables, while a cat's meals be roughly one-third to one-half meat, with grains and vegetables constituting the rest. (For either dogs or cats, a little dairy goes a long way.) Individual animals will have different likes and dislikes, as we do, but basically you can feed your dog and cat the same meal in those different ratios. Don't worry too much about each meal's menu. Lamb or turkey, rice or pasta—any good food will be good for your pet as long as it's of satisfactory quality.

Easy as it is to give your pet real food, it may be harder to make him eat it. Both dogs and cats can become so accustomed to prepackaged food—in part because of artificial flavorings that cause their tongues to tingle, whetting their appetites; in part just out of habit—that a bowl of fresh food can be thoroughly off-putting. Or if they do eat it, real food may provoke some initial sickness, as their bodies react to the change by expelling toxins as healing occurs. In either case, a few commonsense recommendations can ease the transition.

One approach is to mix in a bit of the new with the old. I've known pets who could never quite bring themselves to abandon their commercial-brand fare altogether, and insisted, as the ratios of new and old were gradually changed to favor the new, on having just a dollop of the old spooned in for old times' sake. That's fine. Other pets, cats especially, make the switch but still need to hear the sound of a can opener opening a can of their old food, and perhaps to have its aroma in the air. That's fine, too. Even if you open and discard a small can of Friskies every day while your cat eats healthier food, what are you losing? Fifty cents a day? And you're certainly not throwing out food that would help the world's hungry people. With my own cats, I find that just turning on the electric can opener for a few seconds does the trick.

Another approach, cold as it may sound, is to let a pet who's refusing real food go without—for two or three days, maybe longer. Fasting is another controversial food issue with pets (and you thought feeding your pet was *dull*). My own strong belief is that unless a pet is quite old or suffering from a degenerative disease like cancer, fasting is a natural way for him to clean out his system, regain his health, and marshal new energy—along with an appetite. For Arnold Ehret, my nineteenth-century hero, only fasting made possible the thorough expulsion of toxins and the restoration of radiant health. So it does for animals, and indeed the fasting process for them is more natural than most of us realize. When an animal in the wild gets sick, what does he do? He goes into isolation—to *fast*, until he regains his health by repelling his toxins. The time he goes without food doesn't do him harm. Quite the opposite. As with a human being during a fast, the animal draws sustenance from bodily fats in which many cellular toxins are stored, and by using those cells and flushing out the toxins, he reaches a higher state of health than he had before he got sick. Cats, even more than dogs, have extraordinary powers of self-sustenance without food. Locked inadvertently in closets for weeks, they've been known to jump out with no less energy—indeed, with far more—than when they were locked in. Yet in our society, when a pet refuses to eat for a day or two, we rush him to the clinic, where he's promptly force-fed. In doing so, we ignore his own instincts, and potentially worsen his condition.

A caveat on fasting for animals, however. Animals in the wild can fast as long as they need to; their immune systems are strong and can withstand it. Domesticated pets *may* survive an inadvertent fast of days or longer. But because their immune systems are likely debilitated, they also may not. So fasting as a means to induce a pet to change its diet or improve its health should be monitored, and not allowed to go on for more than a week. During the first day or two, you can serve him a reduced amount of his old food, perhaps with real food mixed in. For the next few days, put out no food but be sure he drinks liquids: steam-distilled water, or a chicken or beef broth (if from a good source), and also fresh-squeezed vegetable juices (carrot is the most popular) or even fruit juices. Then, to break the fast, ease him onto modest amounts of fresh foods for a couple of days before moving him to full portions. But not even all holistic veterinarians agree on this regimen; some insist that a pet should fast for no more than twenty-four hours. Again, common sense applies. See how your pet does in twenty-four hours. If he's lethargic or seems to be in pain, abandon the fast; if he doesn't eat, bring him into a clinic.

I don't do that much fasting in my practice, only because so many of the pets I see are too weak and debilitated to withstand it, and because I've had such success with my program of supplements and homeopathic and herbal remedies.* But occasionally it seems the right choice, not so much for dietary reasons as to help the body regain health. I fasted a five-week-old kitten once that had chronic diarrhea. Another veterinarian had put it on Kaopectate with a bland diet, antibiotics, and then Lomotil, an almost narcotic suppressor intended to stop the intestines' reflex action. And that didn't work either. When I told the owner to put his cat on a fast even after homeopathics failed, he balked: the cat was so young and thin already. What he didn't understand was that the food going in was sustaining the diarrhea. It's called the gastrocolic reflex: the stomach fills, the colon empties. After a three-and-a-half day fast, the cat was able to hold down bland food; the fast had stopped his intestinal reflex and broken the cycle.

At home, I fast my own pets one or two days a month, not to adjust them to a healthy diet, which they already eat and love, but just to clear out their systems a bit. I'll give them dinner Sunday night, then nothing except water until Tuesday morning. By Monday night, they're zipping around like loose electrons. By Tuesday, they're thrilled to eat, but the energy they've gained stays with them for weeks. Fasting for pets is a personal decision, but you should certainly consider trying a one- or two-day fast every few weeks and see how your pet responds.

I'd love to think that my argument is so persuasive that every last person reading this book will stop buying prepackaged pet food today and start cooking for his pets. I'm good, but I'm not *that* good. Some owners do lead lives so busy or stressful that they cannot coordinate a real-food diet for their pets. And some owners, as much as they love their pets, simply aren't going to be bothered. Fortunately for them (and their pets), a number of excellent prepackaged pet foods have come on the market in recent years.

The new prepackaged foods are mostly produced by small companies. (One can only assume that the large pet food companies have chosen not to produce healthy products because good food costs more.) They're hard to find at supermarkets, though some of the sleeker new markets carry them. And if you live in or near even a small American city, you may be within driving distance of one of the natural

---

*This is especially true with cancer. Although the natural tendency of sick animals is to fast, cancer is the ultimate confusion of nature. With cancer, fasting aggravates the wasting that is so common with the disease. At that point, force-feeding becomes appropriate.

pet food stores that have sprung up in the last few years, or the good pet foods and related pet health-care products now available at most health food stores—cheering signs that the lousy major-brand fare may not dominate the market forever.

This may come as a surprise, but the good new choices I'm alluding to here do *not* include several brands promoted aggressively in recent years as ideal pet foods. Iams and Science Diet, to name just two, may be better than some brands, but they're not nearly as noble as their packaging suggests. Iams' Original Formula for cats claims on its front side to contain "high quality chicken," yet lists as its first, chief ingredient "chicken by-product meal." Though "chicken" is the second ingredient listed, several by-products, digests, and meals follow. Science Diet's dog food for large breeds includes front-of-package claims that it "promotes healthy skin & coat," and "builds strong bones and teeth," yet its first ingredients, in the order in which they appear, are: "Ground corn, poultry by-product meal, corn gluten meal, dried beet pulp, animal fat. . . ." And what does this brand of Science Diet add to preserve its animal fat? Ethoxyquin.

The better new brands tell you without qualification which kind of meat they contain, for starters. Here's how Innova's ingredient list for dog food begins: "Turkey, chicken, chicken meal, whole ground barley, whole ground brown rice, whole steamed potatoes, ground white rice. . . ." Doesn't that sound like food *you* could eat? "Whole raw apples . . . whole steamed carrots, cottage cheese, sunflower oil, alfalfa sprouts, whole eggs, whole clove garlic. . . ." I'm getting hungry just typing the list out! In both its dog and cat food brands, Innova also includes natural probiotics that promote good health, including acidophilus, and vitamins E, C, and A, as well as selenium, zinc, and manganese, all good antioxidants. And what it doesn't have is just as crucial: no artificial colors or preservatives. Dr. Wendell O. Belfield, a prominent holistic veterinarian, helped Innova shape its recipes and product lines, including California Natural, as did one of his most respected colleagues, Dr. Larry Chaulk. Now *this* is pet food.

On my short list of other first-rate brands, I include Solid Gold, Natural Life, Wysong's, Cornucopia, Precise, PetGuard, and Abady. All use chunks of real meat, lots of whole (not processed) grains, essential vitamins and minerals, and no preservatives. But with pet food, as with vitamins, the newest and highest standard of excellence is being set by my brother Bob. Call me biased, subjective, a shameless family shill—I don't mind. The fact is that Bob—Dr. Bob, that is—has just come out with the first-ever wholly organic food for dogs and cats. Together with his wife, Susan, he's worked up recipes for pets that are so natural, with such good *real* food, that the results are more nutritional than what most Americans eat for dinner every night. Dr. Bob's Earth Animal food, as it's called, contains free-range, organic chicken meat (with no by-products or meals), whole organic grains (brown rice, millet, and oatmeal), a full complement of uncooked vegetables with loads of chlorophyll and active enzymes, vitamins and minerals from natural sources only, and friendly bacteria for healthy digestion. All of this makes Dr. Bob's more expensive than the low-grade commercial brands—but a lot more reasonable than stinting on pet food and then having to pay for veterinary care when your pet's health deteriorates from malnutrition.

In my practice, and whenever I give lectures on animal care, two questions inevitably come up by the time I've finished describing what good pet food is and isn't. One is: How much should my dog weigh? The other question is: How *much* of the good food should I feed my pet?

The truth is, I'd rather be hit with the first question than the second. The answer is that there is no easy answer, since even dogs of the same breed vary so much. How much should you feed your pet? It depends! On weight, metabolism, temperament, breed. And probably the weather, too. I'll never forget the elderly little lady who came into my clinic one day with a grossly fat beagle. This twenty-one-pound dog literally left a trail on the floor with her wet stomach. When I pointed out that the dog was obese, her owner uttered the two statements classic in these cases: "Well, you told me to feed her a can a day" and "But she only weighs twenty-one pounds!" Of course, this "standard" amount of food was a meaningless recommendation; the dog's appearance was the telling factor, as anyone but her owner could plainly see. In fact, the dog should have weighed fifteen pounds. From that incident, I learned my lesson: I never tell owners how much their pets should weigh, but describe how they should look. What the beagle owner had to do, as I gently told her, was trust her eyes, then cut her dog down to half a can a day.

For puppies and kittens, I generally advise two to three feedings a day, with the food left out for twenty minutes each meal, then withdrawn. (Most pets will finish a meal in far less time than that.) Good water should be left out all day, but ideally should be removed a half hour before meal time, and not put down again until an hour after the pet has eaten. That's because water tends to dilute the concentration of stomach acids needed for the initial digestion of protein. At six months, I'll drop a healthy puppy or kitten down to two meals a day. If the pet is a finicky eater, however, I'll recommend leaving the food out; of all the sins we can commit against our pets, leaving food out has to be one of the most trifling, and with cats may actually be advisable. Dogs whose owners leave food out all day seem no worse off for that; nor do cats.

And, of course, when my dogs and cats do convene for dinner, I also insist on a full report of what they've done all day. What's dinner, after all, without civilized conversation?

One final note on mealtimes.

Every day, beside the bowl of food, you also put down a bowl of water. Chances are, it's tap water.

Worrying about the ill effects of tap water in the U.S. might seem more a preoccupation for Chicken Little than for the rest of us. Unless we're in restaurants where the waiters intimidate us into ordering bottles of Pellegrino, many of us drink tap water without any seeming harm. New York tap water, indeed, is reputedly as clean and sparkling as any water in the world. Why worry about it for our pets?

Unfortunately, our faith in tap water is direly misplaced. I call it the silent killer, and by that I mean for pets *and* people. No matter how pure the mountain stream and how clean the reservoir, by the time tap water reaches your sink, it's filled with chemicals like Strontium 90, and heavy metals like lead and cadmium, the products not only of groundwater pollution here and there but of the pervasive pollution by acid rain. In the Smith Ridge office, before I had a water filtration system, I steam-distilled several gallons of water for our own and our patients' consumption—only to be shocked by the result the next morning upon cleaning the distiller: brown sludge. Now imagine that residue collecting over time in your pet's body. The results may include arthritis, spondylosis, and cancer.

If you do nothing else as a result of picking up this book, put your pet on a healthy diet and buy a water-purifying system for your home. Bottled water can be healthy, but I prefer a good home filtration system. Go with the system: it's one of the best investments in your future, and that of your pet, you'll ever make.

At the risk of sounding paranoid, I have to add that the milk you give your cat is likely no better than the tap water you give your dog. The biological function of cow's milk is, after all, to help turn a calf into a heifer, which means putting several hundred pounds on the animal in its first six months of life. So cow's milk is chock-full of natural growth hormones, protein, and food factors to accomplish that. In both cats and dogs, this overabundance of proteins can react badly with proteins in the body, bringing on allergies or asthma.

For your cat's health, switch to goat's milk or soy milk, perhaps gradually by mixing a small portion of either with cow's milk, then changing the proportions as your cat gets used to the new taste. Better yet, strike milk from your cat's diet altogether. My cats almost never get milk. They don't seem to miss it, and I think they're fitter and healthier for not having it at all.

CHAPTER FOUR

The Dubious Legacy of Vaccines

The links are invisible and, so far, unproven. Even to suggest they exist is to be heaped with scorn from the U.S. medical establishment. Yet a growing number of holistic and now even conventional veterinarians are convinced, from sad experience, that vaccines as they're administered in this country to pets are doing more harm than good. I myself think that's a *conservative* view. I think that vaccines, justly credited as the tamers of disease epidemics, are nevertheless the leading killers of dogs and cats in America today.

The links may be subtle, but they're also pervasive. I can't tell you how often a pet has been brought into our clinic with a history of telltale symptoms: fever, stiff or painful joints, lethargy, or lack of appetite, as if the pet had the flu, but it's not the flu. "Did your dog by any chance get vaccinated several days before this started?" I'll ask. The owner will look at me as if I'm a mind reader. "Just a week or two before," he'll say. "Why?" Less frequently but not rarely, a pet may have a serious anaphylactic reaction, essentially an allergic shock. This is a condition that can be fatal if emergency treatment is not administered quickly enough. When it occurs right after vaccines have been given, the link is all too clear.

More subtly, after a week or two, a pet may show other serious symptoms: bleeding gums, enhanced allergies, seizures, and hemorrhages. Months, even a year later may come kidney or liver failure, degenerative arthritis, and, among other life-threatening conditions, cancer. Are the vaccines to blame? I can't prove that they are. But when I began long ago to suspect the connection and changed my practice accordingly, an amazing thing often happened with those telltale symptoms.

They began to go away.

Vaccines have a complex and often contradictory history—if they didn't, they wouldn't be so controversial—but in theory, they do a simple thing. Each contains a small, modified dose of an infectious disease, ostensibly not enough to infect the person or animal to whom it's administered, just enough to activate the body's immune system and imprint the memory of the disease upon it. That way, if the body is later infected with the disease for real, the immune system will be prepared to fight it off. Without the vaccine, the immune system will remain "naïve"—unimprinted by the infectious disease and so, in theory, less prepared to take it on. The result with no vaccines: worldwide epidemics. The result with vaccines: most of the world's most horrifying, infectious diseases contained or wiped out by the late twentieth century.

Except it's not as simple as that.

The use of vaccines to promote human health goes back two centuries, far longer than the use of vaccines in animal health care, and so provides any number of instructive case histories. Unfortunately, most are more troubling than the story of vaccines we learned in grade school. In 1796, Edward Jenner, an English doctor, observed that dairymaids who contracted a minor disease called cowpox on their rounds seemed not to succumb to the scourge of smallpox. He took a sample of diseased skin from one of the maids and applied it to the cut arm of a healthy eight-year-old boy named James Phipps. The experiment worked just as Jenner hoped: the boy contracted cowpox, but when injected more than a month later with smallpox, he remained impervious to it. The concept of vaccinations was established, and others soon followed. In his enthusiasm, however, Jenner revaccinated the Phipps boy for smallpox twenty times; the boy died at the age of twenty. Moreover, Jenner's own son, who was also vaccinated repeatedly, died at twenty-one. Both fell victim to tuberculosis, which some modern-day researchers have associated with the smallpox vaccine.

Since then, vaccines *appear* to have played the dominant role in vanquishing several infectious scourges, among them diphtheria, polio, and influenza. The problem is, no one knows for sure if vaccines were responsible; the connections are too tenuous. Did a vaccine injected in February prevent a patient from contracting a disease that swept his village the following November, or did some other factor play a role? Perhaps something in his diet strengthened his immune system enough to ward off the disease. Perhaps he had some genetically passed immunity that made the difference. Maybe he was just lucky.

What we do have, in retrospect, is an alarming number of historical correlations between vaccines and disease to suggest that vaccines may have done as much to precipitate disease as to prevent it—a misperception, if true, of epic proportions.

Take smallpox. By the mid-nineteenth century in England, vaccinations had been made mandatory, yet more than forty thousand people a year died from the disease, most of them vaccinated. If the vaccine merely failed to work for some people but protected the rest, that would be one thing. But in several countries over the next century, mandatory smallpox vaccines were introduced after a long, steady decline in the incidence of the disease. Soon after the vaccine programs began—in India, Italy, Japan, Mexico, and Egypt, among others—the number of cases *increased*. In Australia, on the other hand, a mandatory smallpox vaccine program was curtailed after the deaths of two children, apparently from their shots; over the next fifteen years, only three cases were recorded. Vaccine advocates could say that other factors were likely at work in the countries where the number of smallpox cases increased after vaccinations, and that without the vaccine, *more* people would have died. But with other vaccines, the links are just as disturbing.

Pertussis, or whooping cough, was a widespread killer of infants in the nineteenth century, and a serious, though rarely life-threatening, disease among adults. A vaccine was not developed for it until the mid-1930s; over the previous three decades, however, the death rate from pertussis declined 79 percent in the United States and 82 percent in England. The disease continued to decline at the same rate after the vaccine was introduced; when outbreaks occurred, most victims turned out to have been vaccinated.

The pertussis vaccine may be worse than ineffective, however. Researchers have shown that it produces encephalitis, or inflammation of the brain, in animal testing. In humans, encephalitis has been linked to seizures, retardation, and learning disabilities from dyslexia to autism. The first cases of autism in the U.S. appeared in the 1940s as the vaccine became available. Both here and in Europe, the rise in incidences of autism neatly matched the widening use of the pertussis vaccine.

Coincidence? Perhaps, but Neil Z. Miller, author of *Vaccines:*

Are They Really Safe and Effective?, reports a further wrinkle. Initially, autism appeared almost exclusively among the children of well-educated parents, leading researchers to wonder if the disease might not be linked to high genetic intelligence, or perhaps to emotional restraint among upper-class mothers. During the 1970s, however, the disease grew to affect all socioeconomic classes. In retrospect, researchers noted that when the pertussis vaccine first appeared, it was a medical luxury that only families with private doctors could afford. By the 1970s, the vaccine was being distributed free to middle- and lower-income families through public health clinics.

The most dramatic correlation, both in the United States and Europe, appears in the case of polio, along with the most persuasive voice of doubt: the man credited with the creation of the polio vaccine, the late Dr. Jonas Salk.

For most of us, the overriding image of polio remains Franklin Roosevelt, tragically paralyzed in middle age. Polio does result in partial paralysis for some, and even death. The fact is, though, that most who contract this virus suffer far milder symptoms even as it moves to the nerve cells of the brain and spinal cord: headache, a sore throat, or vomiting may occur, or, among worse cases, stiffness of the back or neck, weak muscles, and joint ache. And these sufferers are the unlucky 10 percent: the remaining 90 percent of people exposed to the polio virus exhibit no symptoms or illness at all.

Until the advent of the Salk vaccine in 1955, the only prescription for extreme cases of polio was years of physical therapy and bed rest. Yet even so, in the three decades preceding the vaccine, the death rate from polio declined in the United States by 47 percent and in England by 55 percent. When mass inoculations began in the U.S., accompanied by stirring stories in *Life* magazine on Salk as the great healer of the century, the incidences of polio increased sharply. In Massachusetts, to take an extreme example, there were 273 cases of polio in the year leading up to August 30, 1954, when the vaccine was introduced statewide. One year later, there were 2,027 cases.

The correlation in other states and in England, though more modest, was striking enough that doctors at the National Institutes of Health in the 1950s declared the vaccine "worthless as a preventive and dangerous to take." They also refused to take it themselves or give it to their own children. Yet the pharmaceutical companies that produced the vaccine had the clout to stifle the naysayers and induce the

U.S. Public Health Service to declare the vaccine 100 percent effective. Not until 1976 did Dr. Salk acknowledge publicly that his vaccine was likely "the principal if not sole cause" of all reported polio cases in the U.S. since 1961. More recently, the Centers for Disease Control admitted that 87 percent of all polio cases in the U.S. between 1973 and 1983 had been caused by the vaccine, with *all* cases between 1980 and 1989 attributable to it. By then, tens of thousands of people may have contracted polio needlessly, even as the drug companies that marketed the vaccine made windfall profits.

Today, polio has virtually been wiped out in the United States. But so has it from those European countries that voiced doubts about the vaccine in the 1950s and chose *not* to institute mandatory inoculations. Why? Perhaps because only a few unlucky people had the physical predisposition to contract it naturally in its extreme, debilitating form, and so the disease "self-limited" as it ran the course of possible victims.

That may also explain, in part, the long, prevaccine decline of infectious diseases of the nineteenth century. In large part, as any doctor would agree, those declines occurred as a result of improved standards of sanitation and nutrition. It's hard even to appreciate the ignorance of the era: surgeons were unaware of the need to keep open wounds from getting infected, city planners didn't know to rid the streets of pestilent garbage and horse manure, restaurant owners didn't understand the necessity of serving uncontaminated food. As people began to live in cleaner surroundings, their immune systems were no longer besieged and they grew healthier and better able to keep disease from infecting them. Until, that is, the vaccines arrived.

It's a shocking perspective, but as one goes down the list of other vaccines—diphtheria, measles, mumps, rubella—every last one's history bears out the same disturbing correlations. Low rates of vaccine effectiveness. Suspicious upticks in disease incidence after the vaccines' introduction. And for women, an added threat: the likelihood that vaccinations may thwart these usually mild diseases in childhood but then wear off, leaving them as adults without the natural immunity they would have acquired from getting sick—the immunity they need to pass on to their babies as protection while their immune systems are developing.

So are we better off for having curtailed epidemics with vaccines if in the long run the vaccines leave us weaker as a species than we were before? At the least, such doubts cast troubling shadows on the once bright case for human vaccines.

For pets, the picture is far, far darker than that.

Ask your veterinarian what he thinks of vaccines, and you'll probably get a quizzical look, as in: *Do you have a problem with them?* Or the disapproving frown that means: *How dare you challenge my knowledge and experience?* Followed, if you persist, by a short speech on the extraordinary good that vaccines have done in taming canine and feline distemper, infectious hepatitis, parvovirus, leptospirosis, feline leukemia, parainfluenza, and coronavirus, not to mention rabies. Yes, your veterinarian will say, vaccines are completely safe—so safe that a whole battery of them can be given to your pet in the first six months, then repeated on a yearly basis. Adverse reactions are virtually unheard of; your pet's continued good health, on the other hand, is vaccines' best advertisement.

The history of animal vaccines is not nearly so sanguine. One of its most troubling aspects, in fact, is how little of it there is. When I became a veterinarian twenty-five years ago, there were four vaccine strains commonly given. Three of them were administered in a combination, or polyvalent, vaccine called DHL. The "D" was for distemper, an all-too-common disease in dogs that in extreme cases leads to fatal pneumonia or encephalitis. The "H" was for canine viral hepatitis, which attacks the liver or kidneys and was, like distemper, a widespread and potentially fatal threat. The "L" was for leptospirosis,* technically a spirochete, not a virus, which attacks the kidney and can also be lethal. A vaccine for rabies, given separately by injection but commonly at the same time, completed the list. These were awful, heartrending diseases to witness, and like all veterinarians I was terribly grateful for the vaccines that kept them at bay. Soon, we all hoped, vaccines would eliminate these scourges altogether.

Though none of those four threats is extinct today, reports are rare indeed. Perhaps the vaccines helped; perhaps the diseases self-limited. In any event, the vaccines for all four are still given. Is that a good thing? Let's reserve judgment. Meanwhile, the list of

---

*The ingredient used to combat leptospirosis is actually a bacterin, which contains antibodies injected directly into the bloodstream (known as passive immunity), as opposed to a vaccine, which provokes the immune system to create antibodies of its own (known as active immunity).

standard vaccines has more than doubled, with various others recommended, depending on the part of the country in which one lives.

What happened in the last quarter century to make that list of inoculations grow? One answer, clearly, is that the number of infectious disease threats increased in that time. Parvovirus, which produces severe gastrointestinal reactions in dogs and which at its most virulent can kill a dog in forty-eight hours, went from benign virus in the mid-1970s to raging epidemic a decade later. Coronavirus, which produces vomiting and diarrhea that can lead to dehydration in both dogs and cats, was first noticed at about the time parvovirus was in the early 1970s, and often appears concurrent with it. I remember warning audiences in lectures at that time to watch out: surely in the Northeast, given the way diseases were appearing, some local benign organism would turn virulent soon enough. In 1975, the first incidences of Lyme disease, borne by deer ticks and infecting people and pets alike, were recorded in Old Lyme, Connecticut. Why then? Jean Dodds, a Los Angeles–based veterinarian whose ongoing, brilliant study of vaccines is finally beginning to change the way they're perceived by the American veterinary medical establishment, is fascinated by those historical correlations.

"What happened by about 1975 to make the world allow highly infectious agents to come to the fore?" she muses. "Was it the accumulation of nuclear fallout? Toxic waste? A thinning ozone layer?" One thing is for sure, she says: it wasn't coincidence. "The fact that human parvovirus was discovered at about the same time as animal parvo is very telling. Usually, you see the effects in animals sooner because their life spans are shorter. Something cataclysmic arose in the world environment if animals and people got it at the same time, something that made the immune systems of both less strong." That AIDS arose at the same time, she adds, seems only more evidence of that lurking "something."

Whether or not such a change occurred, animals, like humans, may have been rendered more vulnerable to viral diseases by the very vaccines used to combat them. Certainly the more vaccines we've developed, the more viral diseases we've seen. The history is too new for comparable correlations, but one disturbing pattern is clear: over the last twenty-five years, not only the variety but the *volume* of inoculations given to animals, of new *and* old vaccines, has increased dramatically.

An owner tends not to notice how many vaccines his pet receives—

partly because several each visit are bundled in "combo" vaccines, but more because he's assured that vaccines are "good," and that besides, they "must" be given. But consider with a skeptical eye, just as an exercise, the standard schedule of vaccines to which a kitten is subjected today at almost any veterinary clinic in this country. At six to eight weeks old, it gets its first combo, known as FVRC+E: feline viral rhinotracheitis (an upper respiratory infection), calici (also upper respiratory), and enteritis (also known as feline distemper or panleukopenia). The same combo is given at nine to eleven weeks, then again at twelve to sixteen weeks. Interspersed with the combos are two feline leukemia vaccines spaced two weeks apart; at sixteen weeks comes a rabies vaccine. Then, at the one-year mark and often every year thereafter, comes one more of each inoculation. That's the *standard* schedule. A kitten may also be subjected to vaccines for feline infectious peritonitis, coronavirus, and ringworm, among others. In its first sixteen months, then, the cat probably receives inoculations for up to twenty highly reactive agents.

A dog will receive a comparable lineup, but often in greater number, on the assumption that he spends more time outside than a household cat and is more exposed to germs, especially from other dogs. The vaccine for parvovirus typically is given three or four times in the first year. So are vaccines for canine distemper, parainfluenza, and coronavirus. And dogs, unlike cats, get vaccines for bordetella (kennel cough) and Lyme disease. Hardest hit are show dogs, who get more vaccines than household pets in their first sixteen weeks, then more before each show. (Why don't the people being exposed to other people at the shows run off to *their* doctors to get vaccinated?) Not long ago, an eleven-month-old yellow Labrador puppy was brought in to me having been recently purchased from a very responsible breeder. At six weeks, the puppy had been given his first DHPP combo (distemper, hepatitis, parvovirus, and parainfluenza), followed by another two weeks later, a third one month after that, a fourth one month after that, a *fifth* one month after that. Plus leptospirosis, rabies, bordetella, corona, Lyme, and heartworm medication. More than thirty different highly concentrated organisms had gone into this dog before he was even a year old!

That the old vaccines are given more often than they once were might suggest they don't work as well as they used to. Not true. Two of them, indeed, have worked well enough that they need not be given to every pet. What's disquieting is that they are. Infectious canine hepatitis doesn't exist anymore, so why bother to vaccinate for it? (In fact, a commonly given combo vaccine of ingredients for other diseases addresses hepatitis anyway, so the hepatitis vaccine is not only unnecessary but overkill.) I've seen one case of distemper in fourteen years—a dog from Puerto Rico—and frankly feel that the distemper vaccine is no longer necessary for adult dogs. Even though leptospirosis has reappeared after a long absence, the bacterin used to combat it is ineffective for protection, and has been associated with more adverse allergic reactions than any other ingredient of the typical DHL combo. The rabies vaccine remains crucial in areas where rabid animals have been reported, but does it really require a booster every year of a pet's life, or even every three years, as some states require?

As for the new vaccines, they have a mixed record at best. The parvo vaccine appears to have succeeded in containing outbreaks, though the disease, like polio, may have self-limited. In any event, parvo remains a serious canine threat, which is also to say that the vaccine doesn't always work. (It has side effects, too, but we'll get to those later.) Kennel cough vaccines offer so little immunity as to be virtually worthless, as do the vaccines for feline upper respiratory viruses, like rhinotracheitis and calici. The coronavirus vaccine is generally ineffective, and unnecessary in any event—coronavirus, akin to kennel cough, is a mild condition best addressed with proper diet. Even less necessary is the Lyme vaccine, since most dogs in Lyme-infested areas acquire Lyme antibodies without ever exhibiting symptoms of getting the full-blown disease.

Why, then, are all these vaccines being given? And why so often?

By no coincidence, over those same twenty-five years, the manufacturing of animal vaccines has become a multibillion-dollar industry for drug companies like Pfizer, Intervet, Peska, Fort Dodge, and Solvay. Initially, those companies may have responded to health epidemics in an admirable fashion. Over time, they've evolved as any business does, pushing all the products they can, vying for market share, and creating new markets, sometimes by creating a market for vaccines to fight mild diseases better addressed with treatment. And veterinarians, well intentioned as they may be, have shared in the profits. "It's the vets' fault, really," says Jean Dodds, the veterinarian whose research on vaccines I admire so much. "We stopped practicing medicine and started pushing vaccines and pills." Vaccines, after all, could be "retailed" at sizable markups, with an extra twenty-five-dollar or more profit from the inevitable office fee. Eventually, they came to account for a major chunk of any veterinarian's income.

By the early 1970s, as a result, a new tradition had been established: annual revaccinations. Veterinarians reasoned that the protocol provided a chance to conduct basic checkups of pets whose owners might not otherwise bother to bring them in. In that they were half right: annual checkups *are* important, and owners were prone to neglect them without the goad of "obligatory" shots. But even if one assumes for argument's sake that vaccines have *no* adverse effects, the annual booster made no medical sense. Few if any vaccines lose their efficacy—such as it is—in just a year or two, as proved by various studies. At the least, then, administering annual boosters is redundant and unnecessary. But redundancy isn't the only criterion. *Giving too many vaccines makes pets sick.*

A recognized ambassador between the homeopathic and allopathic worlds, Jean Dodds is more inclined than I am to credit vaccines for containing epidemics in the past. But that, she feels, shouldn't keep us from recognizing the problems they've created since. "We have the luxury to be concerned with the adverse effects of vaccines more than we did before, because we *have* reduced diseases that were killing animals and people," she says. "And vaccines did play a role: they provided protection during heights of infectious outbreaks. Now, as a result, diseases are more contained, and we can look at the incidences that remain and say that vaccines do sometimes seem to play a role. With distemper, for example, the incidence of disease from vaccine is higher than from the disease itself. But we wouldn't have that if pets were dying from a rampant outbreak of the disease for which we had no vaccine.

"So vaccines were necessary to save the population in the face of epidemics. But it doesn't matter what *was*. The fact is that now we have too many adverse reactions."

Richard Pitcairn, one of the country's most prominent homeopathic veterinarians, takes a harsher view that echoes my own. "If I may venture to make a prediction, it is that fifty or one hundred years from now people will look back at the practice of introducing disease into people and animals for the purpose of preventing these same diseases as foolishness—a foolishness similar to that of the practice of bloodletting or the use of toxic doses of mercury in the treatment of disease."

. . .

With a subject as controversial as vaccines, it's best to find one's way to reason by starting with assumptions that all sides accept. Vaccines do clearly fail to protect certain pets in a group. And sometimes they're followed almost immediately by certain adverse reactions. Why?

Conventional wisdom holds that vaccines are pretty much effective unless wrongly prepared or administered. To be sure, preparing vaccines is a tricky business and things can go wrong, not that that's terribly reassuring. Vaccines are made in one of two ways, both of which involve doctoring the protein coats of a real disease virus so that its infectious agents are rendered harmless. A modified-live virus vaccine (or MLV) has, as its name suggests, living agents that actually replicate in a pet's body, provoking a strong and enduring response from the host's immune system. With any living pathogens, doctored as they may be, there's some risk they may revert to virulence; hence the preference on the part of some veterinarians for "killed virus" vaccines, which are safer but less long-lasting, as killed viruses can't multiply in a host. But even killed virus vaccines can be contaminated during production. Dodds observes that a commercial canine parvovirus vaccine was contaminated not long ago by blue-tongue virus, a cow disease. Administered unwittingly to pregnant dogs, the vaccine resulted in abortions and death.

Far more commonly, as both allopathic and homeopathic veterinarians acknowledge, vaccines fail because they're given too soon. In their first weeks of life, puppies and kittens are protected from disease germs by a temporary immunity acquired from their mother's first milk (called colostrum). This "maternal immunity" of antibodies comes either from the mother's experience of fighting disease or from vaccines that stimulated those antibodies. As a result, it varies from case to case. A mother vaccinated just prior to pregnancy will pass on stronger immunity than one vaccinated a year or more before conception—a rationale for many veterinarians to inoculate animals before breeding. During the weeks when maternal immunity is in effect, it does ward off disease, but also blocks vaccines.

The now standard schedule of immunizations for a dog begins at six to eight weeks with a combo vaccine containing canine distemper, adenovirus, and parvovirus. That's when maternal immunity starts to wear off. But it can last up to eleven weeks—or longer. That wouldn't be a problem if veterinarians chose to do what's called "titering"—

having blood samples from the mother examined at an outside lab so as to determine how long her maternal antibodies will be effective in her pups (an extrapolation called a normograph), and scheduling vaccines accordingly. But titering isn't yet taught in veterinary schools as a standard procedure, or routinely used in conventional practice. Easier—and more profitable—to revaccinate often and hope for the best. If the animal gets sick in the meantime—well, the vaccine was "bad." This isn't just the conventional view, by the way: Ronald Schultz, a much admired veterinarian and professor at the University of Wisconsin, advocates multiple vaccinations—three or four in all—to address the maternal immunity problem. "Vaccinating at six, nine, or twelve weeks, or at nine and twelve weeks, is probably adequate to immunize greater than 95 percent of all pet cats and dogs."

Vaccines may also be given too *late*. A pet, that is, may have contracted the disease by the time he's inoculated, in which case the vaccine will have no effect. Titering can detect disease as well as it does immunity, but since it's rarely done, these incidences persist. Even if the vaccine takes, there's a "window" of time before it becomes effective (if it becomes effective at all). For canine distemper, the window can be two to four weeks. For canine parvovirus, it can be as many as ten weeks. A puppy already adopted can be kept away from other dogs (and their feces) easily enough, but the parvo "window" is a real problem for kennels and animal shelters. The standard course in those cases is to revaccinate even *more* often.

There's no doubt that maternal immunity plays a large role in blocking vaccines, that a disease can be incubating when a vaccine is given, and that a vaccine can fail to protect a pet during the "window" of time it's becoming effective in the body. But I think lack of efficacy is the least of vaccines' problems.

My doubts about vaccines begin with the way they're delivered to the body. Injecting a concentrated foreign substance into the bloodstream is not only a shock to the system—it's unnatural. With the exception of rabies and Lyme, none of the diseases addressed by that standard regimen of vaccines enter the body directly by injection. Distemper, parvovirus, viral hepatitis, leptospirosis, coronavirus, parainfluenza—all are absorbed via the oral and/or respiratory systems, where they encounter the immune system's first lines of defense: the skin itself, saliva and mucus membranes in the mouth and throat, powerful stomach acids, and enzymes and bacteria in the gastrointestinal tract. Obviously, diseases sometimes break through those defenses;

still, the rest of the immune system is warned that a viral threat is coming, and given time to rally its white blood cells and antibodies. Where is there a dog or cat in nature who's exposed to seven or eight diseases at the same time by injection? Yet we subject a pet to exactly that shock with injected, polyvalent vaccines. The immune system isn't designed to withstand that onslaught. (How would *you* feel getting vaccinated for chicken pox, polio, measles, mumps, whooping cough, smallpox, and the flu all at the same time, year after year?) Hit with repeated injections, especially combinations, it can lose its strength.

Vaccines are intended, of course, to *boost* the immune system, but even if given individually, I believe they cause harm. If we artificially stimulate one aspect of the immune system to prevent a particular disease, we weaken some other aspect. The body is the ultimate zero-sum object: any gain by one part of it diminishes another part. And that changing balance, I believe, is proportional: the more you boost the immune system with vaccines, the more you weaken it—*somewhere*, perhaps later rather than sooner, but with the inevitable result of ill health.

When the immune system is compromised, it's open to attack by germs from all sides. That's the main reason why establishing links between vaccines and subsequent disease is so difficult: the results are as random as the germs are. Still, in certain group situations, a pattern emerges. One early warning sign about vaccines came from a study in the 1960s and 1970s of Australian aborigine tribes whose rates of infant mortality had skyrocketed to 50 percent. The infants were dying of all manner of diseases, which utterly mystified researchers. Finally, the researchers realized that the government had recently instituted a nationwide mandatory vaccination program. The vaccines appeared to suppress the infant aborigines' immune systems so that they succumbed to the nearest germs they encountered. When the vaccinations were stopped and the infants' diet was supplemented with good nutrition, the mortality rates quickly dropped to that of white Australians.

More than a century ago, a homeopathic doctor named J. Compton-Burnett coined the term "vaccinosis" to describe a wide array of subtle, *chronic* conditions he felt resulted from various vaccinations. Compton-Burnett felt that these conditions actually made people more susceptible to the disease they were vaccinated against, rather than less so, predisposing them to an *acute* form of it in later life.

In a fascinating adaptation of Compton-Burnett's theories, Richard

Pitcairn has applied the same logic to animal vaccines and their aftermath. Vaccines containing a modified acute form of a given disease engender a low-lying, chronic form of that disease in the host, he believes; the results may account for as much as 80 percent of the illnesses veterinarians treat. (Obscuring the connection further, a vaccine for one disease may provoke symptoms of another, or simply lead to manifestations of generally sluggish health.) Pitcairn has even identified "chronic" counterparts to the acute symptoms of various diseases, sort of like "Column A" and "Column B" on a Chinese restaurant menu. With feline distemper, or panleukopenia, for example, he draws these comparisons:

ACUTE SYMPTOMS	CHRONIC SYMPTOMS
Lassitude; indifference to owner or surroundings	Lazy cats, not active, inclined to lie around most of the time
Inappetence	Appetite problems, finicky, not wanting to eat well
Fever	Chronic fever for weeks, with few symptoms except for cervical gland enlargements
Rough, unkempt coat	Poor groomers (or cats that never groom)
Dehydration	Chronic dehydration leading to cystitis and bladder calculi formation; chronic interstitial nephritis
Rapid weight loss	Emaciation; thin, "skeletal" cats; hyperthyroidism
Vomiting; profuse, watery diarrhea (often blood-tinged)	Inflammatory bowel disease

These symptoms, reinforced by more immunizations, lodge perma-nently in the cat's body, Pitcairn suggests, producing not only chronic conditions but also growths of all kinds. In time, they may bring on the disease the vaccine was meant to guard against. They may also bring on a troubling array of extreme, often fatal conditions. Patterns may not serve as proof to a skeptic, but pile up enough case histories and the sheer weight of them becomes persuasive. Consider these from Smith Ridge:

• Not long ago, a two-month-old Maltese puppy was brought into the clinic. He was the cutest dog I'd seen in months. But he was blind, walking in circles, his eyes clicking back and forth as he pushed his head against the wall. Three days before, he had had his first round of vaccines. Temporary blindness with encephalitis (swelling of the fluids around the brain) is just one of many potential short-term reactions. With homeopathics and specific supplementation to his improved diet, we managed to restore his sight *and* his health. Needless to say, he did not receive any more vaccinations in his recom-mended series.

• I saw a three-year-old terrier not long ago who had been treated over the course of half his short life with antibiotics and steroids for chronic colitis—bloody diarrhea. The dog's condi-tion had not improved, so the owner sought out alternative therapy at Smith Ridge. While working up the terrier's case, I noticed that he had been treated for his initial symptoms of colitis just two weeks after receiving his yearly vaccinations: DHLPP (distemper, hepatitis, leptospirosis, parainfluenza, and parvo), corona, rabies, and Lyme—eight ingredients given at the same time. Plus heartworm medication, all in the same visit. Coincidence? I highly doubt it.

• A four-year-old corgi with epilepsy was brought to me because his antiepileptic drugs, phenobarbitol prescribed in combination with Dilantin, failed to stop his frequent seizures. I weaned the corgi from his medication while initiating his metabolic and homeopathic support program. The seizures stopped—for nine months. Then one day I got a call from the dog's owners, an older couple. The dog was suddenly in "status epilepticus," a state of constant seizures that could only be bro-ken by anesthetizing him. When at last he pulled out of the seizures, he was blind. What had happened? The owners had brought him in to their regular veterinarian after receiving a reminder about annual vaccinations. Two days after the vaccines were given, the seizures had begun.

The owners actually wanted the dog put to sleep—they said they were too old to deal with the problem, and felt so sorry— but I just couldn't do that, so I took the dog in at the clinic myself. After several days of steady detoxification, he became severely diarrhetic, so I isolated him in the back room of the clinic. The next morning, I arrived to find the floor covered with bloody stool. But the dog's vision was back! And no more seizures. This was, in fact, a healing crisis (see Chapter Six). Within a week, we'd found the corgi a new home, with stern instructions for his new owners: *no vaccines*.

• A five-year-old domestic short-haired cat named Rusty was brought to me in terrible condition. Her gums were rotting, her muscle tone was shot, she had flaky skin and several small lumps, and she'd begun vomiting everything she ate. And all of these symptoms had come on rather suddenly. Had the cat eaten anything unusual? I asked. No, the owner said. Had she *done* anything unusual recently? No, the owner said. In fact, Rusty had left the house only once in recent weeks—to go to her local clinic for her annual checkup. When I asked for her medical report, my fears were confirmed: Rusty had been given four separate injections, one for feline distemper, rhinotracheitis, and calici virus; one for feline infectious peritonitis; one for feline leukemia; and one for rabies.

In her own research, Jean Dodds has found evidence that all of these symptoms and more were vaccine-induced. One focus of her work is the onset of muscular atrophy, incoordination, and seizures—known collectively as polyneuropathy—as a result of vaccines for distemper, parvovirus, and rabies. I'm particularly intrigued by another link she's established: the association between liver and kidney failures and a canine vaccine for Lyme disease.

The vaccine, known officially as Borrelia burgdorferi bacterin, was rushed onto the market in 1990 by the Fort Dodge Company and has been mired in controversy ever since. The U.S. Food and Drug Administration approved it after examining the results of a lab test on only eighteen dogs. As the *Wall Street Journal* reported, the vaccine was then advertised aggressively across the country, even though nearly all the cases of canine (or, for that matter, human) Lyme disease had occurred in the Northeast. In an ad (no longer in use) that appeared in medical journals, children were seen cavorting with dogs over a legend that read, "Lyme Disease plays rough . . . so why play around?"— implying that children could contract the disease from dogs, which scientists said was not the case. The ad also featured a map of the United States and the claim that Lyme disease had been "confirmed" in forty-four states, though in fact the Centers for Disease Control could only confirm it in seventeen states. The campaign worked: in Nebraska alone, where not a single case of Lyme disease had been reported, Fort Dodge sold 18,000 doses in 1990. In that entire year, 2.5 million doses of the vaccine were sold to 9,500 veterinarians in forty-six states.

Had the vaccine worked, or merely *failed* to work, the only result would have been a lot of unnecessarily vaccinated dogs. But by the end of 1991, researchers at Cornell University's veterinary school had counted at least twenty cases of vaccinated dogs who later exhibited symptoms of Lyme disease. The most common symptoms were joint aches that led to limping and eventually degenerative joint disease. The next most common were kidney or liver failures,* as appeared to occur in the case of Annie.

Annie was a feisty, five-year-old terrier mix so energetic that when her owners sat down to dinner, Annie would jump higher than the table, as if propelled by a trampoline, hoping for handouts. Unfortunately, Annie lived in North Haven, New York, a tiny hamlet next to Sag Harbor on Long Island's South Fork which has become notorious as the Northeast's epicenter of Lyme disease, thanks to the epidemic proliferation of white-tailed deer who carry the ticks that carry the disease. Fort Dodge sold a lot of its vaccine in 1994 to the area's unwitting veterinarians; one dose found its way into Annie. Two weeks later, she lost her appetite and drank large amounts of water—a sign, as her veterinarian knew, of kidney failure. These were also signs of Lyme disease, and as her veterinarian observed, Annie might have been infected by the tick-borne spirochete months or even years before. If

---

*In both organs, a "protein-protein" reaction took place. The protein of the organism from the vaccine reacted violently with the organs' antibody protein, immunoglobulin, precipitating the disease rather than provoking a successful rout of the agent by the immune system.

so, however, the spirochetes had remained dormant—until the vaccine delivered enough reinforcements to activate them. When intravenous fluid therapy failed to restore her kidney function, Annie was put to sleep with an injection from the veterinarian who had injected her with the vaccine just five weeks before. The veterinarian wasn't to blame; he'd had no idea the vaccine might do such harm. All he could do was note the suspicious chronological link between the vaccination and the onset of Lyme disease, and quietly stop administering the vaccine to other dogs soon after Annie's death.

How many other cases of canine Lyme disease may have arisen from the Lyme vaccine? As of mid-1998, Professor Richard Jacobson of Cornell's veterinary school remained wary of drawing any overt conclusions. But Jacobson, who has studied more than a thousand dogs vaccinated for Lyme disease that became symptomatic with all the clinical signs attributable to Lyme, does acknowledge this telling statistic: 52 percent of those dogs were found to have antibodies only to the vaccine, not to the disease itself. "We can't prove the vaccine *caused* the disease," he notes carefully. Perhaps, that is, some of these dogs simply failed to develop disease antibodies even though infected by the disease. However, he adds, every time he's challenged a dog with actual Lyme disease, the dog's antibody count has "gone through the roof." To me, it seems fairly obvious that the vaccine caused the disease—obvious enough that if I were a conventional veterinarian and heard this account for the first time, I'd immediately discontinue using the vaccine. Why has Jacobson not been able to prove and publish his assumptions as yet? "There was no good way to control the study," he says, "out in the field where it needs to be done."

Meanwhile, various Lyme vaccines remain on the market, though some veterinarians have chosen not to use them. Dr. Mark Davis of the South Fork Animal Hospital in Wainscott, Long Island, for example, distributes an explanatory memo when clients ask if their dog should be given the vaccine. "Our observations during the last four years have shown some preventative effect from the vaccine," the memo reports. "However, we have also seen a number of dogs who have been vaccinated develop Lyme symptoms. Side effects seen during the last four years include fever, soreness, lethargy. Most recently, we suspect but are unable to prove that several dogs have developed kidney disease from the vaccine. This is of major concern. Because of the side effects, we can no longer recommend the use of this vaccine. Perhaps in the future a safer and more effective vaccine will be available."

In fact, a major pharmaceutical company called Meriel has come out with a new recombinant vaccine that seems promising, though as Jean Dodds observes, not enough testing of it has been done to be sure it doesn't have side effects, too. But even an effective vaccine may be unnecessary. As Jacobson points out, only 5 percent of nonvaccinated dogs that he's infected with the Lyme organism have gone on to develop any clinical disease. So even a vaccine that claims to be 90 percent effective is only addressing the needs of five dogs out of a hundred. If it's 90 percent effective, it's merely helped four of those five dogs—possibly at the cost of rendering many of the other dogs sick.

With cats, a similarly suspicious link cropped up between a new vaccine and increased incidences of hyperthyroidism. The correlation was especially compelling because hyperthyroidism isn't a virus or bacteria that might be spread any number of ways. It's a glandular malfunction. The thyroid gland controls metabolism; a cat with a hyperactive thyroid is one whose metabolism is speeded up, so that he loses weight and at the same time acquires a faster heartbeat, rendering him prone to heart disease. For this condition to appear suddenly at epidemic levels—one in a thousand or more—was odd, to say the least. If no contagious organism has been associated with this disease, what is the agent causing the epidemic? Logically, you look for some new environmental factor that may be responsible. With hyperthyroidism, a logical factor was a new vaccine for feline distemper.

The distemper vaccine is, for both kittens and puppies, an important one that should be given. The key is moderation. When it first appeared, veterinarians simply added the distemper vaccine to others to make a combo. The result, I feel, is that the immune system in some cats broke down. Nutrition-poor commercial pet food and the overuse of antibiotics almost certainly played a role in these cases as well, but the vaccine seems to have tipped the balance. Today, it remains part of a combo, and cats continue to get hyperthyroidism more often than they once did. The pity is that the distemper vaccine could easily be modified to be administered on its own and, if given once, be effective for life without incurring much of a risk.

Less often, but no less serious a problem for that, vaccines appear to induce any of several autoimmune diseases. When a vaccine antigen is introduced, it may not provoke the immune system into generating antibodies as intended. Instead, it may sneak under the radar, so to speak, and insinuate itself into the body's white or red blood cells. Eventually, it will cause a change in the cells' outer membrane. The host's immune system then reacts as if its own cells were foreign, and attacks itself. (*Auto* means "self," as in autobiography.) An autoimmune disease commonly linked to vaccines is systemic lupus erythematosus, or SLE, which causes skin eruptions but also affects the joints, kidneys, and heart, and renders the immune system that much more vulnerable to secondary bacterial infections. Others include AIHA, autoimmune hemolytic anemia; pemphigus, also characterized by serious skin eruptions; and bullous pemphigoid, in which blisters and other eruptions appear in and around the mouth but may spread to the abdomen, groin, and other areas.

It took me years to recognize that many of the conditions I was treating in cats and dogs might be traced to vaccines. The awareness grew slowly, incrementally. *Maybe the eight vaccine components this dog got a week ago might have helped provoke this allergy. Maybe this cat's stiff joints might be vaccine-related, too....* The most critical link eluded me the longest, even though it was staring me in the face every day at the clinic. It just didn't occur to me that the cancers I was seeing might also be caused, in part if not completely, by overaggressive vaccine regimens.

Eventually, the coincidences simply became too obvious to ignore. I had animals all over the country responding beautifully to holistic treatment for one cancer or another. Then I'd get the panicked calls. A tumor had just appeared. Or with those who'd had tumors removed, the tumor was back, worse than before. I'd ask the owner, "What in the dog's environment changed?" Nothing. "Did you put him back on commercial pet food? Stop giving him the supplements?" Nope. "In fact," the owner would say, "our local veterinarian told us just two weeks ago how great our dog was doing when we brought him in for his annual vaccines!"

I suppose it should have been obvious from the start. Cancer, after all, simply doesn't occur in hosts with strong immune systems. Vaccines, given as copiously as they are to pets, stress the immune system; the pets get cancer; the vaccines cause cancer. Call it a corollary to classic Aristotelian logic: If A creates B and B creates C, then A creates C. Any doubts about the connection have by now been crushed under the sheer accumulation of telling case histories.

By the time I treated Wesley, a three-year-old Jack Russell co-owned by the actress Jennifer O'Neill, he had a long history of overvaccination. Some months before, he had developed a tumor on his abdomen that another veterinarian removed surgically. When I studied the medical report, I was amazed: while under general anesthesia, Wesley had been given a combo vaccine of DHLPP (distemper, hepatitis, leptospirosis, parvovirus, and parainfluenza) plus a coronavirus vaccine, plus rabies. Seven agents in all, while the poor dog's immune system was already struggling with the general anesthetic and the cancer! Surprise: Wesley had soon grown another tumor, this one in the genital area. The second lump, too, had been removed under general anesthesia. Two weeks later, Wesley was brought in "shaking and breathing hard," with a 103-degree temperature, swelling, and trauma. Only to be given antibiotics and cortisone. That was when O'Neill decided that another approach might help. Unfortunately, too much damage had been done. Cancers continued to grow all over Wesley's body, no matter what we did; within a short period, the dog was dead.

Not long ago, I saw an older terrier mix named Missy with a tumor on her back already diagnosed as mast cell cancer. We chose in this case not to traumatize the dog by removing the tumor surgically, as the owners' local veterinarian had recommended. Instead, we tried a nutritional program. The program worked; the tumor began to shrink, then stabilized for several months. Suddenly it grew much larger. Again, the owners' local veterinarian made the case for removing it. Instead, I stuck an exploratory needle in. Clear fluid oozed out; the new growth had converted to a cyst. For two years, Missy did fine. Then last winter she had an eye problem, and her owners took her to their local veterinarian. The veterinarian took her off to a treatment room to examine her eye under a special light. "For a fourteen-and-a-half-year-old dog she's doing fine," the veterinarian reported as he returned Missy to her owners. "But I noticed from her medical history that she was long overdue on her vaccinations, so I brought her up to date." The owners, who'd expressly avoided vaccinations at my behest, were appalled. Within six weeks, Missy developed an almost inoperable cancerous tumor surrounding her ankle joint. The tumor was removed, but only with difficulty. And at what cost to Missy's overall health? Only time will tell.

Most vaccines are still given by injection, and only one oral vaccine for animals—given to wildlife for rabies—is available. The vaccine for bordetella, or kennel cough, can be administered "intranasally," with nose drops. Unfortunately, intranasal vaccines sometimes seem to precipitate on-site problems. My own suspicions were first raised in the mid-1980s, when I obtained ownership of the small clinic that became the genesis of Smith Ridge today. Part of the business was a boarding kennel, which I began to manage along with my practice. In order to be as responsible as possible, I made sure that every dog who checked in was up to date on his bordetella, or kennel cough, vaccine. For any dog who wasn't, I'd administer an intranasal vaccine, which was said to start being effective as soon as it was given, so that the dog could be boarded without delay. Within a few months, I realized that several of the dogs given intranasal vaccines were emerging from their stay at the kennel with flu-like symptoms—among them kennel cough! As owners began muttering that their dogs had "caught" bordetella at our kennel, I quietly stopped giving intranasal vaccines. The incidences of kennel cough dropped to virtually none.

Unfortunately, intranasal vaccines may also lead to other, more serious problems, including, in my experience, nasal cancer. One sad case was Wilhelm the Great, a wire-haired Jack Russell, who by the time I saw him had suffered for years with chronic sinusitis—an ongoing runny nose, in effect. A look at his medical history confirmed that the sinusitis had flared up right after the first intranasal vaccine he'd been given for bordetella bronchiseptica. Bordetella is a mild condition, hardly life-endangering, and easily addressed by isolating the afflicted puppy from other dogs and putting him on a good diet with supplements and homeopathic remedies. The vaccine, moreover, is often useless. But every puppy who gets the intranasal bordetella vaccine has to absorb the shock to its immune system of those disease antigens (sometimes at as young as two weeks old, if the puppy was born in an area where bordetella is prevalent). Often that shock produces sinusitis. Occasionally, as the sinusitis worsens and is medically treated, nasal cancer appears, especially when a patient's medical history includes frequent administration of combo vaccines. That was Wilhelm the Great's latest plight.

Along with nutritional supplements, we gave Wilhelm regular doses of Blue Earth Dragon, a Chinese herb combination found to ease sinus problems in both animals and people (Blue Earth Dragon comes in pill form; see Chapter Five). As it happens, the herb combination contains a controversial herb called ma-huang which works as an antihistamine, but which to some doctors looks suspiciously like a narcotic stimulant. My own feeling is that if the herb is natural (as it is), rather than synthetic, and if it's not actually toxic (which it isn't), then we ought to use it for its beneficial properties, and not let it be outlawed by the medical establishment or its regulatory agencies that created the vaccines whose unfortunate consequences we're trying to address. At any rate, the herbal treatment, in conjunction with the rest of the program of supplements we put Wilhelm on, worked: his nasal cancer receded, along with his chronic sinus problem.

If Wilhelm had not just been "the Great" but a Great Dane, the odds against him would have been greater. Great Danes are among several breeds that Jean Dodds's research has determined to be especially vulnerable to cancer and other extreme adverse reactions from vaccines. A key factor may be their dilute, or whitish, coat color: weimaraners, Shetland sheepdogs, and albinos of any breed also appear to have extrasensitive immune systems that combo, or polyvalent, vaccines can more easily overwhelm. Diet can play a role too, Dodds believes: Akitas may be at increased risk because they were brought only recently to this country from Asia, and remain accustomed, biologically, to a fish-and-vegetable diet they no longer receive. As well, a breed may be susceptible to one particular disease, increasing its apparent requirement for one vaccine. Such is the case, tragically, with Rottweilers and the parvovirus vaccine.

Ever since parvo began afflicting dogs in the 1970s, Rottweilers have been recognized as being unusually vulnerable to it. Rottweiler pups, as a result, have been put on what veterinarians call accelerated vaccine schedules for parvo—which is to say that they've been blitzed. After the first standard inoculation at six weeks—too early, in my opinion—a Rottweiler pup will often get additional parvo vaccines *each week or two* until he's sixteen weeks old, then again at six months and a year old. Conventional wisdom holds that vaccines are harmless, so the protocol is rarely questioned; indeed, it's seen as that much greater a guarantee of good health. But vaccines *are* harmful! And the more of them you inject into an animal's body—"modified-live" or "killed" as the antigens may be—the more of them the animal's immune system has to combat. It's as if someone asked you to store boxes of radioactive waste in your basement, after assuring you that it's no longer radioactive. How does anyone really know it's safe? Even if it is, you've still got a basement full of very unappealing waste. And you'll still expend a lot of physical effort getting rid of it. You may also find, as you do so, that it damages your health in some unexpected way—causing anything from allergies to cancer—as the radioactivity "leaks out" and the vaccine gains access to the rest of the body. With Rottweilers and the parvo vaccine, the side effect was cancer.

Every month now, I see an average of five desperately ill Rottweilers from around the country. Many have bone cancer, a very painful kind and probably the most difficult of all the cancers to treat successfully, or lymph cancer, not painful but also very aggressive. We've had an unusual degree of success in treating both kinds with the methods I'll describe in Chapter Eight. But when you start with cancers that have historically resulted in overwhelming fatalities, success is relative: a lot of dogs still die.

Cats, unfortunately, have vaccine-induced cancers of their own. When a feline leukemia vaccine first appeared in the spring of 1985, it was welcomed as a godsend, for the virus had killed thousands of cats since its emergence two decades earlier. FeLV, as the disease known, is especially insidious because it can be carried by cats who show no visible symptoms of the disease yet infect other cats—through saliva via mutual grooming. When it eventually manifests, it provokes an immune deficiency condition coupled with rapid destruction of red blood cells, and is usually considered fatal. (In very young cats, the same virus may instead hit the anterior, or front part, of the chest, leading to a large mass associated with the thymus gland, and the subsequent filling of the chest cavity with fluids.) Most veterinarians were thrilled to receive the vaccine, and administered it to so many cats they treated. I would have done the same if I hadn't been "holisticized" by then. Instead, I began seeing cats with immuno-suppression diseases whose medical histories bore a depressing similarity: many had been given the leukemia vaccine in the recent past. Some of the conditions seemed bizarre. I saw young cats with stomach and kidney cancers; before the vaccine, I'd hardly seen any. As for the sharply higher incidences of feline peritonitis in cats three to four weeks after administration of the feline leukemia vaccine, that, too, raised suspicions.

The FeLV vaccine is now refined enough that cats no longer die from it . . . *directly*. In certain cases, however, it may precipitate leukemia *in*directly. Sometimes, that is, it is possible that the leukemia virus is residing passively in a cat's bone marrow, as if in a bottle on a sunken ship. Administering the vaccine may stir it up, just as disturbing a shipwreck might break the bottle. Spilling into the bloodstream, the virus may cause full-blown leukemia before the vaccine can stop it. Of course, FeLV, even if in the bone marrow, can be detected in cats by testing for it. If the antibodies are not present, neither is the virus. Then the vaccine may be more safely given, and will probably protect the cat for life. But I think that the only rationale for doing this is if the cat is in imminent danger of exposure.

Unfortunately, while testing can minimize the risk of having the leukemia vaccine lead to the disease, recent case histories that Jean Dodds has studied suggest the vaccine occasionally provokes *another* disease, the often fatal disease called feline infectious peritonitis, by compromising a cat's immune system and thus rendering her more susceptible to it. Worse, it appears to be one of two vaccines that engender highly aggressive fibrous tumors called fibrosarcomas at the *exact site* where a cat was injected.

In incidences frequent enough now to constitute an epidemic, the vaccines for both feline leukemia and rabies are providing more than a pattern of seeming cause and effect between vaccines and cancer. If seeing is believing, what they're providing is proof. Both are typically injected between a cat's shoulder blades or the other flank areas. In case after case, a fibrosarcoma grows exactly where the injection was given. Remove the tumor, leaving nothing but healthy tissue behind, and it grows right back, right at the incision site or just adjacent to it. It's like some surreal energy-field disruption from the vaccine. I've seen dozens of these cases; right now, I'm working on six of them. Although I've occasionally had success with this type of cancer, if I save one of these, I'll be happy: basically, fibrosarcoma kills, either directly or by forcing a veterinarian to make the humane choice of euthanasia.

More than visual proof implicates the rabies vaccine in this hideous cancer. I've sent the tumors out for biopsy by a pathologist. The verdict: vaccine-induced fibrosarcoma. At the University of Pennsylvania, a veterinary pathologist named Mattie Hendrick recently conducted a broad study of similarly afflicted cats and found links definitive enough for her to formally name the condition vaccine-associated feline sarcoma. Hendrick stopped short of recommending that cats not be given the two implicated vaccines. Both leukemia and rabies, as she observed, are lethal diseases, and the risk of contracting either without vaccines is greater than that of developing a fibrosarcoma from the vaccines. The issue, she said, is not whether cats should be vaccinated but how often. While that's under debate, she said, veterinarians can reduce the risk of mortality from vaccine-induced fibrosarcoma by following this handy tip: vaccinate in the left rear leg for feline leukemia, and in the right rear leg for rabies; then, if a tumor develops, the cat can be saved by amputating one leg or the other, and you'll know which vaccine was to blame.

Excuse me? Is this really how we solve vaccine-induced fibrosarcoma—by cutting off the cat's leg? That's medical progress?

I think we can do better than that.

In July 1997, the first Veterinary Vaccines and Diagnostics symposium of some five hundred veterinarians, scientists, physicians, immunologists, and epidemiologists convened at the University of Wisconsin and reached a landmark conclusion. These specialists—as many of them conventional as alternative in their outlook—agreed that vaccine boosters should not be given more often than every three years, and that annual titer testing be performed in the interim to confirm protection.

Considering that nearly all of the country's sixty-five thousand veterinarians still promote annual revaccinations, and mutter darkly of the dangers of not adhering to that schedule, the new three-year recommendation is a major change and won't be embraced overnight. "The recommendations are filtering down," says Jean Dodds, whose research was critical to the conference. "And that will take some time. We're in the transition phase, gathering data." Dodds acknowledges that the new recommendations are actually more modest than they could be. "We don't want to appear too radical here," she says. "We want to take it a step at a time. But in fact, those of us who've done vaccine research for years know how much longer many vaccines last than advertised." Indeed, Ronald D. Schultz, a well-known professor of veterinary science at the University of Wisconsin and the organizer of the conference, wrote more recently that when there is no interference from maternal immunity, immunized puppies are protected for *life*, just as children are.

I should preface my own recommendations by saying that Jean Dodds, forward-thinking as she is, views *me* as a radical. Frankly, I look forward to the day when *no* vaccines need be given. Several of the ones I do give now are administered to protect my practice from being targeted as unethical or, in the case of the rabies vaccine, to conform with the law. Those few that I feel are necessary now—because generations of decline in pet health have left so many patients more vulnerable to disease than they need be—can be given, I believe, just once. Both before and after they're given, I also do all I can to strengthen a pet's immune system, and to educate his owners, so that the vaccines do minimal harm to the little beings they're infiltrating.

When a puppy is about eleven weeks old, and not before, I give him a distemper vaccine. A single vaccine, on its own, unbundled from the standard combo vaccine. On a separate visit, I give him a parvovirus vaccine. *One.* Your veterinarian may think that he can only get these vaccines bundled in a combo, but that's not the case with distemper and parvo for dogs. Manufacturers will comply if he asks. With a kitten, I'll give a distemper vaccine (feline rather than canine), also at about eleven weeks. With both puppies and kittens, I also give homeopathic remedies and vitamins to counteract the vaccines' immunosuppressive effects.*

With one important exception, I give none of the other vaccines claimed to be so crucial to a pet's well-being. *No* to the Lyme vaccine for dogs, to canine hepatitis and bordetella, parainfluenza and corona, all of which either don't work or aren't needed, and may cause harm. (Safer, in each case, is to give antibiotics—or, better still, homeopathic remedies—should disease occur.) *No* to a new canine rotavirus vaccine that is about to hit the market, despite the fact that there's virtually no incidence of the disease. A big *no* to the existing leptospirosis bacterin, which has caused more allergic reactions than any other single ingredient in the standard canine DHLPP combo.† With cats, for the same reasons, *no* to feline infectious peritonitis and feline leukemia and ringworm, feline rhinotracheitis and calici (although the last two are still included in most feline vaccine combos). The exception, about which certain qualifications need to be made, is rabies.

*A good program to follow is to give pets the following vitamins beginning two to three weeks before vaccinations, and extending two to three weeks thereafter. Vitamin A: 10,000 IU a day for a fifty-pound dog; 2,500 IU a day for the adult cat. Vitamin E: dog, 400 IU a day; cat, 100 IU a day. Vitamin C: dog: 2,000 milligrams a day; cat, 500 milligrams a day. Start the C at 500 milligrams a day and increase every second day until the recommended dosage is reached. Give the dosage in stages two to three times a day. I also give a dose of 30c thuja just after vaccinating.

†The combo's other ingredients come as powders. The leptospirosis bacterin comes as a liquid, so it was traditionally used as a diluent—mixed with the powders to create an injectable mix. So apparent are the reactions to it, however, that even conventional vets have begun to put the leptospirosis liquid aside and mix the powders with sterile water instead. As it happens, leptospirosis has reappeared in my area in scattered cases after a long hiatus. I haven't seen any cases myself, but some of my colleagues have. Most agree that the preferable course of action is to avoid the bacterin, as it's reported not to be effective in protecting against this new strain, and simply to use antibiotics when the disease is confirmed; it responds quite readily.

One might observe that any debate about whether or not to give the rabies vaccine is beside the point: it's required by law in most states. But laws can change if enough logic and political clout are set against them. In New York, for example, the rabies vaccine was once an annual requirement; now it can be given once every three years. Better, then, to reason one's way to the best answer about the rabies vaccine and hope the law follows suit.

Rabies among pets and people is rare, but it's also a very serious disease that does have a way of cropping up unexpectedly. A virus borne by saliva from a rabid animal's bite, the disease may take anywhere from a week to a year to incubate. Once it reaches the brain, the disease produces severe mood shifts, followed by encephalitis—some animals grow frenzied and violent at this point, as the popular image of rabies suggests; others become paralyzed—and, inevitably, death. Unlike other animal diseases, rabies can be passed on to people, who experience the same progression of dreadful symptoms if the disease incubates. Fortunately, the rabies vaccine has been remarkably effective in protecting pets—and their owners—from the disease. The handful of human cases each year in the U.S. are, therefore, almost always the result of bites from rabid wildlife, such as bats in the case of a girl in Greenwich, Connecticut, in 1996 and a New Jersey man in 1997.

This is not to say, however, that the rabies vaccine need be given every year, as Florida and certain other states require. Indeed it should not, given its potential to produce aggressive or destructive behavior, random barking, and paranoia-like fear—as well as damage to the thyroid and endocrine systems, skin irritations, a general compromise of the immune system, and, as noted above, feline fibrosarcoma. I vaccinate a puppy after three months of age, then revaccinate at the one-year mark, and then again every three years, as New York state law requires. If I could, I'd amend the law to require revaccination once every five or six years, and even then mandate titering to see if the reinoculation is needed. Titering can disclose astounding—and cautionary—results. I am currently treating a ten-year-old dog named Maggie who has been in remission for a year from mast cell cancer. The dog was legally due for a rabies vaccine; instead of complying immediately, I did a rabies viral titer. The dog turned out to have an immunity ratio of 1:4,600. Which is to say that due to all the other rabies vaccines she'd been given over the years, her immune system was better able by many multiples to combat rabies than if she'd had no vaccines. By comparison, a Lyme titer of 1:64 would suggest there was probably enough Lyme vaccine still in the animal to protect against the disease; a ratio of 1:128 would suggest ample protection (with the other common canine diseases, a titer over 1:5 indicates a positive response to vaccination—no need, in other words, to revaccinate in the immediate future). The dog I was treating had the protective equivalent of a nuclear arsenal. And with all that reaction in her system, I was supposed to give her more of the same? In my judgment, giving that dog another rabies vaccine would have been a criminal act: conspiracy to murder.

Cats are legally required to have rabies vaccines, too, though often they seem to have even less need of them than dogs. What are the chances of an indoor cat getting rabies? One in a billion? What are the chances, on the other hand, of a cat developing fibrosarcomas from the rabies vaccine? Greater chances than I'd like to take. For now, the law prohibits me from doing what I think is best; perhaps the law will change.

With an issue as complex as vaccines, the decisions merely begin with which ones to give. These questions are crucial, too:

- *Should the virus antigens be modified-live—the ones that multiply in the host—or "killed"?* When I started out in practice, I used MLVs—the stronger the better, I thought. But as I grew wary of the whole notion of vaccines, MLVs began to seem particularly risky. Though they confer more sustained antibody protection than killed vaccines, their challenge to the immune system imposes too great a strain. Now, after all I've seen in the way of adverse reactions to vaccines, it scares me to put any potentially live infectious agent into the body. Does that mean "killed" vaccines are preferable? By process of elimination, yes. But this is hardly to say that "killed" vaccines are always harmless. Because they're less virulent than MLVs, they're also less effective. As a result, manufacturers routinely boost them with powerful adjuvants, or additives, to provoke a more sustained immune response. But these adjuvants can also cause adverse effects. My preference, overall, is still to give *no* vaccines.
- *Should the same dose size of vaccine be given to a Chihuahua as to a Saint Bernard?* If you're not familiar with veterinary science, you're probably thinking, "Gee, that's an easy

THE NATURE OF ANIMAL HEALING

one—of course not." Guess what? That *is* the way vaccines are administered. And to most veterinarians (and all drug companies), "one dose fits all" is such common practice that it's simply never questioned. Press the point and you'll get a vague rap about the vaccine antigens being such minuscule agents in an animal's bloodstream that dose size is of no concern. Ergo, a one-pound Chihuahua puppy and a 150-pound full-grown Saint Bernard both get 1-cc vaccine doses that contain not only viral agents but various chemicals used to inactivate the pathogens, plus the chemical "vehicle" used to carry the organism into the bloodstream, plus a preservative to keep the whole toxic mix potent, plus a colored dye agent (typically red) to make it look pretty as it enters the body.

I've long felt that even a Saint Bernard doesn't need all the antibodies that a 1-cc dose size produces, let alone the extra chemicals, and that a puppy's health is endangered by that amount, especially when injected right into his body. But now Jean Dodds has learned something truly mind-boggling about vaccine dose size from sources in the drug industry. To ensure efficacy, manufacturers for years have made vaccines *ten times more potent than what is needed to challenge the immune system.* After all, if vaccines are harmless, what's the downside? If you can, persuade your veterinarian to give smaller doses, but understand that even if he's sympathetic, he may not feel he can oblige. In theory, he could lose his license for not administering the full 1-cc dose, or might have to recall all of the pets to whom he gave a substandard dose and revaccinate them at full dosages, meaning that those unfortunate "victims of the law" would be getting even more overdosed with antigens. That's how controversial vaccines are—and will remain, until attitudes, and laws, begin to change.

• *Should you buy over-the-counter vaccines for your pet and administer them yourself?* That's an easy one: no. Eager as I am to see owners rely less on veterinarians than themselves in matters like this, vaccines are too dangerous to be handled by people with no medical training. The over-the-counter brands emerged, ironically, from the drug industry's unbridled growth. Enough people were turned off by the costs of ever more aggressive vaccination schedules that do-it-yourself, cut-rate vaccines appealed to them. But cut-rate vaccines only benefit *other* drug companies. The ones who lose—by not getting vaccines properly administered, and by missing out on the checkup that a vaccine visit, at least, provides—are the animals.

• *Should your veterinarian administer vaccines to animals who are ill, malnourished, or on drugs?* The answer is obvious—no!—but because most veterinarians view vaccines as benign, they administer them as standard procedure in some of these circumstances. Commonly, they even give a whole battery of vaccinations while a pet is under anesthesia for surgery, oblivious to the possible consequences of inundating a pet's body with highly concentrated antigens while his immune system is already under siege. The cases that beat all, in my experience, are those of pets whose cancers are so terribly aggressive that they've been given just a few months to live. Yet their veterinarians diligently bring them "up to date" on their vaccines, and start dogs on heartworm preventatives despite the fact that it takes five months for the bite of an infected mosquito to produce clinical heartworm in a dog's body. I don't understand the rationale for giving a pet a chemical to prevent diseases that can't even surface until months after his supposed demise. If anything, the vaccines will shorten these pets' remaining life spans. Where's the sense in *that*?

Looming over these issues is the most important and controversial one of all: *When to revaccinate?*

With my own dogs and cats, the answer is: Never. I *will* titer them and, in the event of any reported incidence of a certain disease in the area, consider giving a weight-related dose. I think these vaccines last for life, as human vaccines do, and I've been given no reason to revise that view in my more than two decades of living holistically with pets. The standard procedure of revaccinating every year is simply ludicrous. It makes no sense: How can animals of different sizes, given the same dose size vaccine, all need boosters exactly one year later? The vaccination policy at Smith Ridge is continually changing, due to the influx of new information, changing standards, and changing law. My current stance is that I may revaccinate after three to five years, but only after titering to determine if the antibodies generated by the original vaccines are no longer active. In most cases, they *are* active. I never vaccinate pregnant animals, because a mother may "shed" the virus as the vaccine takes effect, leading to abortion or infertility, or infecting her offspring. I never vaccinate females near or during estrus; the added stress of the hormonal activity they're experiencing at that time can provoke disease when a vaccine enters the bloodstream. And I never vaccinate older pets if I can possibly help it.

Of all the unfortunate assumptions about vaccines, those about older pets are, to me, among the most exasperating. A fourteen-year-old golden retriever who comes to a clinic for some minor ailment will be brought "up to date" on his vaccines as a matter of course. The owner may be informed but not . . . *consulted.* Why should he be, when vaccines "must" be given? Indeed, an older pet needs them more than one in his prime, goes the logic, because his immune system is starting to deteriorate and needs the extra help. But that couldn't be more wrongheaded. The last thing an aging immune system needs is the extra *stress.* And how likely is it that a dog near the end of his natural life span will contract any of the diseases for which he's being vaccinated? How much more likely is it that the vaccines will do him enough harm to shorten that life span unnecessarily? Yet the logic persists. I remember a teacher at veterinary school discussing the case of a dog eight and a half years old who was diagnosed as having canine distemper. Usually, my teacher explained, canine distemper affected far younger dogs. In fact, this was the only dog he'd ever seen reported with the disease above the age of eight. Yet today, in our misguided enthusiasm, we're vaccinating dogs twelve and sixteen years old—dogs who'll never get canine distemper, but who may well suffer adverse effects from the vaccines.

Saddest of all are the older pets who've had to endure a whole battery of vaccinations to be admitted into a kennel. In our overlitigious world, some kennel owners apparently worry more about liability than about the lives of the pets they board (though, in fairness, they're likely to be unaware of the health ramifications of demanding that pets of any age be completely "up" on their vaccines). Recently, we treated a nineteen-year-old domestic short-haired cat who had been boarded at a kennel for two weeks so that her owners could take a much needed vacation. The kennel rules about vaccines were inflexible, so the cat's veterinarian dutifully gave her the full FRVC+E before she was checked in. When her owners picked her up two weeks later, the cat was emaciated, her immune system wiped out. It's as if a one-hundred-year-old woman had planned a two-week stay at a seaside hotel, only to learn that before she checked in, her doctor would have to vaccinate her for chicken pox, smallpox, polio, and flu—at the same time! If this was your grandmother, would you let that happen to her?

Finally, you may want to consider the homeopathic alternative to vaccines, called "nosodes." Like vaccines, nosodes contain an infinitesimal bit of the disease against which the host is to be immunized. The differences are subtle but profound. A far smaller amount of the disease is isolated and prepared as a tincture, then diluted with nine drops of water or alcohol and shaken exactly 108 times, so as to add kinetic energy to the dilution. After several more dilutions with exponentially more water or alcohol (ninety-nine drops for the second dilution, 999 drops for the third, and so on, with the dilution shaken 108 times at each stage), the nosode is then said to be "potentized." This means that it retains none of the actual isolate of the disease, only the isolate's "energy memory," which can provoke the immune system into producing antibodies without any risks of virulence.

If this sounds a bit like witchcraft—well, it *is* arcane, but only to those who've never heard of nosodes or seen them work. In fact, nosodes have been used in Europe since the nineteenth century, and are championed by a growing number of homeopathic veterinarians in this country. John Fudens, D.V.M., has written about them, and offers the analogy of a car's combustion engine to explain the "energy" that nosodes impart. "We don't use gasoline to power our cars," he observes. "The gasoline is mixed with air and exploded by a spark. It is the energy released by this process that drives our car, not the raw gasoline." By the same logic, he adds, "we do not use natural gas, coal, or diesel fuel that power stations consume to heat, cool, and light our homes. We use the energy of those materials broken down by the stations. The energy is called electricity. We cannot see this energy directly, only indirectly, in our homes and offices. The same principle is made with homeopathic nosodes."

One of the great appeals of nosodes, Fudens observes, is that they're benign. They're taken orally, so the trauma of injections (both viscerally and to the patient's immune system) is avoided. Not only are nosodes virus-free, they also contain no antibiotics or chemicals. And, says Fudens, "they work. There are hundreds of reports in the literature of homeopathy stopping human epidemics and saving lives when conventional medicine, with or without injectable vaccines, could do nothing." Currently for animals, nosodes are available for canine distemper, parvovirus, heartworm, Lyme, feline leukemia, feline infectious peritonitis, and kennel cough, as well as other diseases.

I include nosodes here because Fudens is not alone in his enthusiasm for them. In my own practice, I've used them as a backup to vaccines, even as a substitute. Though, as it happens, my mentor on vaccines, Jean Dodds, still views nosodes rather warily. "There's strong experimental data," she says of nosodes, "but no real evidence of efficacy. Many people are happy giving pets nosodes. But the absence of a reaction doesn't prove that what you did worked. It may just prove that one particular animal doesn't need vaccines because he has natural immunity." And indeed, I'm happier not using them. Partly it's due to the emphasis I choose to put on health rather than disease. Health unleashes such a powerful form of energy, both physical and psychological, that neither nosodes nor vaccines should be necessary, in most cases, as adjuncts.

Ultimately, the best alternative to vaccines, the one that allows us to keep our use of vaccinations to a bare minimum in a pet's youth and repeat them rarely if at all, is neither arcane nor complicated. Indeed, it couldn't be simpler, yet it's the concept on which my whole practice is based.

Good health!

CHAPTER FIVE

The Tools of My Trade

I magine you're a dachshund, maybe five years old, coming in for a checkup. You know what to expect: the cold linoleum floor of the waiting room, that jumble of scents from other animals who've left trails of fear in the air, and then the uniformed technician who pulls you by the leash into a tiny room and shuts the door behind you. Suddenly *up*, there you go, onto a steel examining table. And out come those hypodermic needles again. . . . But imagine this time your owner has taken you to a different clinic. Hmm. Nice old carpeting, sort of like home. The other patients seem oddly cheerful—none of that gallows humor you usually hear. Uh-oh: that technician again. Taking you . . . where? Into a nice room with pictures on the walls. And what's that music on the stereo? Mozart! You *like* Mozart. Okay, *up*. Now why is this doctor smiling? And why's he wearing those funny dog and cat pins on his lapel? Ah, he's feeling your spine. You know how it is with dachshunds: show me a middle-aged dachshund who doesn't have a bad back and I'll show you a stuffed—but wait. Whatever he's doing feels *good*.

With a holistic veterinarian, treatment really does begin in the waiting room. Putting pets at ease with comfortable decor, soothing them with gentle music and a friendly touch—these aren't mere niceties. They're efforts made in recognition of the fact that in animals as much as in people, physical illness has a psychological dimension. In short, animals do sense what's going on in the waiting room, and in the examining rooms beyond, with a sensitivity, I'm convinced, that's more complex and acute than ours.

To skeptics, "holistic" connotes New Age, flaky, unscientific, and unproven. But holism has a clear and simple dictionary definition: "the view," to quote *Webster's*, "that an organic or integrated whole has a reality independent of and greater than the sum of its parts." Holistic veterinary care begins with the premise that a pet's whole being must be healthy in order for him to be well, because the physical and psychological parts, which are equally important, affect each other. And that when a pet is ill, his whole being needs treatment.

When a new patient comes in, I try to learn as much as I can about him, to understand him *wholly*. To me, it's just common sense. The more you know about a pet, the more clues you have to guide you to proper treatment. If physical illness prompted the visit, I'll pay as much attention to the way the owner describes the symptoms as to the symptoms themselves. What attitude does the owner seem to have about the illness? How do owner and pet interact? Might a dog's dermatitis be a manifestation of anxiety he's absorbed from his owner or his home environment? Along with the symptoms that brought him in, are there other less obvious ones that the pet exhibits—chronic ones, perhaps, that may put his condition into context? Certainly I'll look at his medical history to see how he was treated before: the chronology of vaccines, the ailments reported and drugs given in response, the pattern, perhaps, of worsening health. I'll ask about his diet. I'll learn what I can about his genealogy, looking, if he's full-bred, for indications of genetic disease. Then I'll take a blood sample to have its values measured in what I call a Bio Nutritional Analysis™ (BNA).

That's when my own holistic approach begins to get a little different.

The Bio Nutritional Analysis

All veterinarians study blood values: the enzymes, proteins, electrolytes, and metabolites that indicate the function of various internal organs. How they read those values, and how they react to them, is where the fork in the road lies. Most veterinarians focus on significant deviations from what is considered normal, then address whatever organ is implicated, so often with cortisone and antibiotics. What I do, in essence, is to look at all imbalances, even moderate ones, and try to see them in context—in the whole. Why *is* that one organ so out of balance? Are other organs implicated? If so, how? And what can be done to restore all of them, not just to passable medical health but to a fine-tuned *metabolic* balance so that the body is wholly healthy and can take care of itself? This approach, and the Bio Nutritional Analysis that makes it possible, are the framework for much of what we do at Smith Ridge.

The metabolic organs, should you have forgotten from Biology 101, are the ones that metabolize food the body can use into energy and process the rest out as waste. Metabolism involves some obvious suspects: the stomach, which helps break down food; the pancreas, which produces enzymes to aid in digestion; the liver, which converts food into "fuel"; and the kidney and colon, which pass waste. But it also involves the adrenal, next to the kidney; the thyroid, in the throat; and in the brain, for example, the pituitary, which regulates these others.

The metabolic organs that the BNA tracks all have established "normal" ranges. The mystery that led my brother Robert and me to design the BNA for veterinary medicine, however, was that many pets in advanced stages of illness appeared to have normal blood values. So often, a very sick pet would be brought to us for a second opinion and the owner would tell us that his regular veterinarian had conducted a blood test that showed "nothing abnormal." Perhaps, we thought, the problem lay in how "normal" was defined.

A "normal" range for a certain value—an enzyme in the liver, say—may be 20 to 150, meaning that a lab technician can expect to find that concentration of enzymes in a certain small amount of blood. But by that standard, a reading of 149 is considered just as normal as one of 80. Only if the reading comes back under 20 or, more significantly, over 150 will a diagnosis be made, such as hepatitis. Out of curiosity, we began using nutritional supplements to try to bring the high-normal and low-normal readings closer to an ideal median. Our thought was that an animal's health might improve enough to allow him to marshal his own immune system to check the advance of—or even ameliorate—his disease.

We've since come to realize that virtually every condition of ill health, from skin inflammations to chronic diarrhea to diabetes, can be addressed by enhancing metabolic organ function. Fine-tuning each value is the objective. So is achieving an overall balance. What we do, in effect, is to restore pets to the level of health their ancestors enjoyed. Wild animals simply don't get degenerative diseases to the degree we see them in our domestic pets. They don't take nutritional supplements either, but they don't have to because they're eating the metabolic organs of their prey—the pancreas, the thyroid, and so forth—from which they absorb the needed support that supplements could provide. When animals are domesticated and put on a low-grade commercial pet food diet, their health declines and their metabolism becomes unbalanced. By giving them supplements that realign them with nature, we can often get them well. With pets not yet diseased, the BNA works even better, offering strong indications—not diagnoses, not certainties, but indications—of disease that may occur later on if not addressed now. With its metabolism fine-tuned, a pet has an excellent chance of living a long and relatively disease-free life.

To appreciate the BNA in action, let's start with its most basic premise: that a single organ can function optimally when its blood values remain within a strict median, not within the wider "normal" range. To offer a good example, there are three values that medically indicate how well the kidneys are functioning. These are blood urea nitrogen (known as BUN), creatinine, and inorganic phosphorus. All are waste products from different parts of the body which the kidney is responsible for eliminating.* Different labs have different measuring systems; at the one I use, normal BUN for a dog is 8.0 to 25.0, normal creatinine is 0.5 to 2.0, and normal phosphorus is between 2.0 and 6.0. Conventional medicine teaches us to ignore imbalances that fall within those ranges. Unfortunately, by the time the values become "abnormal," a dog will sometimes have begun manifesting symptoms of kidney disease (sometimes considered irreversible). A conventional veterinarian will treat this condition first by administering intravenous fluids to the pet to diurese the kidney, then by putting him on a special diet that contains high-quality proteins in low concentrations.

When any of these three values is even slightly elevated or depressed, I start right in with a program of nutritional supplements geared to correct the imbalances. I don't know for sure that a kidney problem exists yet. The values in this case, because they originate from sources outside the kidneys, may actually indicate other problems, especially if only one of the three is elevated. And even if all three are rising unduly, the kidney may not be diseased yet, but rather a likely target of disease in the near future if the imbalances are left uncorrected. The need for treatment will be no less real for that, merely pre-

---

*The blood urea nitrogen is a by-product of protein metabolism, the creatinine is a waste material produced by muscle metabolism, and the phosphorus is a product associated with bone metabolism and glucose utilization.

ventative rather than curative. My choice of supplements will depend in part on how well other organs are functioning in relation to the kidney, but as a rule they'll include what are called "glandulars," as well as vitamins, enzymes, antioxidants, and herbal and homeopathic remedies.

I'll discuss all of those in detail later, but perhaps I should say here that glandulars, probably the most important of the bunch, are just what you might suspect: concentrates of raw animal organs.* I believe, as do many holistic veterinarians, that glandulars supply pets with nutrients that wild animals get from eating the glands and organs of their kills, and so strengthen them against disease. (As discussed later, in the section on glandulars, I also believe that an autoimmune reaction is involved.) I had some trepidation about trying out glandulars nearly two decades ago, and was aware that they had provoked fierce controversy in the medical literature. (Indeed, they still do.) So at first I used them only as a backup treatment. But over time I've seen them work so effectively—not merely remedying minor organ imbalances but actually reversing organ damage—that I now rely on them as my first line of defense with nearly all metabolic imbalances. Fortunately, there's a commercially available glandular for every metabolic organ we treat.

Correcting minor imbalances in a single organ is certainly helpful, but in applying the BNA, it's just the beginning. Imagine the metabolic organs as a solar system of balls linked to one another by sticks. What happens when you push one ball up or down? The rest are pulled from their original positions, probably with those nearest to the ball you're touching moved the most, and those farthest from it the least. Though conventional medicine remains set on addressing the symptoms of the most affected organ and ignoring the rest, the fact is that all of

---

*The glándulars come from chemical-free livestock, not from other dogs and cats! And lest the word conjure up grisly images of a veterinarian feeding bite-sized chunks of animal kidney to his patients, the glandulars come as encapsulated powders, liquids, or pills. It's worth noting, too, that animals are not killed for this purpose. They're slaughtered by the meat industry, and their organs are then distributed to the companies that manufacture glandulars. If you're a vegetarian, as I am, that may seem a Faustian pact, but it's one I can live with, given how much good I've seen glandulars do. And remember: Dogs and cats *are* carnivores by heritage, so that their systems benefit from glandulars as naturally as their forebears benefited from eating raw animal organs and glands.

these organs are linked to one another—and so, inevitably, are their problems.

Consider the organ that lies just above the kidney: the adrenal, or, to give it its new medical name, the suprarenal. (*Ad renal* means "toward the kidney"; *supra renal* means "above the kidney.") Is it so radical to suggest that even modest imbalances in the adrenal may in time get worse and affect the kidney, too?

Here's how.

Simply put, two of the adrenal's basic functions are to handle stress and inflammation. For the first, it releases adrenaline to speed up the heart rate, stabilize blood pressure, and get you ready for "fight or flight," which is what stress tended to involve if you were a caveman, and which in different ways does today, too. For disease purposes, we're more interested in the other of those two adrenal missions. To deal with inflammation, the adrenal dispatches natural cortisone (the name comes from the gland's outside layer, the adrenal cortex). Over time, natural cortisone—the more exact term is "cortisol"—has the side effect of drawing sodium out of the cells. Sodium is half of what constitutes salt. As it's flushed through the body toward the kidneys to be excreted, it in turn draws water from the cells it passes by, just as table salt draws water from hot humid air on a midsummer day. The pet or person to whom this is occurring feels thirsty as his bodily water is diminished, and urinates more often to pass that water. The outgoing water and sodium, as a result, also overwork the kidneys. So in short: the harder the adrenal cortex is pressed to make cortisol, the harder the kidneys are forced to work, too.

To me, the main indicator of metabolic function for the adrenal is an enzyme called alkaline phosphatase. If its value is even slightly elevated or depressed, we go in with glandulars and the rest of our arsenal of natural remedies. In most cases, as the alkaline phosphatase eases back to the median, so too will the pet's increased water consumption and urination. This in turn will lower the stress on the kidneys, preventing future kidney problems.

Unfortunately, by the time we do a BNA that discloses adrenal imbalance, the situation has likely been complicated by outside forces—namely, conventional medicine. When an inflammation appears, help (of a sort) tends to come first from the administration of synthetic cortisone to address the problem, be it allergies, "hot spots," or, as often, arthritis. Chemically close to natural cortisone but not derived from it, the man-made version suppresses inflammation. When applied topically, it filters through the skin's cellular structure; when administered orally or by injection, as cortisone is much more often given, it enters the body directly. As the cortisone imparts its effect on the body, you see the two common side effects described above: increased thirst and more frequent urination, just as is the case when the body creates too much natural cortisone, though to an exaggerated degree. The adrenal, as a result, is thrown out of metabolic balance.

Due to its anti-inflammatory effects, synthetic cortisone is one of the drugs most commonly prescribed in veterinary medicine. Frequently, dogs on synthetic cortisone have elevated levels of alkaline phosphatase, as compared to the "normal" amount. A conventional veterinarian will see that value from a blood test but feel that it's justified, because the dog is on all that cortisone. I'll see it and feel that no matter what, it's not normal. What are the effects of such a high level of alkaline phosphatase on the body? They'll be a mirror of all the side effects of cortisone stated in the medical books. I say, let's get the body's own adrenal gland functioning efficiently so that it can make its own natural cortisone and heal itself. So we put the pet on natural supplements, ease him off the synthetic cortisone if he's still on it, then watch his alkaline phosphatase come down to normal—*our* version of normal. Soon enough, his inflammation either lessens or disappears, addressed by his own natural healing process.

In our practice, almost all animals do get put on an adrenal supplement, because most BNA returns disclose an adrenal imbalance suggesting stress, inflammation, or both. That's not to say that all get put on the same one. In fact, we use half a dozen different adrenal supplements; the choice depends on what other organs are implicated in the BNA. Mil Adrene (Miller Pharmacal) is raw adrenal, a direct and potent choice. If the calcium value in the blood appears low, we'll use a supplement called Drenatrophin (Standard Process Labs), which combines both adrenal support and the needed calcium. If sodium is low, we'll use Adrenochelate (Nu Biologics). And if the adrenal's alkaline phosphatase is especially high, I also try to balance the body's alkalinity with acidity, which means using ascorbic acid, which is vitamin C. The adrenal supplements, by the way, are all as readily available over the counter in health food stores as vitamin C is. So are most of the supplements we use.

Using remedies that neatly address a metabolic imbalance of two or more organs makes holistic sense. It's also a practical matter: supplements are expensive. If we ask an owner to buy too many different kinds, he may refuse, or buy only some of them. Even if he takes them all, the expense will surely increase his anxiety about his pet's condition, and an owner's stress, as we'll see in Chapter Nine, is sensed by his pet in very real ways. Then, too, getting an animal to take a whole list of different supplements becomes an exercise in futility. Typically, a BNA will reveal several metabolic imbalances. Unless they're severe, I may use just a few metabolic supplements that address them. Strengthened by those, and backed up by enzymes and a good multiple vitamin, the body can usually take care of the other imbalances itself.

Over the years, as we've refined the BNA, the problems of one organ have come to be seen as affected not only by those closely associated with it but by more distant organs in the metabolic system. Of those few veterinarians who consider the adrenal's influence on the kidney, for example, I'd doubt that any consider the pituitary in reaching a diagnosis. Most veterinarians rarely deal with the pituitary at all. Yet this tiny, crucial gland in the brain is the one that, among other jobs, governs the release of cortisol by the adrenal. If it's malfunctioning, the adrenal may appear to be the organ with a problem, although it's not.

Think of the pituitary as the top of a genealogical tree, with the adrenal down one branch. Another branch is the thyroid, the gland adjacent to the windpipe which regulates metabolism. The pituitary's in charge of it, too. It tells the thyroid to secrete its hormone L-thyroxine, as needed by the body. One result of a low value for L-thyroxine, usually in dogs, is sluggishness; other effects are excess weight and symmetrical hair loss. If the value gets abnormally low, a conventional veterinarian will put this pet on a synthetic thyroid drug, the most typical of which would be either Synthroid or Soloxine. But again, what if the problem is in the pituitary? If it is, you have a situation that's analogous to a toaster with a severed cord. When it fails to heat bread, do you conclude that the toaster is broken? Or simply that it needs a new plug? The toaster in the analogy is the thyroid; the severed plug is the pituitary. Unless the pituitary function is corrected, a pet will be subjected to increasing doses of Synthroid or Soloxine, with less and less effect, to fix a thyroid that doesn't need fixing. The end result may be an atrophy of the thyroid gland tissue as the pituitary, through what is called the "negative feedback mechanism," detects all the synthetic thyroxine being administered, and therefore shuts down the natural thyroid function. With the BNA, on the other hand, the pituitary's own imbalance will be taken into account. And if that imbalance is what's affecting the thyroid, then as it's corrected you'll see a dog restored to his energetic self naturally, and his values normalized.

A very similar situation occurs with the adrenal when synthetic cortisone is used. The cortisone, through this feedback mechanism, leads to an atrophying of the adrenal cortex. If chronic cortisone administration is cut off abruptly, the result can be life-threatening. Therefore, when I see a patient in this situation, I start him immediately on natural supplements which have a cortisone-like effect that enables me to wean the pet off the synthetic cortisone. This process usually takes one to two weeks, and should be monitored well.

Remember the three key values for the kidney? Not long ago, I got a frantic call from an out-of-state owner whose dog I'd been treating in consultation with her local veterinarian. The dog, who had a tumor, appeared suddenly to be suffering kidney failure. At least that's what the owner's local veterinarian said. Why? Because the dog's blood urea nitrogen (BUN), one of those three key values, had spiked up to four times its normal level. That's kidney failure, all right—if you only look as far as the kidney. But curiously, the other two key elements, creatinine and phosphorus, were still at "normal" levels.

To me, that suggested the kidney was still working. If so, it wasn't the cause of the BUN buildup. Perhaps something else in the body was generating an awful lot of BUN, more than the kidney could handle. Where does BUN come from? It's a by-product of protein metabolism. What is a tumor made of? Protein.

When I stood back and looked at the larger picture—made clearer by a BNA—I realized that this was, in fact, a case of an animal trying to heal himself. The tumor was dissolving, and the body, as a result, was expelling the toxicity associated with its breakdown. The dog did feel bad, and his BUN reading looked dire, but he was on the verge of restoring himself to health. By waiting until that process had concluded—and not trying to tamp down the kidney BUN with medical therapy—we allowed him to regain his health, which in turn restored his BUN to normal levels. Soon enough, the owner reported that the tumor had shrunk in size.

Granted, the big picture provided by the BNA can be confusing, too. Certain values may appear ideal at first. Months later, after putting a pet on supplements to balance the others, the "normal" ones may start to rise! Presumably, the cat or dog has been getting healthier in the meantime. Why should his liver enzyme, for example, be rising now? I was mystified by that until I saw such belatedly high values begin to go down again, and figured it out. The liver had been so unhealthy when we began the program that it hadn't worked well enough to generate its enzymes, which would have produced the higher values expected. As it became healthier, it woke up, in effect, and began working harder until it could reestablish normal function. Suppose you had cirrhosis of the liver and then did something to damage it further. Your liver readings would appear as normal or depressed because of the cirrhosis, which is also to say that your liver wouldn't be working well enough to put up a fight and generate higher values. Its normal liver cells, containing the liver enzymes needed to wage that fight, would have been replaced by scar tissue. Eventually, my brother and I realized that that was also part of the reason why cancer patients tended to show such "normal" readings. Hard-hit by cancer but also by the chemotherapy and conventional drugs used to combat it, their metabolic organs had simply given up.

Though the BNA has evolved considerably over the last two decades, it remains in essence what it was when we conceived it for veterinary medicine: a different way of looking at standard blood values. What makes it so useful is the significance it attaches to even modest imbalances, and, as important, the emphasis it places on relationships *among* those values. Yet along the way, we've come to appreciate certain values, enzymes in particular, that if not undiscovered might as well be.

One, already stated, is alkaline phosphatase, which tells us how the adrenal gland is doing. Alkaline phosphatase is traditionally associated with the intestine, bone, and liver, which when diseased spill high levels of this enzyme into the blood. Conventional medicine looks to alkaline phosphatase simply as an indication that the intestine, bone, or liver is unwell. We saw that it also suggested a metabolic imbalance in the adrenal, whose job it is to control certain aspects of those bodily parts in the first place. Another is an enzyme called SGOT—serum glutamic oxaloacetic transaminase. In people, SGOT is found both in muscle and liver cells. In animals, oddly enough, it's found mostly in muscle. So its usefulness is specific. Yet it's rarely noted unless a pet has, for example, acute heart disease; by then, all it does is indicate the obvious. Then there's LDH—lactic dehydrogenase—which unfortunately is no longer included in most standard blood tests. LDH is closely involved with lactic acid, which builds up when carbohydrates from food are not being metabolized properly. Carbohydrate metabolism is handled primarily by the pancreas. So the LDH is an especially good indicator of pancreatic function. And because of its link with lactic acid, it also tells us whether the blood is too acidic or too alkaline—a crucial yardstick for metabolic balance.

The BNA also includes scrutiny of a gland that almost never gets considered: the thymus. In very young pets, the thymus plays a central role in managing the immune system, delegating tasks to various lymphoid organs. Soon, however, the thymus begins to wither, and management of the immune system shifts to the lymph glands, the spleen, and especially the bone marrow. This evolution is accepted as natural, but somehow it doesn't seem nature's style to let such an important gland atrophy as we grow. I've long suspected that the thymus of a young pet nurtured on nutritional supplements may continue to function, helping the immune system into old age, and that *this* is what nature intended.

In living creatures, it's difficult to tell just how long the thymus does remain intact (though I use one blood value, globulin, as a barometer of thymus function; when it's unusually high or low, I'll use a thymus glandular). Not long ago, however, the owner of a dog I'd treated called with an intriguing report. Her dog had had cancer and had not been expected to live more than a few weeks when I first saw him. I'd managed to extend his life two and a half years beyond that expectation, partly by putting him on a thymus glandular. Over the course of therapy, I related to her what I believed to be the role of the thymus and how it atrophied with maturity. As it happened, she lived near Cornell University, and when her dog died of more old-age-related causes, she had the dog autopsied at Cornell's veterinary school. "I can't believe it," she called to tell me. "And neither can they. They found active thymus tissue." The pathologists were flabbergasted: How could a grown dog still have active thymus tissue? My theory, though I have no scientific proof to support it, is that we did more than reverse the cancer. By restoring the dog to health, the thymus that had atrophied in his youth *began growing back*.

We developed the BNA, my brother and I, because it seemed bizarre that so many degenerative diseases should have no effect on the internal metabolic organs as represented in blood tests. Now we know they do. In fact, the success we've had in treating all degenerative diseases metabolically has convinced me that *visible, outward symptoms almost always have some relation to the internal organs*. It's a relationship that works in both directions.

By fine-tuning the organs, we've found that improvements in visible symptoms soon follow. Which is also to say that when we balance the body's internal mechanisms, the body heals itself. This is the inverse of what we've seen over and over in conventional medicine: that when outward symptoms are *suppressed*, there are internal consequences. A dog treated with large doses of cortisone for a skin inflammation may develop kidney failure later on. A cat treated similarly may develop diabetes. In conventional medicine, no connection will typically be made between the external and internal conditions, so they'll be treated separately—both with suppressive drugs. Over the long haul, both will worsen.

It would be convenient if all visible signs of ill health had clear and consistent links to certain internal organs, like buoys in the water, attached to anchors below. Toxicity, alas, isn't that predictable; it seeks the path of least resistance from wherever it is in the body. And visible symptoms, as a result, may be traced to any number of internal problems. Chronic colitis, or diarrhea, for example, may as likely be traced to an enzymatic imbalance in the pancreas or liver as it may to a spastic colon. That's one of the reasons we developed the BNA; to get a better sense of which of many internal organs may be implicated by the visible symptoms common to so many pets.

Still, certain resonances between external symptoms and internal conditions remain as intriguing as when Chinese doctors noted them thousands of years ago. Kidney problems often seem to provoke disturbances of the ear, for example. The eyes and the liver, according to Chinese tradition, are linked as well. Not long ago, a dog was brought to me with liver cancer. The first thing I noticed was that she was missing an eye. The owner explained that two years before, the eye had been surgically removed because the dog had glaucoma. Ever since, the dog had been on drugs to keep the glaucoma from blinding her other eye. In retrospect, the cause of the tragedy was clear: the dog's glaucoma had been treated as a root cause, when to me it was merely a symptom of the internal problem, namely liver disease. And in reviewing the dog's medical history, I noticed that she had elevated levels of liver enzymes going years back when she was initially diagnosed with glaucoma. The eye was, in effect, the messenger. What used to happen to messengers in ancient Rome who brought bad news? They got killed! Worse, the anesthesia used in the operation, and the drugs prescribed afterward to arrest the glaucoma in the remaining eye, were specifically toxic to the liver! So two years later, the dog had full-blown liver cancer. We've been treating the dog for several months now; so far, so good.

If I'd seen that dog when her glaucoma first appeared, I would have suspected that the liver was implicated upon examining her, but not known for sure. I certainly would have felt for the acupuncture point on her back associated with the liver, and likely detected a weakness (as shown by the dog's obvious reaction of discomfort). A metabolic analysis of her blood would then have established the link. Medically, the dog's liver function may have registered only slightly outside the "normal" range. But the levels of a number of her enzymes would have seemed abnormal to me—enough so that the dog's metabolism needed restoring. I can't tell you that that particular dog's glaucoma would have cleared up as a result, or that she would have remained free of liver cancer. In medical science, conclusions as clear-cut as that require years of double-blind studies: three groups of animals afflicted with the same condition, one-third of whom would be treated with a promising alternative, one-third treated in a conventional way, and the last third given placebos, with the whole process monitored, written up, and published in the *Journal of the American Veterinary Medical Association*, followed by years of acrimonious debate. I can only say that of the pets treated at our clinic within the framework of the BNA, nearly all respond better than with just conventional medicine—from which most have been brought like refugees by their stressed-out, baffled owners.

Encouraged by all these good results, my brother Bob and I have computerized the BNA to make it available to other veterinarians. The plan is to create a computer database that instantly interprets pets' blood samples and prints out a list of supplements tailored with specific measurements for each patient. The combination of those supplements, when added to a regular healthy diet, will give all but the sickest pets the fuel and energy needed to correct gland imbalances and nutrient deficiencies, to reestablish and to maintain wellness. We have established a toll-free number so that we can issue updates and answer inquiries. The number: 1-800-670-0830, or access bnaweb.com.

Supplements

The results of a BNA provide a sort of connect-the-dots outline of a pet's overall state of health. His *holistic* state. Now I will turn to the natural supplements that help me correct the flaws in the picture—or, to put it more accurately, to help the pet correct them. A cautionary word, though, before you read on.

Every book I've seen on holistic veterinary care for the layman carries a stern advisory on its opening page to the effect that nothing the reader is about to learn is meant to substitute for real veterinary care, and that if his pet is sick, he should take him to a veterinarian and not try to cure the pet himself. That said, the authors go on to offer detailed lists for treatment of every conceivable condition: how many milligrams daily of vitamin A or C or E; which potencies of arnica, nux vomica, and other homeopathic remedies to administer; and so forth. I don't mind that the messages are mixed. I know the prefatory warnings are there for legal reasons to protect the authors; this book is no exception. My gripe is that the "cookbook" approach, with all its recipes for treatment, contradicts an essential premise of holistic medicine: that each patient is an individual. Indeed, the whole point of taking the holistic view is to size up an individual's particular health profile, his *whole* health, so as to treat him that much more effectively than conventional medicine, with its tunnel-vision focus on fixing the obvious symptoms in the same unvarying way, patient to patient.

The recipes in holistic veterinary books look impressive, of course, and no doubt help many animals. The problem is that readers sometimes take them too literally, prefatory warnings notwithstanding. The other day a woman marched her dog into my examining room, shut the door, and spent the next forty minutes detailing all the treatments she was using for her dog's squamous cell cancer. She knew she should be giving him 25,000 units of vitamin A daily, she said, so she'd added together the number of units of A contained in one over-the-counter supplement she'd bought and those contained in another, and turned to a third supplement because it had the right dosage of vitamin A to supply the rest of the units. She had lists of numbers, all balanced to make the number of milligrams come out to the exact total recommended by one of her holistic "cookbooks." And perhaps the dog was getting the right amount. But even if so, his metabolic organs clearly weren't processing it well.

"Let's do an analysis, individually test this animal, and come up with a regimen that is more accurate," I said. I made some quick decisions based on what I knew of the dog's case, then added that in a week we would adjust them, depending on the blood results. The woman looked at me aghast. "But the book says . . ." Right—the book *said*; she'd done what it said; and yet her dog's blood results would indicate significant imbalances not being addressed by the supplements she had chosen.

I used to deal more in "recipes" myself, until I came to rely on experience, aided by the BNA and, for cancer patients, Immuno-Augmentative Therapy (IAT), which I discuss in Chapter Eight. Now I adjust my treatments case by case, individual by individual. I take into account a pet's size, weight, metabolism by blood result, and age, not to mention his immediate health needs and tolerance, then readjust treatment as I assess the pet's reactions to it. Practicing medicine that way helps—a lot.

Moreover, while not every holistic veterinarian would admit this, the fact is that natural supplements don't need to be meted out in such exact doses as, say, the dose of a highly toxic chemotherapeutic in conventional medicine. They're mostly benign, after all; usually the worst result of giving too many of them at any given time is that the body eliminates them (i.e., diarrhea). At the same time, they do work. Which is what this is about.

I *am* thrilled that so many owners in the last few years have come to use holistic "recipes" rather than timidly accept the dictates of conventional medicine. This is a giant step in the right direction, especially when an owner has been told that his pet's condition is hopeless. But if I can reach those owners with just one message, it's that there's another step to be taken, from "recipes" to an understanding, with one's holistic veterinarian, of the need to treat each pet individually. It is, quite simply, the difference between a neophyte in the kitchen who slavishly follows a recipe and a confident cook who understands all the ingredients well enough to decide, if it's summer, that he'll substitute fresh basil for the dried variety, and maybe throw in some fresh vine-ripened tomatoes while he's at it.

So you won't see recipes in the descriptions that follow. You *will* see basic indications of dosage, which readers can definitely use for treatment, adjusting those dosages as common sense suggests for the needs of their particular pets. Nearly all the supplements described are readily available over the counter in health food stores or through veterinary suppliers (and those few that are harder to get aren't that much of a challenge); I've listed manufacturers and other pertinent information in the source guide at the end of this book. My hope, though, is that owners will be motivated less to treat their own pets than to ask their veterinarians to apply these approaches—and, if they encounter closed minds, to search until they encounter open ones. My hope for my colleagues, if they've read this far, is that they give these ideas a try.

Glandulars

These concentrates of raw animal glands are the most effective supplements I've found to address imbalances of all the metabolic organs. Though they sound arcane, in fact the concept of glandulars was promising enough at the turn of the century for numerous medical studies to be done about them. The idea behind them was almost embarrassingly simple: that "like cells help like." The diseased cells of a human liver, that is, might be boosted by administration of liver cells from another host. Moreover, the cells need not be species-specific, only organ-specific, which was to say they could come from the liver of a cow or pig.

The first great success for "organotherapy," as it came to be called, was with the thyroid. In 1912, animal thyroid cells were injected into children suffering from cretinism and myxedema (bloating of the body), conditions caused by an underfunctioning thyroid; the glandulars brought dramatic improvements. Over the next several years, other successes were reported. Undersized children benefited from concentrates of animal pituitary glands; and a test group of children who had reached sexual maturity too quickly were helped by extracts from animal pineal glands, which apparently supplied the melatonin that healthy pineal glands secrete in children to inhibit sexual maturity until puberty.

How animal glandulars worked in the human body remained a mystery, however. Frustrated, researchers began searching for the distinct element that might be the key. In 1922, Frederick G. Banting and his graduate student Charles Best began focusing on the pancreas. They knew the pancreas was somehow involved in dispatching blood sugar as energy for the body. They knew that when too much sugar built up in the blood, it meant that the pancreas wasn't doing its job, and that for the patient, diabetes would follow. They also knew that extracts of animal pancreas taken orally seemed to help. But how? Eventually, they succeeded in isolating insulin from the pancreas of a sheep. They won a Nobel Prize for their work, and when therapeutic insulin followed, a lot of diabetics were able to live longer and more comfortably as a result. Still, the breakthrough steered science decisively away from the use of glandulars as they appear in nature—a decided loss, because a whole pancreas contains various other substances called intrinsic factors which are discarded in the process of extracting insulin, and these factors are integral to the proper overall functioning of the pancreas. In retrospect, that may have constituted as much of a wrong turn as the one that led to vaccines.

One of the few contrarians who resisted the trend was Dr. Royal Lee, the father of glandulars as we use them today, and the founder of Standard Process Labs, a large nutraceutical supplier in Palmyra, Wisconsin. In the 1940s, Lee theorized that most organ failures are so-called autoimmune diseases, in which the immune system mistakenly attacks its own host's organ. Why would the immune system do that? Perhaps, Lee theorized, the organ begins to deteriorate naturally, perhaps from malnutrition. When it does, it sloughs off nucleoproteins—Lee's term was "protomorphogen," derived from the Greek and meaning "primary cell organizer"—that the immune system targets for destruction as useless waste material. But the nucleoproteins are "marked" genetically as being part of the organ from which they've broken off. Sometimes, as a result, Lee theorized, the immune system turns to attacking the organ itself.

Borrowing from organotherapy, Lee developed a concentrated extract of bovine nucleoproteins that could be taken up by the body as a sort of "decoy" target—or, in effect, an antigen of very similar proteins, one which could distract the immune system from the diseased organ, absorb its firepower, and give the organ time to heal. The more the organ healed, the fewer nucleoproteins it cast off, suggested Lee, and therefore the less the immune system targeted it. With enough glandular decoy action, the organ would regain its metabolic balance, the immune system would leave it entirely alone, and—voilà, full health restored. When his findings were published in a medical journal in 1946, Lee was condemned as a crackpot, and his theories were left to languish, though in the 1950s, Watson and Crick relied on this work to help them define the structure of DNA. These nucleoproteins contained the genetic markers that were the cornerstone of their research.

Though he continued to practice into the 1960s, Lee today is one of those forgotten seers, like Arnold Ehret, whose work will need more than a book like this one to be revived. In the intervening decades, however, a few curious researchers have experimented with glandulars and made intriguing, if little-recognized advances. Dr. David Trentham of Beth Israel Hospital and Harvard Medical School has found that the pain and swelling of rheumatoid arthritis in human patients is eased by doctoring their morning orange juice with a collagen solution made from chicken cartilage. Since rheumatoid arthritis is now thought to be an autoimmune disease, the solution fits Lee's theory perfectly, with the cartilage "distracting" the immune system from attacking its host's own cartilage. Trentham's work has led the way for Eli Lilly, the huge drug company, to invest tens of millions of dollars in research on animal glandulars to treat multiple sclerosis (with cow brain protein) and the eye disease uveitis (with cow eye protein), as well as rheumatoid arthritis (with the chicken cartilage Trentham used). In health food stores, meanwhile, a number of over-the-counter glandulars have appeared that simply use the whole desiccated gland, reduced to a powdered or liquid concentrate, in the hope that the concentrate will retain the organ's nucleoproteins in potent form. These are the glandulars that I've used to such good effect.*

My brother and I began more than twenty years ago with glandulars from a company called Nutridyne, now defunct, which produced an extensive line of them. We found them useful, often dramatically so, and gradually made them a more and more important part of our therapy. Now we get our glandulars from a wide array of companies—including Standard Process. The one I use most often is the adrenal, because so many health problems in both dogs and cats involve the adrenal's two realms of stress and inflammation, and because the adrenal glandular also appears to boost the immune system and counter allergies and allergic reactions. Indeed, the supplement regimen for

---

*I've found that these preparations in concentrated form are more effective than just feeding an animal chunks of raw glands.

almost every sick animal includes one of many available adrenal supplements.

Ironically, the disease we've had many of our greatest successes with is associated with the insulin producer: the pancreas. In diabetic emergencies, of course, we use injectable insulin, and are grateful to have it. We continue to use insulin as each patient's condition dictates, but when a diabetic pet's blood starts to regulate itself more normally on metabolic supplements, we start to wean him from it. In doing so, we're not just trying to prove a point. Giving insulin gets the blood sugar moving, to be sure, but only rarely appears to cure diabetes. In most cases, the patient—person or pet—is left utterly dependent on insulin injections for the rest of his life. By using glandulars and other supplements, we've been able to ease the pancreas back into producing its own insulin again. By fine-tuning the diabetic patient's other metabolic organs at the same time, we've been able to get his metabolic system working as a whole.

What I'm saying is that we haven't merely treated diabetes, we've stabilized or lowered the dose of insulin needed—and in some cases even eliminated the need for insulin altogether. In so doing, we've restored a pet to *health*.

Vitamins

Wendell O. Belfield, one of the best-known and most respected holistic veterinarians of recent times, treated virtually every form of serious illness in dogs and cats by administering massive doses of vitamin C. Because vitamin C helps support the immune system, Belfield's approach had an elegant simplicity to it: pump up the immune system dramatically enough, he reasoned, and it can do the rest. Most veterinarians, especially myself, assign C a less central role in their therapies today. But combined with glandulars and other natural supplements, the collective power of vitamins is crucial.

As soon as they're weaned, I like to put young dogs and cats on chewable multivitamins—a regimen that, if combined with a healthy diet, ought to keep them disease-free within the first year of life. Any number of over-the-counter brands will do; I happen to use the one my brother created, Dr. Bob's Daily Health Nuggets (see Earth Animal in source guide). The nuggets contain optimum levels of B vitamins (B_{12}, PABA, riboflavin, pyridoxine), minerals (chelated, trace, and essential), friendly bacteria, digestive enzymes, and fourteen ground-up enzyme- and chlorophyll-rich vegetables. They're great for the skin because they're rich in lecithin, which is composed of inositol and choline, both of which aid in liver function. (A healthy liver leads to a healthy body, so that the skin—the third kidney—has fewer metabolic waste products to eliminate.) The nuggets are nothing more or less than good food distilled.

The nuggets certainly provide more than enough normal vitamin content for a healthy pet. Only in cases of ill health do I resort to higher doses of one vitamin or another, and even then, with vitamins as with all things, moderation is best. (With serious illness, of course, other measures are also needed, as indicated by the blood values of the Bio Nutritional Analysis.) Generally, when vitamins are needed in extra strengths, I'll use the following dosages for a thirty-pound dog: vitamin A, 5,000 IU daily; vitamin C, 500 to 1,000 milligrams daily in split doses; vitamin E, 200 IU daily.* For a cat, I'll cut these dosages in half. But remember: Doses vary from individual to individual, condition to condition. A cancer patient is going to get supplements two to three times a day. Depending on his needs, the next cancer patient might get *different* supplements twice a day.

I do give the same kinds and brands of vitamins to dogs and cats both. And with both, I cut back on these higher doses soon after I begin to see improvement. The essential list:

Vitamin A The builder of body tissue, both externally and internally. Dry, itchy skin and a dull coat are typical signs of an A deficiency, and the most easily addressed by supplemental doses. Often, gum and teeth problems are also A-related. Internally, vitamin A is like motor oil for the lining cells of the liver, kidney, and lungs. It keeps those organs working smoothly, and helps ward off the diseases common to them (like hepatitis and pneumonia). Since the liver is the main metabolic and detoxifying organ in the body, as many as half of my patients will show an elevated value of serum glutamic pyruvic transaminase, or SGPT, the enzyme that shows the liver is overtaxed.† (The high SGPT means that more of this enzyme is leaking from the liver cells, where it is primarily found, into the bloodstream than should be the case,

---

*Vitamins are measured in varying ways. Some, like A, are measured in international units, or IU's. Others, like C, are meted out in milligrams or grams.

†SGPT is now known by a new name, alanine aminotransferase (ALT).

which means there's some liver cellular inflammation or damage.) For liver problems, vitamin A is one of the treatments of choice, along with liver glandulars. Because of its role in tissue integrity and liver function (vital to the immune system), A can also be helpful in supporting many cancer patients.

The most popular source of vitamin A is probably beta-carotene, which is derived from vegetable sources. Because cats and dogs are basically carnivores, however, I prefer to give them the vitamin A that appears naturally in fish liver oils.* The most common way to administer it is in gelatin capsules; the oils from cod liver and halibut liver are the two I use most often. If a pet refuses to eat a capsule with his meal, simply poke a hole in the capsule and squeeze the oil onto his food, then mix it in. Most cats will lap it up happily, fish lovers that they are.

Vitamin B   The "Bees" help boost the immune system, rendering cell membranes more permeable to various immune components of the blood. More immediately, they impart a jolt of energy. Every day, I use injectable B complex vitamins, plus injectable B_{12}, because they make sick animals feel better, which helps them *get* better. The "Bees" also stimulate the appetite, a boost to most sick and debilitated pets. And since within the B family there are acid B's and alkaline B's, I've used either kind to counteract elevated acidity or alkalinity in a patient. When a BNA discloses a high-alkaline phosphatase value associated with the adrenal, for example, I'll include acid B's in treatment. A particularly helpful member of the family is B_6, which has antiallergy effects. B_6 also enhances use of magnesium in the body, which is good for pituitary function in the brain (and as we've seen, the pituitary is the control center for other metabolic organs, among them the thyroid and adrenal). And when used in conjunction with L-carnitine,† another natural supplement, B_6 has proved very useful in enhancing proper fat metabolism in pets suffering from fatty tumors (lipomas) and obesity.

---

*Horses, on the other hand, should be given vitamin A from a beta-carotene source, because they're herbivores.

†On its own, L-carnitine also enhances heart muscle function, so dramatically that conventional veterinarians are now using it to strengthen weak hearts and mitigate certain forms of degenerative heart disease.

Vitamin C I rely, as all doctors do, on C, but with a few qualifications I wouldn't have made years ago. There's no doubt that C's ascorbic acid is a wonderful tool against any viral or bacterial condition because it boosts the body, which can then mobilize its forces as needed. As a preventative, C can help deter hip dysplasia and other joint inflammations by enabling the body to properly mobilize calcium, which helps keep bones and joints from deteriorating. And as Belfield showed, cats injected with 12 or more grams of vitamin C daily for three or four days can boost their immune systems enough to start reversing leukemia and other cancers, as well as feline lower urinary tract disease (FLUTD) and other degenerative diseases. Administering C intravenously gets it into the bloodstream immediately and enables us to give high doses that would normally cause diarrhea when given orally. But such dramatic improvement, in these cases, has a cost.

Belfield's work was based on the recognition that animals in the wild produce their own vitamin C, and that domesticated pets often show C deficiencies that suggest they've lost the ability to make their own. Give them the C they're missing, Belfield reasoned, and all will be well. When Belfield came out with his findings, I tried injecting megadoses of vitamin C, too, and saw some of the impressive turnarounds he'd seen. The problem was that when many of the leukemia-stricken cats were taken off their megadoses of C, their leukemia would return. Like insulin, in other words, C was a treatment but not a cure.

As my brother and I honed the BNA, we began using other supplements, along with more modest amounts of C, on pets with cancer and other degenerative diseases, focusing more on correcting their metabolic and immunological imbalances than on just reversing their actual symptoms. That enabled them to produce their own vitamin C, strengthen their immune systems themselves, and ultimately put their cancers in remission.

For other, less dire conditions in cats or dogs, I'll leave C out of the mix altogether, unless specific values in the patient's blood chemistry indicate an alkaline condition (because C in its ascorbic acid form will buffer alkalinity). And since young, healthy dogs and cats do still manufacture their own C, especially if on a diet of any commercial food fortified with the vitamin, we now give young animals as little as one-tenth the vitamin C we once did, and only if the blood work indicates a need for it—to cats, perhaps 125 milligrams once or twice a day, to large dogs perhaps 500 milligrams once a day in tablet form—and let them provide the rest themselves.

Vitamin D The "sunshine vitamin" is so called because the sun's ultraviolet rays on the skin activates D, which increases calcium uptake for bones and joints. In older pets, as discussed in Chapter Two, it helps stave off arthritis, hip dysplasia, and other inflammations; a deficiency of D in a young animal can inhibit the growth of bones, muscles, or teeth. The amount of D contained in multivitamins or Dr. Bob's Nuggets, however, is more than sufficient to allay these problems. (Most vitamin A supplements are complexes that also contain D.) I've not found a use for D in megaquantities—bone and joint inflammations are both addressed more quickly by injectable C or a glandular—and so as a vitamin on its own, it's not part of my standard lineup.

Vitamin E This is the oxygen facilitator, as well as a hormone enhancer. For either of those needs—or both—I use it in supplemental doses on about 80 percent of the dogs and cats I treat.

As an oxygen facilitator, E promotes circulation of the heart and arteries, so I use it whenever a BNA discloses elevated values such as potassium and the muscle enzyme creatinine phosphokinase, or CPK. (The more oxygen, the less *oxidation*—literally, the process by which oxygen is diminished, causing cellular decay, a sort of biological version of the process that rusts iron.) Vitamin E also helps keep connective tissue—skin and muscle primarily—from losing its elasticity. Thus I'll use E when I see an elevated value for SGOT, an enzyme associated with muscle function. Fortunately, dogs and cats are rarely afflicted with arteriosclerosis, a hardening of the artery walls, or muscular dystrophy, with its progressive wasting of the muscles, but generalized heart disease involving the cardiac muscle has become all too common in dogs and cats. Vitamin E has been used successfully with cattle for a condition called white muscle disease, which is almost identical to muscular dystrophy except that it affects the heart directly. As a result, I'll use E as one of several supplements to treat any muscle deterioration or disease, especially of the heart.

The energy and vigor that E helps generate are hormonal as well. We know hormones vaguely as those things that make people grow, give them sex drives, and cause mood swings in women at times of estrus, pregnancy, childbirth, and menopause. Actually, a hormone is a messenger, dispatched by one organ or tissue into the bloodstream to carry orders to another to effect some physiological activity, such as growth or metabolism. Mostly, they're fatty in nature. If they become unstable—in part because they're not getting enough vitamin E from ingested food—they turn rancid, just like butter or vegetable oil (which is also to say that they begin to undergo a process of oxidation). When that happens, they grow toxic to the body, imparting messages not of growth and vigor but of aging and deterioration. Middle-aged and older people can benefit enormously from taking regular doses of E, which works as an antioxidant, keeping the hormones from becoming rancid. So can aging, weak, and diseased pets, all of whom can be improved by rejuvenated hormones. Of course, a pet who's being neutered or spayed loses a lot of important hormones when its sexual organs are removed (testes for males, ovaries for females), so I sometimes recommend high doses of E before and after the procedures to help offset some of the negative effects of hormone loss. I've also used it with valuable breeding dogs to reverse incipient sterility. And because hormones are also produced by other metabolic organs— among them the adrenal, kidney, pancreas, and liver—E can help rejuvenate them as well.

Like vitamin A, E comes most commonly in the form of oils— wheat germ oil, in the case of E, rather than fish oils—and so is usually contained in gelatin capsules. With larger animals, particularly horses, E is often given in liquid form, mixed in with feed; it can be ordered as wheat germ oil by the gallon. And for large animals, E does come in injectable form.

When I first studied vitamin E, by the way, I learned that in substantial doses, E and A compete for absorption in the intestines. The point was that the two should not be given at the same time. Yet other studies declared the opposite, that the absorption of vitamin E was enhanced by the presence of vitamin A! Until medical researchers sort this one out definitively, however, I'll stick with the conservative view, just to be safe, and so avoid giving E and A together whenever possible. (The amount of both vitamins in most multivitamin preparations is too modest to raise any concern.)

Vitamin F You haven't heard of it? Actually, vitamin F is just a nickname for essential fatty acids, which energize the cells of dry skin and, with pets, add luster to the coat. You can find F in various commercially available oils. I tend to use safflower oil, which has a particularly high concentration of it, but sesame oil is another good choice. So, for that matter, is flaxseed oil, which contains the recently popularized omega fatty acids. Flaxseed oil has stirred a lot of attention of late as an immunosupportive agent in people, and as a possible counter-measure for chronic skin conditions like psoriasis. In people or pets, the F oils are ingested orally, either in liquid form or in gelatin capsules (they are not applied topically on the skin, as one might think). I include one or another of them among the supplements for most of the animals I treat, since skin symptoms tend to be associated with degenerative disease. But I'll also usually recommend it as maintenance for healthy animals: a little F oil poured into food twice a week is the easiest way to keep your pet's skin and coat healthy and vibrant, as they say in the shampoo commercials. Also, make sure the labels state that these oils are mechanically pressed, not processed, and always keep them refrigerated after opening.

Enzymes

In layman's terms, the body has three major kinds of natural enzymes, three kinds of soldiers that effect changes to keep the body functioning and healthy. First come those that help in the breakdown and digestion of foods (in the mouth, stomach, pancreas, and intestines). Then come those cellular enzymes that help the blood and organs metabolize food and process waste. Third are the antioxidants, also cellular, that help keep cells from the oxidation process that we recognize as aging and degenerative disease.

A deficiency of the first kind is the easiest to address: for that, we just give oral supplements. The pancreas is the chief enzyme producer of this group (a task it manages to accomplish even as it produces insulin). The usual suspect is a nutrient-poor diet of commercial pet food which can wear the pancreas down and so rob the body of enzymes. Along with lethargy and poor growth, that can degrade the immune system, the skin, and the coat. Problems of the second kind— enzymes produced within the internal organs—are addressed by the organ-supportive supplements indicated by a BNA. As for antioxidant enzymes, they can be supplemented orally, too, though in cases of serious depletion, they can be administered by injection as well.

The first measure most holistic veterinarians will take with an enzyme-deficient pet is to put him on a natural diet rich in raw foods.

Uncooked food, especially meat and vegetables, is brimming with enzymes, so much so that as it breaks down in the digestive tract, the enzymes actually help digest the food they're in. *That's* efficient. I appreciate the enzymatic power of raw food, and I recognize, too, that many enzymes are lost in cooking, since heat easily destabilizes them. I feed my own pets raw *and* cooked food; either way though, I mix in a bit of enzyme powder. This way, I know for sure that the enzymes are getting into my pets' systems. (If a pet's pancreas isn't doing a sufficiently good job of producing enzymes, for example, uncooked food will not solve the problem completely.) As it happens, raw food is often of little help to the kinds of patients I see more often than any other: those with cancer. Their systems are simply too weak to process the foods properly. For them, I've found after years of experience that cooked food and enzyme supplements are the only way to go.

Young pets, puppies or kittens, go right on enzymes along with their multis or nuggets. Nearly all older pets do, too, even if their pancreas function is strong; more enzymes mean greater digestibility, and therefore more energy pumped through the body. In most cases, pets will accept enzymes better in powdered form than in capsules, and the enzymes will be absorbed readily enough. With a severely debilitated or emaciated animal, I'll recommend sprinkling the enzyme powder onto a pet's food ten or fifteen minutes before he eats it. Upon contact, the enzymes start to break down and digest complex foods into simpler ones just as they do in the body, so that when the animal eats the food, he's actually eating partly predigested fare that his body can take up as energy that much more readily.

My favorite brands are Prozyme, which has enzyme extracts from the plant kingdom, and a product line of enzymes with more specific formulas from a company called NESS. V1 is NESS's general food enzyme for dogs, V2 is for cats, V3 is for hair and skin problems, V4 is for immune system support, and V5 is for cats with urinary problems (particularly urinary blockages that appear to occur in part due to a lack of enzymes, which allows improperly digested protein waste to build up in the urinary tract). The V4 formula is especially interesting. It contains "proteolytic" enzymes, which digest protein. Since cancerous tumors are composed of protein, I've sent these enzymes in like so many Pac-Men to help break the tumors down, and also given them between meals to enable them to be taken up most directly. Other therapy for cancer is certainly needed, as I'll explain in Chapter Eight, but enzymes do their part.

I should note, here, that as useful as enzymes are, I don't rely on them as heavily as I once did, simply because I have a wider array of therapies for cancer, and my success rate has improved by incorporating enzymes into an integrated program, rather than using them on their own.

Antioxidants

As the third kind of enzyme, antioxidants are so important that they merit separate consideration. As a pet grows older, cells become diseased or die, resulting in the various conditions associated with aging, from graying or thinning hair to arthritis, skin disease, and, most notably, cancer. These diseased cells acquire an electric charge and break free, bouncing off other cells and imparting charges to them, too. Hence their name: free radicals. In fact, this is the process called oxidation. To counteract it, the body has stores of antioxidants—special clusters of enzymes, principally SOD (superoxide dismutase), and vitamins and minerals, including vitamin A/beta-carotene, vitamin C, vitamin E, and the mineral selenium. All too often, though, these are diminished by antibiotics and other drugs (most dramatically by chemotherapy for cancer), as well as by radiation from various sources, all of which hasten the aging process. To shore up the body's natural supply, we give reinforcements in the form of supplements.

Generally, I don't give antioxidants to young pets, though I do recommend them to ease the side effects brought on by X rays, anesthesia, and surgery. For older pets, however, especially those beginning to suffer from degenerative illnesses, antioxidants are one of the treatments of choice; they're also anti-inflammatory. In fact, I'll put most sick pets on them, whatever their condition. They're nonprescription, readily available at health food stores, and terrific as all-around health promoters. (I take them myself.) I'll vary the amount I give according to weight and condition; basically, most antioxidants are one-a-day tablets. One that I've used for years with great success is a wheat sprout concoction from Hawaii called Dismutase, which is SOD, one of the body's primary natural antioxidants.* It's distributed by a company called Biovet, which has a whole line of antioxidants. Another favorite is AOX/PLX—a bit more effective than Dismutase,

---

*The body's natural antioxidants include superoxide dismutase, peroxidase, reductase, and catalase.

as it contains the three other antioxidants. It was originally marketed for people (and still is) as "Ageless Beauty," because of its capacity to retard the aging process. It's a wonderful supplement for both people and pets with arthritis, because arthritis, after all, is really just an inflammatory or oxidative reaction in the joints. I've learned that four AOX/PLX tablets have a physical effect equivalent to 2.5 milligrams of prednisone, the most commonly prescribed synthetic cortisone. Biovet also has products called Canine Support and Feline Support which bundle most of these four antioxidants into one pill for general support. Another natural antioxidant is Pycnogenol, made by any number of companies and widely available. Pycnogenol is derived from the bark of a European coastal pine tree and a grape seed extract, among other natural sources. Benign as these ingredients seem, Pycnogenol is considered one of the most powerful of the antioxidants.

I've been using antioxidants for two decades or more. Finally, they're being written about in the mainstream press, and a number of other veterinarians are trying them. Great! Now, though the mention of antioxidants still raises its share of eyebrows, I can launch into my explanation of "free radicals" without having owners and veterinarians alike think I'm an unhinged radical myself.

Calcium

An imbalance of calcium in the bones and especially the joints precipitates inflammations, including arthritis and hip dysplasia, in a heartbreaking number of dogs, especially large-breed dogs.* (In my experience, far fewer cats suffer calcium problems and their consequences.) In the BNA, calcium shows up as one of the significant values that, if unaddressed, can lead to problems. Often a calcium problem is the result of poor diet, exacerbated by aging and poor intestinal absorption of nutrients as food is processed into waste. For holistic veterinarians, calcium supplements are a logical choice, and widely used. But here's one alternative therapy that I'm not so crazy about.

Calcium is trickier to deal with than most people realize. There are, in fact, five major forms of it in the body: calcium magnesium, calcium oratate, calcium gluconate, calcium lactate, and calcium phosphate.

---

*There is a reciprocal relationship between calcium and phosphorus, regulated by a small gland attached to the thyroid called the parathyroid. The complexity of this relationship is beyond the scope of this book.

What I've learned over the years is that if you have an imbalance of one kind and happen to administer the supplement for another, you can further off-balance the one that's out of whack to begin with. So subtly different are the various calciums that choosing the wrong one could be a real concern. I'd rather not take the risk.

When I see low calcium, I consider the cause. More often than not, it's a deficiency of those pancreatic enzymes that "combust" food into energy. That, in turn, inhibits the absorption of calcium across the intestinal wall. So instead of giving extra calcium, I give enzymes to boost natural pancreas function, which enhances intestinal absorption; put the animal on a good diet; balance his metabolic problems with specific glandulars; and get him on a daily regimen of alternating multis and Dr. Bob's Nuggets. It's a matter of going for metabolic balance, as in most cases, and enabling the body to use calcium from its natural diet. If calcium levels are high, I give supplements to enhance fat metabolism, as calcium plays a role in the absorption of fats and proteins.

Homeopathic Remedies

All too often, I hear the words "holistic" and "homeopathic" being used interchangeably. The truth is that they are quite different from each other.

A holistic veterinarian, which is what I am, employs an array of therapies to keep an animal wholly healthy in body and spirit. Homeopathy is one of those therapies. There *are* homeopathic veterinarians who feel that health is best maintained with homeopathic remedies, usually unaccompanied by other approaches except in dire circumstances. In my experience, other therapies can and do help, often in conjunction with homeopathy, and ought to be used as long as they do. Homeopathy is also based on the premise that a single remedy, the one that best appears to fit a patient's needs on every level, should be administered once, then not again until the homeopath can see if it has worked—an interlude of one week, maybe two. My problem is that many of my patients don't have two weeks to wait! They have diseases that allopathic medicine has failed to alleviate; they need all the supplements, and all the therapies, that may be useful to them *as soon as possible*. But homeopathy is one of those therapies, and the fact that it seems to defy common sense, that no one in the two hundred years of its practice has ever been able to prove it works by the standards of modern medical science, and that as a result conventional doctors see it as little more than quackery, bothers me not at all. I don't know exactly how it works, either, although I have a pretty good inkling. But I've *seen* it work, again and again.

In other branches of medicine, conventional or otherwise, knowledge has accumulated from a long line of experimenters. Homeopathy is different. Its founding father, a German doctor of the late eighteenth and early nineteenth centuries named Samuel Hahnemann, single-handedly arrived at its radical premises, carried out the years of testing of natural elements which proved essential to it, and eventually wrote its encyclopedia of homeopathic remedies and their applications. If no one since then has been able to prove Hahnemann's findings, no one applying them has had any cause to revise them, either. Two hundred years later, his extraordinary achievement stands.

In 1796, Hahnemann was a forty-year-old physician and chemist, and the author of medical papers renowned throughout Europe. Yet he was in despair. For all the brilliance and sophistication of the arts of his time, medical science relied on medieval practices—bloodletting for one, leeches for another—that killed many of its patients, and Hahnemann had come up with little to improve its record. One day, while translating a distinguished Scottish doctor's *Materia Medica*, or summary of medical knowledge, Hahnemann found the Scotsman's explanation of how quinine abetted malaria so wrongheaded that he ingested the stuff himself just to see what it would do. To his surprise, the quinine appeared to bring on all the symptoms of malaria, though not the disease itself. That was when Hahnemann had his eureka moment. If quinine in large quanities triggered a semblance of malaria in a healthy person, maybe a smaller dose would *repel* malaria from a person who actually had it. Like will be cured by like, as Hahnemann theorized, and so it was.

Over the next fourteen years, Hahnemann engaged in feverish research, testing one natural substance after another on groups of healthy volunteers he called "provers." Every time the provers reported symptoms similar to one disease or another, Hahnemann would try the substance in question on people who actually had the disease. Time and again, the "homeopathic" remedy, as he came to call it, repelled the disease. In the *Materia Medica* he published in 1810, he detailed sixty-seven such remedies (a sum greatly amplified by subsequent work). Two years later, as the starving survivors of Napoleon's army straggled back from Waterloo, a typhoid epidemic broke out among them and

Hahnemann was able to test his theories on 180 desperate cases. All but one patient recovered.

To doctors and pharmacists who saw Hahnemann's success as a threat to their own practices, the remedies presented easy targets. Extract of mountain daisy? Fool's parsley? Aloe and garlic, gum tree and rose apple? Poppycock, surely! Had the remedies been applied directly—seeing was believing, after all—Hahnemann in time might have turned back the skeptics. But "like cures like" was accompanied by a far stranger premise: that the more diluted his medicines were, the *more potent* they became. Why? Because at each stage of dilution, Hahnemann would shake the remedy vial vigorously; the shaking, or "succussion," would disseminate the "energy" from the original drop of remedy to the diluent; and the more dilutions and succussions that occurred, the higher the "potency" of the vial's contents. Hahnemann called it the "law of infinitesimals." Specifically, he started with one drop of remedy to nine drops of alcohol, and shook the vial containing this mixture, holding it against the palm of his hand, 108 times. That "succussion," he said, imbued it with a 1X potency. When he put one drop of this 1X mixture in with nine more drops of diluent, the original drop was now $\frac{1}{100}$ of the solution, but after succussion, it became twice as potent—or 2X. More potent remedies could be 6X, or 10X, or even 30X. Never mind that the original drop of remedy was now undetectable; its energy in the diluent, Hahnemann believed, had only grown.

Only slightly less radical were Hahnemann's theories about how to prescribe his concoctions. Simply matching a remedy to a patient's physical symptoms wouldn't do. Hahnemann felt that the whole patient had to be sized up, as much for his psychological as his physical condition. A woman with flu symptoms who appeared shy and self-critical would get one remedy; a second woman with the same flu symptoms who showed anger or bitterness would get another. When Hahnemann thought he had the remedy that matched a patient's whole being, he administered a single dose. Then he waited a week, perhaps two, to see how the patient reacted. If the patient's symptoms had vanished but returned, he might give another dose of the same potency; if the symptoms were worse, he might increase the potency or change the remedy; if the symptoms had not reappeared, he would give nothing.

Incredibly, Hahnemann's remedies seemed to work. But as homeopathy's popularity spread through Europe and over to America in the nineteenth century, its critics grew ever more determined to discredit it—so irrational did it seem, so scientifically unprovable. The American Medical Association was formed in 1846, three years after Hahnemann's death at eighty-eight, and one of its aims was to stamp out homeopathy. The number of homeopathic colleges grew anyway: at the turn of the century, there were twenty-four hundred of them in the U.S. alone! But by 1923, as conventional medicine progressed and became more established, and the AMA declared that doctors found to be practicing homeopathy would be drummed out of the organization and have their reputations ruined, the number of homeopathic colleges dwindled to two.

In Europe, despite parallel advances in modern medicine and the proliferation of quick-fix drugs, homeopathy never really fell out of favor. In England, Queen Elizabeth for years had a homeopathic physician. Prince Charles has championed the cause, and indeed nearly half of British doctors refer some patients to homeopaths. Nearly as many doctors do in France as well, and almost every French pharmacy has a wall of homeopathic preparations, while lesser but significant numbers of doctors and patients have embraced homeopathy in Germany and the Netherlands. Recently, the pendulum has begun to swing back to homeopathy in the U.S. Not only at health food stores but at mainstream drugstore chains, homeopathic remedies for flu and sinus relief, allergies and arthritis, stress and depression now generate sales of more than $200 million a year—and rising, at a rate of 20 percent a year. One big reason for homeopathy's newfound legitimacy here is that holistic veterinarians discovered it, used it successfully on their patients (an open-minded group), and got the word out to other pet owners. Our pets *can* help us lead healthier, happier lives, if only we're willing to listen!

Homeopathy *is* a strange science, I can't deny that. In a sense, it's almost more of a religion: it requires a leap of faith. And yet the notion of a medicine that has only the "imprint" of a substance in some intangible way, whose potency comes from its "vibrating energy," isn't quite as outlandish as it seems. For me, it began to seem entirely logical after a three-week bout of acute respiratory congestion. I'd experienced a lot of stiffness in my neck muscles and upper back. Despite taking a whole battery of supplements, standing on my head for long periods of time (seriously!), and exercising to try to sweat it all out, the condition stayed with me. I figured I'd just have to give it more time to subside. One day, as I was driving to work, singing scales to try to clear my throat, I pulled into an intersection as the light turned green. From another side, a car ignored the light that was now red, barreled across the intersection toward me, then screeched to a halt, avoiding a head-on collision by just inches. I felt an instant of severe tension, followed by giddy exhilaration. All my stiffness and congestion of the past three weeks were instantly gone! Some form of energy shift occurred here. We are at the frontier of a new "energy age" of medicine; this is what happened to me and is, I feel, the level on which homeopathy works.

A proper homeopathic veterinarian works from exhaustive lists of remedies, from Abies canadensis (Canadian pitch fir) to Zizia (meadow parsnip, wild rice). Like Hahnemann, he sizes up a patient's whole being—admittedly more difficult with a pet than with a person, though various indications of character and mood can certainly be inferred—prescribes one ingredient, and waits to judge its effect. My own approach, given how sick many of my patients are and how little time I have to save them, is necessarily more abbreviated. I go for the combinations.

Though classic homeopaths use only "single" remedies, a growing number of others have come to espouse combination remedies that mix a number of ingredients to be given together, usually at low potencies. Since the ingredients are benign, I side with the homeopaths who argue that there's nothing wrong with administering more than one at a time, and that this "shotgun" approach may lead to faster responses. The product line I use most often is called Biological Homeopathic Industries (BHI), a subsidiary of the Germany-based company Heel. A typical BHI homeopathic is called simply "Calming." Its contents, just to give you an idea of what these combinations are: chamomilla 2X, humulus 2X, paciflora 2X, valeriana 2X, veratrum 4X, ignatia 8X, coffea 10X, moschus 10X, sulfur 12X, and nux vomica 30X. Some of those are flowers (chamomilla), some are trace elements (sulfur), others are plants (veratrum is white hellebore). One is actually a poison: nux vomica, from strychnine, or poison nut. But part of homeopathy's strange, inverse reality is that certain poisons, if diluted enough, repel "like" toxins, or states of "disease," in the body. In sizable doses, strychnine would cause vomiting as its poison entered the body. Nux vomica, an infinitesimal amount of strychnine, *prevents* vomiting and eases the stomach. Hence its place in "Calming."

BHI produces a whole line of combination remedies I use, from "Cough" to "Hair and Skin." So does Boiron, a company based in Lyons, France, that does a large and growing business in homeopathic remedies for people, which we use for pets. A company by the name of ProV Line, based in Sewickley, Pennsylvania, and distributed by Nutritional Specialties, makes several combination remedies we use, including "Motion Sickness," "Ligament Repair," and "Post Surgical." (Their own "Cough," for example, contains alum 6X, laurocerasus 12X, adrenaline 4X, belladonna 3X, ipecac 3X, drosera 3X 10X 30X 200X.) Dr. Goodpet Pet Pharmacy Remedies has a "Flea Relief" remedy, another called "Scratch Free," as well as Dr. Goodpet's "Good Breath" and "Diar-Relief," all of which I've used to good effect—and sometimes in combination with one another. (See the source guide for a more complete listing of companies that distribute homeopathic remedies.)

All these preparations are taken orally, though not all come in the same form. Some are pills. Most are bottled liquids with instructions that call for putting ten drops on the tongue two or three times a day; in those cases, the medicine is absorbed through the outermost cells of the tongue and the lining of the mouth. Often I'll provide a sort of jump start by giving a pet his first doses by injection; putting a substance almost directly into the bloodstream usually has more immediate effects than oral administration. But the daily regimen of drops makes the more enduring difference. Usually, combination homeopathics are taken twice a day, but the administration is so variable, depending on the condition and its severity, that it's best to follow the instructions—and then use common sense.

Combinations, in my experience, are best used for treating *symptoms* of disease. If a dog has diarrhea, I give him BHI's "Diarrhea"; soon enough, the diarrhea abates. (To quote from a BHI handbook: "Intestinal excretion should never be suppressed by antibiotics or chemotherapeutics, as the intestines are the one great tube through which toxins and metabolic wastes may be eliminated. This toxic aggression should be treated by homeopathic stimulation of enzymes, and not by chemical destruction of bacteria.") A classic homeopath will persist with the remedy and hope to reverse the cause of diarrhea as well. I've seen that happen often enough to have enormous faith in homeopathy's power to "cure," not merely to treat. However, I've also found I can get faster results by combining homeopathy with my other efforts to restore a pet's metabolic balance: a good diet, vitamins, enzymes, and the appropriate glandulars. These measures generally work faster internally. Homeopathic remedies tend to work faster symptomatically, and so the two approaches complement each other beautifully.

At the same time, for painful conditions that may not be curable, but only treatable, homeopathic remedies can be the more important of the two approaches. With arthritis, for example, I'll have an owner give his pet a homeopathic called "Zeel" from BHI three times a day until the pain seems to diminish, then have him cut back the frequency. If the symptoms recur, simply give the homeopathic more often again. I know this seems no different from the approach of conventional drugs—treating the symptom rather than the cause—but it is different. In most cases, the ingredients in a homeopathic remedy go deeper than the symptom, gently working on the cause if not actually reversing the disease. How they do this remains unquantified by conventional medicine, so I have no proof, no laboratory studies or medical journal papers, to brandish. I only know that I've seen these remedies produce an easing of illness, time after time, that is far more profound than the mere relief of symptoms.

Sometimes, too, homeopathy can actually address internal imbalances more effectively than glandulars and the rest. If an animal with arthritis, say, has a malfunctioning pancreas or liver so that the food given him isn't being properly metabolized, the homeopathic prescription for arthritis may contain an ingredient that helps restore metabolic balance. If that sounds capricious, I don't mean it to: how the body reacts to disease and treatment really is, to a greater extent than conventional doctors like to acknowledge, unpredictable. One body will respond better to a remedy than another, though both have the same disease condition. A preparation for arthritis may contain an ingredient that unexpectedly also handles a bladder problem. I can't promise you the reaction will occur in the next animal. I've just seen it happen before.

Though the list of homeopathic ingredients is exhaustively long, a dozen or so of the most common are in most combinations, so fundamental and far-ranging is their use. Most arthritis remedies, for example, will have Arnica montana, from the plant leopard's-bane, which soothes inflammations, cuts, or almost any other symptom associated with trauma or physical injury. Arnica's multiplicity of uses, unfortunately, cannot be represented on packages that contain it: the FDA requires that the labels of homeopathic remedies list one use each, and impose such stringent standards for proving that use, that none but the most informed consumers are aware of the various other ways a remedy might help them. The homeopathic thuja, for example, has long been known to counteract the undesirable effects of vaccines. Yet the label on any vial of thuja can make only one FDA-approved claim of use: for warts.

While I rely on combinations for arnica and most other homeopathic ingredients, there are a few "single" remedies I use on their own. To a classic homeopathic veterinarian, these are merely a start; there are literally hundreds more, and the reader interested in learning more about them is encouraged to seek out one of the many comprehensive books on the subject, a few of whose titles are listed in the source guide. But frankly, I've found that along with the combinations, these are the principal ones I need:*

Calceria fluorica (flourspar or flouride of lime)   This mineral has been known to be successful in treating tumors of the mouth.

Calendula (extract of marigold)   Used topically, calendula is incredibly soothing for all sorts of skin irritations, burns, or suppurating sores. I've also used it topically to good effect for diseased gums.

Chelidonium   From the plant greater celandine, chelidonium is an excellent remedy for sluggish liver action and jaundice. It appears as an ingredient in certain products like Hepaticol (Professional Veterinary Products), but sometimes I'll use it in its pure state; if it happens to be the remedy that works with a patient, it *really* works.

Conium   Older animals, especially males with weakness in the rear legs (i.e., German shepherds), sometimes develop a condition called degenerative spinal myelopathy. It's an almost unstoppable and irreversible spinal cord degeneration. Conium can help; in fact, I've had a couple of startling successes. Like most homeopathics, it comes in pellet form, and is held in the pet's mouth until dissolved, or made up into a liquid preparation.

---

*A personal note: Most homeopaths I know dilute their homeopathic remedies with a 20 percent vodka solution to prevent spoilage. (The brand of choice, I'm told, is Stolichnaya.) In my experience, pets seemed to dislike the alcohol, so I use pure distilled water and refrigerate.

Estrogen (estradiol) Effective for female urinary incontinence, which is usually caused by an estrogen deficiency brought on by spaying. The estrogen helps regulate the muscles in the bladder which control urination. Conventional medicine would put a female dog on the *hormone* estrogen, which like the birth control pill in humans has been shown to have carcinogenic implications, or phenylpropanolamine, also used in such diet pills for people as Dexatrim and Ornade. (Common side effects include irritability, tremors, rapid heart rate, cardiac arrhythmias, hypertension, and urine retention.) I get the same results from the homeopathic form of estrogen, which has no side effects.

Nux vomica The essential homeopathic for vomiting. Recently, I've begun to use a rectal suppository combination instead, called "Vomitus Heel" (from BHI). Pets for whom single remedies of nux vomica have had no effect on their nausea are showing dramatic improvement in minutes. Amazing stuff.

Phosphorus Excellent for bleeding. At the end of the first parvovirus epidemic, I began to use it in conjunction with high levels of intravenous vitamin C and fluids to maintain hydration. It was effective in treating the severe bloody diarrhea that accompanies parvo. More to the point, it kept sick dogs from dying and produced dramatic improvements in so many more of them, so much more quickly, than did the conventional medicine I'd been taught to use. Parvo has mostly receded as a threat—for now at least—but I still use phosphorus with bladder and nasal cancers, two diseases which have considerable bleeding, and also on tumors of the spleen in cases where pet owners have chosen not to have the spleen removed surgically because the animal is too weak or old, and the tumor begins to bleed into the abdomen. BHI also puts phosphorus in one of their formulas called—what else?—"Bleeding."

Silicea (silicon oxide) Classically, silicea is used at high potencies to clear up abscesses, accumulations of pus, or other disruptions of the skin. Strangely enough—and homeopathy *is* strange—I've found it useful in addressing cancerous bone tumors. (More on that in Chapter Eight.)

Thuja occidentalis (arbor vitae) As early as the mid-nineteenth century, Dr. Compton-Burnett published a paper titled "Vaccinosis and Its Cure by Thuja." I keep a little squirt bottle of thuja in the refrigerator at the clinic. When I give a pet a vaccine (one of the very few he'll get from me!), I give him a squirt in the mouth; usually I'll give him another squirt or two when I next see him.

Valerian (valerian root) In strong doses, valerian acts like caffeine, accelerating the pulse and causing excitability and nervousness. In infinitesimal doses, it acts in reverse, as a calming agent.

If combinations have all but replaced single remedies in my practice, another kind of homeopathic has come to seem even more critical. Question: What do you get if you cross a glandular with a homeopathic remedy? Answer: One of the most exciting therapies I've ever used. *Injectable homeopathic dilutions of organ and body tissue concentrates.* Or, as we jokingly call them at the clinic, "injectable body parts."

When I began incorporating them into my practice, I didn't substitute these dilutions for a proven therapy. Indeed, hardly any of the therapies I've added over the years have taken the place of more established ones. For pets with serious diseases, that would pose an unacceptable risk. As a result, I can't say if my rate of success with such conditions has increased as much as it has solely because of the injectable body parts, or because of the way they work in conjunction with other therapies. Nor is there a two-hundred-year history of accumulated knowledge and experience to draw on, as there is with classic homeopathy. This is radical stuff, regarded warily by a lot of homeopaths, let alone by conventional doctors. My own sense, based on experience, is that any therapy which works orally, such as glandulars and classic homeopathy, will work even better when injected. Anything delivered more directly into the bloodstream is bound to have a more immediate effect than when it has to work through the cells of the tongue, the lining of the stomach, or the digestive tract and be exposed to the factors of dilution and enzymatic action. But now, along with common sense, I have dozens of case histories of pets whose dire conditions appeared to take a turn for the better when these injections were used.

One, whom I treated earlier this year, was a five-year-old Lab named Abigail, owned by a woman named Linda. Abigail was diagnosed with kidney failure secondary to Lyme disease. By the time I saw her, she had had well over $1,500 worth of conventional treatment:

antibiotics for Lyme disease, intravenous therapy, and more. Still, her kidneys were failing. At the Animal Medical Center, where she was treated thoroughly and well, the attending staff finally gave up, literally sending her home to die. Appended to her medical sheet was a note that read: "Abigail is a very sweet patient. Unfortunately our treatment is palliative as we most likely will not be able to stop the progression of her kidney disease." She was sent home on six different medications, one for the Lyme disease, one for blood pressure secondary to kidney failure (called renal hypertension), and so forth. Her legs were swollen as a result of fluid retention, she was intensely vomiting, and her red blood count was dangerously down. The way she became a patient was that Linda's then fiancé was an electrician called in to do work at the Smith Ridge clinic one evening after business hours. I was staying late, as usual. The electrician knocked on my office door. Could I please treat Abigail? She was, he said, in critical shape.

I was due to leave town the next day on a trip, but what could I say? Linda brought Abigail in early the next morning, and I made some fast decisions. First, I said, we'd stop all six drugs she was on. Although I typically don't "cold turkey" a pet, especially one on that many drugs, we had the dubious luxury of being able to do so right away, since Abigail was clearly about to die. I put her back on intravenous fluids, but now including high doses of vitamin C. Then I gave her an injection of homeopathic kidney: a bit of pig kidney called Ren Suis, distilled and subjected to the "succussions" of homeopathy so that it was, in a Western sense, no longer present, though homeopathically, its imprint of energy was "succussed" to three different potencies. While I was gone, my staff repeated this treatment at the clinic for a couple more days. Then Abigail was sent home and her owners were instructed to give her regular doses of homeopathic kidney orally, along with a few key supplements.

By the time I returned four days later, Abigail was literally brand-new, running around like a puppy, playing with her toys, her vomiting and other symptoms gone. Even now, almost two years later, she remains as vibrant as she's ever been. As an extra dividend, several conventional veterinarians well versed in Lyme disease, and especially this aspect of it, have been so impressed by Abigail's recovery that they're interested in adopting this therapy for their own practice.

We now have "injectables" of virtually every part of the body: heart, liver, kidney, bladder, colon, eye, cerebrum, cerebellum, bone, mammary, and more. Often what we do, in association with the results of a BNA, is inject the appropriate homeopathic body part upon seeing the pet, based upon the specific organ implicated in the disease for which he was brought in (the "presenting" disease, as we call it). With severe cases, this is usually done once a day for three days. However, if the pet in question lives far away and won't be hospitalized, we mix the remaining two vials into an oral dilution for the owners to administer.

One other injectable we use very frequently which is *not* homeopathic is an extract of adrenal cortex, also from a barnyard animal, often a pig. (I include it here because we use it so much in conjunction with our homeopathic injections.) Natural cortisone, remember, has an effect similar to, if gentler than, synthetic cortisone, addressing inflammations and other associated problems, but without the side effects that make the synthetic kind the "reliever of all symptoms and curer of none." Almost always, we mix this with a multiple B vitamin and with concentrated B_{12}. The result, which you could call a "cocktail," acts as a "pick-me-up," appetite stimulant, and anti-inflammatory in most pets who receive it. Occasionally, as in the case of Fia, these injectables bring more dramatic results.

When I first treated her, Fia was a four-and-a-half-year-old Persian cat with all four legs fused at the joints, a condition diagnosed as crippling polyosteoarthritis. Cortisone and antibiotics had done little to help, and so Fia's condition had been termed hopeless. For the last month, she had just lain still on a pillow, her owners unable to bring themselves to have her put to sleep. Hearing of Smith Ridge by chance, they brought Fia in as a last resort. I thought she was a difficult case, but was hopeful that over time, we could achieve some beneficial effects alternatively, in conjunction with some form of surgical intervention on the fused joints. First, of course, I took a blood sample to perform a BNA. Then, before sending her home with a couple of supplements to await her blood results, I gave Fia an injection of homeopathic "Zeel" from BHI and a very small dose of an adrenal-B "cocktail" at acupuncture points on her back. She hadn't moved in over a month before I saw her, and the doctors at the major clinic where she had been treated had told her owner that she'd have to be put to sleep within a week. They told her to think carefully about the quality of life Fia would have even if they managed to buy her a little time. Not long after I treated her, I received two slides, along with this note, from Fia's owner, Nicole Pacich:

Enclosed are the slides of Fia before and after we came to your office July 23. The reason I took those pictures of her when she was sick was I was afraid she wouldn't make it, from what the other doctors had told me, and I wanted something to remember her by. When I got them I realized how awful she looked, and how miserable she appeared, and I never want to see them again. Thanks to you! I'll never forget how she walked—two hours after we brought her home from your office.

Three years later she remains in good health, walking normally on all fours.

You'd think that such results would encourage the FDA to allow all of these injectable homeopathics to be sold in this country, but with its usual attention to the trees at the expense of the forest, the FDA has so far not allowed many of them to be imported. Instead, some of these products, manufactured abroad, get detoured through Mexico and Canada to individuals who then bring them across the border—legally and openly through U.S. Customs. So our patients benefit from them, but only after these products have run a course that, though totally legal, makes us feel like drug dealers.

More inexplicably, those same regulations allow an even newer kind of homeopathic matter to be processed and sold in the U.S.: homeopathic *diseases*. From Washington Homeopathic Products, for example, we now receive highly potentized dilutions of various tumors, each kind to be given as a remedy for its canine or feline counterpart on the essential homeopathic premise that like cures like. Tumors are mostly protein of one sort or another; the homeopathic tumor essence has sometimes been effective in keeping our patients from continuing to produce more tumor protein of their own. In the cabinet beside my desk are more such concoctions: homeopathic mast cell tumor, feline oral cancer, and so forth. Recently, I've taken on a very promising line of injectable cancer remedies, also from the Heel company. Although I've just started using them, I've already seen impressive results.

A final word on homeopathy: *miasm*. Two centuries ago, Hahnemann used the term in relation to a hypothesis he couldn't test on any group of "provers," but which had come to seem logical in light of his exhaustive study of human symptoms and their natural antidotes. Just as the "energy" from a single drop of mineral or plant extract seemed to be felt by the body and produce tangible effects, so might the

THE NATURE OF ANIMAL HEALING

"energy" from a chronic disease be felt by an entire population and then passed from one generation to the next, creating an inherited pre-disposition to the disease which couldn't be detected by medical sci-ence but was no less real for that. Over time, Hahnemann came to conclude that three miasms had spread around the world, creating the predisposition in man to the conditions we now know as chronic dis-ease. One he called the "psoric miasm," after *psora*, which means "itch," to denote skin conditions. The second was the "syphilitic miasm," which led to all manner of immunosuppressive illness. The third was the "psychotic miasm," an intergenerational "residue" of gonorrhea which led to all forms of mental instability and illness.

John Diamond, a contemporary homeopathic doctor who has writ-ten extensively on Hahnemann and his findings, suggests that in the intervening time, a fourth miasm had emerged and, like the first three, spread its energy around the planet. The fourth miasm, Diamond thinks, is cancer. Many holistic veterinarians are convinced that among pets, yet another miasm has appeared in recent decades: the rabies miasm caused by annual rabies vaccines. Its low-level, chronic mani-festations: aggressive behavior and—think about it—fear of thunder-storms. Why, they point out, would animals in nature be afraid of something that can't hurt them? In fact, wolves *aren't* afraid of it. Why dogs and cats?

Herbal Remedies and Plant Extracts

I think of herbs and plant extracts as the natural supplements closest to conventional drugs, so rapidly and specifically do they work to ease symptoms. (And many drugs, remember, have chemicals that mimic the active ingredient of an herb or plant.) Used with other supple-ments, they also often seem to tip the balance—the metabolic balance, that is—for an internal organ struggling to be healthy. And as agents of physical and psychological relief, herbs can be quite extraordinary. Among my favorites are the following:

Aloe vera   Every house should have an aloe vera plant, not just for pets but for people. Aloe's power as a soothing agent for burns, rashes, and stings is well known; half the sunburn lotions on the supermarket shelves contain it. The more natural way to use it is just to break off part of the leaf and apply the aloe it contains directly on the hurt. Aloe can be taken orally, too, in which case it's great for intestinal function, either in easing constipation or abetting chronic diarrhea. For these needs, simply ask a reliable health food outlet for its highest-quality commercially available aloe preparation.

Apple cider vinegar   This folk remedy has so many ostensible uses that believers claim there's virtually nothing else a person or pet needs. One of its chief indications is to enhance bowel function. I use it in dilute solution for chronic yeast infection of the ear (a problem that occurs more in dogs than in cats). I'll recommend that owners put a teaspoon of vinegar in half a cup of water and flush it into the ear, which creates an acid environment that kills the yeast.

Astragalus   A literal meaning of this Chinese herb, so I've heard, is "old man's hair still black." It's one of the most effective herbals you can find for immune support. Recent studies have suggested that astragalus is especially promising as an anticancer agent, which stands to reason, since it's immunosupportive. Available fresh or dried, in tablet or liquid form, and also as a principal ingredient in several Seven Forests formulations (available at any health food store), astragalus is an herb I'm using more and more as part of a pet's overall treatment. I also take it myself.

Chamomile   The flower of the chamomile plant has long been recognized as a soothing herb, both for mental stress or irritability and its physical manifestations. People drink chamomile tea, of course, but so do pets: I just let the tea cool and let them drink it. For sleeping disorders, it often works dramatically well. It often appears as an ingredient in the homepathic combination remedies we use for anxiety.

Echinacea   Derived from the purple coneflower, echinacea taken orally promotes the healing of cuts and various skin irritations. Internally, it boosts the immune system, so much so that in Germany, a pioneer in echinacea research, well over one hundred nutraceutical remedies for colds, flus, coughs, and other common ailments contain it. Just in the last year or two, echinacea has gained national attention as an herbal remedy so clearly effective that even the news team of *60 Minutes*, initially skeptical, ended up endorsing its use in a recent story.

Ephedra   Any one of some forty kinds of desert bushes yields this herb, which acts as a bronchodilator, opening up the breathing passages to help ease bronchitis and asthma. As an ingredient in the Chinese herb ma-huang, used for thousands of years as a medicinal tea, ephedra also has a caffeine-like potency to speed the heartbeat and metabolism and increase blood pressure. Those effects have led to its commercial promotion in recent years as a natural energy booster, which the FDA has rightly frowned upon, resulting in warning labels on packages of "Rocket Blast" and other such brands. Since pets aren't given to recreational drug abuse, ephedra used properly poses no risk in veterinary practice. It does help dramatically with pets who have breathing problems. I use it on its own, in capsule form, as in a product called Dr. Christopher's Breathe Aid. It also appears in Seven Forests' Blue Earth Dragon for nasal problems and Pinellia 16 for coughing and asthma.

Garlic   A natural antibiotic and aid in digestion, garlic supplements are widely available as pills, tablets, concentrated drops, and powders. I prefer to add it in its natural form—cloves of the bulb—to the food I cook for my pets, and urge clients to do the same. It's rich in vitamins (particularly A, B complex, and C), proteins, and trace minerals, and is an excellent antibacterial agent and antioxidant. It may also boost liver function and prevent heart disease, cancer, and other degenerative diseases—and basically do everything but make your pet fly. I also use Kyolic—aged garlic. In its liquid form, I've used it for resistant parasite problems. For nonresponsive ear infections, I've reduced its concentration by half with distilled water; a few drops can be put in the ear and massaged gently, with any excess absorbed by a cotton ball.

Goldenseal   An excellent infection fighter, both orally and topically. But I've also found goldenseal to work in diabetic pets as an herbal enhancement for insulin. I happened on this intriguing potential after finding a booklet called *Insulin vs. Herbs and the Diabetic*, by Ladean Griffin. Then I treated a diabetic cat whose owner refused to give injections of insulin to restore her blood sugar balance. I prescribed half a capsule of goldenseal twice a day, and the cat's condition stabilized— for *years*. Its blood sugar never came down to what conventional veterinarians would call normal, but the cat did well clinically, and lived free of severe blood sugar imbalances until its death at an older age.

Kelp   This seaweed product contains iodine, the mineral that supports thyroid function. The thyroid, remember, is the organ that helps control metabolism, especially protein metabolism. So if an animal has thyroid problems and the thyroid glandular combinations for thyroid don't happen to contain kelp, I'll add kelp in powder form to the treatment list.

Milk thistle For liver disease. The seeds of this thorny plant yield an extract called silymarin, which promotes proper liver cell function and prevents toxins from overwhelming the liver. In people, milk thistle has become increasingly popular as a preventative of liver cancer. It's also seen as an antiaging agent, because milk thistle has "flavonoids" thought to capture free radicals. We use it to help restore the liver's metabolic balance in any form of liver disease, or when metabolic liver function needs to be enhanced.

Red raspberry leaf tea Has a salutory effect on all uterine problems. I know of breeders who use it when a dog is about to give birth; it comes as bulk tea or as an encapsulated powder. I too recommend it to enhance proper birthing; I start by putting it in with food two weeks before an expected delivery and continue with it several weeks after birth.

Valerian Extracted from the root of the plant *Valeriana officinalis*, valerian has long been used as a relaxant, both for the nervous and digestive systems. If I get a call saying "My animal is going off the wall!", I say go to a health food store and get valerian root in any of the dozen or more brand-name preparations in which it's likely to appear. And use it at one-third to one-half the recommended human dose.

Yunnan Paiyao Used in ancient Chinese wars to help stop the bleeding of wounded soldiers, Yunnan Paiyao comes in strips of herbal capsules, or as a powder in a bottle. In either form, the herb comes accompanied by a curious red pellet said by the Chinese to have even more potency to stanch hemorrhages. We use Yunnan Paiyao orally in all sorts of conditions associated with bleeding. We also use it topically, breaking open the powder-filled capsules directly over a wound; the powder cauterizes the wound and promotes healing.

. . .

As with homeopathic remedies, herbs for veterinary care often come in prepackaged combinations. The first one listed is for animals only. The rest are for people; we just don't tell that to our patients.

Ar-Ease (Crystal Star)   For arthritis relief. Primary among its many ingredients are alfalfa, yucca, and devil's-claw, all powerful anti-inflammatories for arthritic joints.

BLDR-K (Crystal Star)   An extract to help with bladder and kidney problems, its chief ingredients are juniper berries, parsley, uva-ursi, dandelion, gingerroot, and corn silk. I like it particularly for cats and small dogs because it comes as a liquid preparation.

Essiac   A combination of four herbs (burdock root, Indian rhubarb root, sheep sorrel, and slippery elm bark) which seems to help support the immune system, reduce the toxic effects of conventional drugs, increase energy level, and decrease inflammation. (The nurse who pioneered its use was Renee Caissé; Essiac is her last name spelled backward.) Now it's gaining acceptance as a cancer fighter. A lot of owners come into the clinic these days asking if I've heard of this new wonder product and saying they've used it themselves as well as given it to their pets. At the same time, they're coming into the clinic because their pets aren't entirely well. I'm incorporating essiac into my treatment—it's widely available through many distributors—but haven't yet reached a judgment about it.

Heartsease/Hawthorn Caps (Crystal Star)   For use in heart disease, as its name suggests. Active ingredients are, in addition to hawthorn, heartsease, Siberian ginseng, and motherwort. In my experience, hawthorn is the most effective herbal for heart support, with all the strength but none of the side effects of conventional drugs.

Night Caps (Crystal Star)   A natural relaxant and sleep inducer that contains valerian root, skullcap, passionflowers, kava root, and GABA (an amino acid that has a marked effect as a natural tranquilizer). A similar brand is Relax Cap, which has a distinctive herb, called ashwaganda, first used (and so named) by American Indians. It's also useful for seizures, primarily epilepsy, both because of its valerian and skullcap components. (Skullcap, derived from a kind of mint leaf, helps relax the central nervous system.)

Tinkle Caps (Crystal Star)   For a remedy that addresses urinary problems, is this a silly name or what? But it works, ameliorating conditions of cystitis; it's also effective in treating kidney disease, bladder cancer, and even feline urological syndrome (FUS). Its active ingredients are uva-ursi, parsley, and juniper berries, all of which are known as herbal diuretics that increase urination (and, more of interest to people than pets, help promote weight loss) and flush out excessive fluid or toxic build-up. Its formula is similar to that of BLDR-K, but it comes as an encapsulated powder.

In addition to these combinations, I've had great success with a product line of Chinese herb combinations called Seven Forests. One we use a lot is Blue Earth Dragon, for sinus problems; another is Forsythia, for chronic ear infections. Just as an example of what these formulations contain, here's the ingredient list for Zaocys, a Seven Forests supplement for skin disease: zaocys, agkistrodon, cnidium fruit, schizonepeta, xanthium, astragalus, cicada, red peony, Tang Kuei, siler, dictamnus, and rehmannia. Wow!

Finally, a word on *propolis*. It's not an herb, exactly, it's not a vitamin, it's . . . the stuff you find in beehives, if you're brave enough to look. (Actually, it's a plant product brought to the hive by the bee.) And here's a question: What's one of the only places where you'll find virtually no infections of any kind? A beehive. Because of its level of propolis. So I use propolis in low-grade infections, as a liquid tincture or a pill, to aid a pet's immune system. I've found it particularly useful with bladder infections, when a pet fails to respond to vitamin C; there and elsewhere, propolis kills bacteria, sometimes as effectively as an antibiotic does, but without the side effects. Now I'm also using propolis salve for topical infections. Works great!

Bach's Flower Remedies

If homeopathic remedies are energy medicine for physical ailments, Bach's flower remedies work in the same intangible manner for the emotions. And since the health of the mind and the body are inextricably linked, improvement of a patient's mental state may bring physical improvement as well. Dr. Edward Bach (1890–1936) was an English homeopathic doctor who determined that dilute infusions of flowers and tree buds could be as efficacious in their way as the plant roots, trace minerals, and other natural elements that Hahnemann had used. As part of his research, Bach would go into the woods, choose a flower, and meditate while holding it. He claimed to feel a particular negative emotion from certain kinds of flowers: sadness, say, or anxiety, or fear. When he did, he would compose a homeopathic tincture to reverse the effect, and administer it to patients experiencing these emotions.

Bach's research eventually produced a list of thirty-eight flower remedies, each of which addresses a distinct mental condition, from Agrimony (anxiety behind a "brave face") to Willow (resentment at unfair treatment). The Flower Essence Society of California is dedicated to furthering Bach's work; it provides complete remedy lists along with other pertinent information, and sells remedies singly or in sets. The remedies come in small, dark-brown bottles (that must, like homeopathic remedies, be kept out of direct sunlight and must not be exposed to extreme temperatures); the general dosage is four or five drops put in a pet's drinking water daily, or one or two drops put directly in the mouth.

I've used flower remedies on pets ever since a low period in my own life, when I picked out about five remedies that seemed to fit my state of mind, took them twice a day, and after a week began to experience a definite lift. The problems in my life hadn't gone away, but suddenly they seemed less weighty. I'd gained a new perspective. With pets who have physical problems that appear to involve emotional stress, I'll add a flower remedy to the treatment. For pets who seem physically healthy but act emotionally upset—depressed or lethargic (often with a poor appetite), antisocial or outright hostile (biting or barking), nervous or fearful (often peeing indiscriminately)—I'll try the flower remedies while also attempting to determine if a circumstance at home provoked the problem. I'll discuss the emotional links between pet and owner at length in Chapter Nine; let me just say here that many manifestations of emotional distress which call for flower remedies have their origins in the relationship between owner and pet.

Of the thirty-eight classic Bach remedies, the one I use the most is the Rescue Remedy. That's no surprise to anyone who's worked with flowers. Rescue Remedy is the most commonly called for because it addresses both mental and physical stress. I'll use it with pets who've been subjected to any stressful situation, from weaning and relocation to a new home, to injections to turmoil or trauma in the home. To cats who are sensitive to needles, I'll give a few drops of Rescue Remedy on the tongue; within seconds, you can see the cat relax, enough so that when I ease a needle in to take a blood sample, he barely notices it. When I use it on a pet who's in shock, or has been hit by a car, bitten by another animal, or subjected to some other acute physical trauma, the results can be truly dramatic.

In addition to his internal injuries, a pet in that condition will have the pale, blanched gums of an animal in physical shock. First I'll put him on medical therapy: intravenous fluids to maintain his blood pressure, and high levels of a fast-acting, injectable form of cortisone. Usually, the effects of physical shock are reversed in fifteen to twenty minutes. That's when I take Rescue Remedy and drop it on the gums and tongue. It's amazing: you can actually see a wave of pink color return, instantaneously. The acupuncture point for shock is just inside the upper gum, right above the line that separates the two front teeth. So I'll also stick an acupuncture needle in there and twirl it. The wave of pink extends, bringing the pet further out of shock.

One other wonderful use for Rescue Remedy is as grief medicine. When one pet in a household of several pets dies, I recommend that an owner give Rescue Remedy to the other pets. The star-of-Bethlehem, which is one of its ingredients, is the flower that soothes grief— well enough that I often advise a deceased pet's grieving owners to take it, too.

As distinct from Bach's thirty-seven other remedies, Rescue Remedy is made from five different flowers: cherry plum, clematis, impatiens, rockrose, and star-of-Bethlehem. It comes as a dilute liquid, but also as a cream that can be applied topically after accidents and other emergencies. I use the other Bach remedies as indicated in my Bach flower reference guide. Among them: crab apple (for detoxification; good after vaccines), snapdragon (for biting or chewing), and star-of-Bethlehem (grief and trauma). Though the best results come when the match between remedy and pet is just right, it's hard to go too far wrong here. The remedies are utterly benign, and any one of the thirty-eight has soothing properties. (According to Bach, you can also use up to four at a time without negating their effect.) They're worth a try for your pet; as with most of these therapies, they're worth trying on yourself as well. I usually recommend that a pet owner get a booklet on the remedies, read up on them, and choose a remedy that sounds right for his or her pet. Who knows a pet's moods better, after all, than his owner? Alternatively, I recommend that an owner call an expert on the flower remedies. One whom I've consulted and for whom I have great respect is Barbara Meyers, of Staten Island, New York (718-720-5548).

Acupuncture

I remember reading the *New York Times* one day in 1971 and being blown away: there was James Reston, distinguished editor of the Great Gray Lady, in China to cover Nixon's historic visit, and being operated on with . . . acupuncture! That was the day most of the Western world, myself included, heard of acupuncture for the first time. Though the AMA harrumphed that it made no sense, and skeptics of all stripes ridiculed it as New Age silliness, acupuncture soon made inroads in the U.S. After all, it *worked*. As one of its first converts in the field of veterinary medicine, I was dazzled by what it could do to ease chronic pain and restore the flow of energy the Chinese called "chi." I felt the excitement of a whole new world opening up. But never had I been subjected to such condemnation. I felt like a vampire; I'd start talking about acupuncture and people would pull out their crosses!

The fact is that acupuncturists in ancient China regularly practiced on horses, upon which the country's agrarian economy depended. Gradually they turned their attention to other farm animals, and finally to household pets: dogs, cats, and birds. Adapting acupuncture to veterinary medicine, it turned out, was as easy as could be, since animals possess basically the same network of energy meridians and reflex points as human beings do. And so it acts in all the same beneficent ways: increasing circulation; releasing endorphins (the body's natural pain relievers) as well as hormones; and, at the same time, decreasing inflammation both internally and externally.

I initially studied acupuncture in 1975, when I took a course to be certified to practice. I was astounded by the responses I saw, and as a recent graduate of veterinary school, I was at a loss as to how to square them with the training I'd received. One day a paralyzed basset hound was flown down for us to study. In school, I'd been taught that if a dog is paralyzed for three weeks, he's very unlikely to regain his mobility. The basset hound had been paralyzed for three months. During the treatment my teacher demonstrated, the dog stood voluntarily. The next morning, he was walking—shakily, but walking all the same. I couldn't believe it.

Subsequent demonstrations were no less extraordinary. A Chinese teacher took us to a farm to show us a badly limping horse. According to his owner, the horse had been chronically lame for a year and had not responded to conventional therapy. The teacher located a bulging blood vessel right above the hoof of the injured leg, stuck a thick, 14-gauge needle in, and let a stream of dark, purplish blood spew out. After about three cups' worth had drained, the blood lightened to a normal hue of red. The teacher withdrew the needle; the horse walked off without limping. The horse, as the teacher explained, had had a stagnation of energy in the blood, or "blocked chi." The teacher had merely opened the blockage and let positive chi flow freely again. No more lameness. I returned one month later for my next session to find the horse still walking and running normally.

Ordinarily, acupuncture involves no bloodletting, just the painless insertion of far tinier needles at specific points to unblock the flow of this invisible energy, which eases the pains and diseases that blockages cause. But the results are no less dramatic. Even among some conventional veterinarians, it's now one of the treatments of choice for arthritis, hip dysplasia, and diseased spinal disks. I've found it useful, too, in treating neurological conditions (i.e., epilepsy and some kinds of paralysis) and easing respiratory conditions (such as allergies and asthma), digestive problems (like chronic diarrhea or vomiting), and even problems of the skin. (In my practice, these treatments are always coupled with a supplement-and-homeopathic program that renders the conditions more reversible.) And since the release of endorphins literally brings peace of mind, I will use acupuncture just to calm a nervous or hostile pet.

There's no need to go on at length here about how acupuncture works, or appears to work: what the twelve pairs of energy meridians, or pathways, actually are; where the 365 reflex points associated with these meridians are (one for each day of the year—curious, yes?); whether the chi is actually neural electricity or not; and how this energy of life is enhanced at these points. Books have been written on the subject. What I do want to say is that acupuncture is a critical part of our practice, and that if your veterinarian doesn't at least endorse it and know of an acupuncturist to refer you to when your pet exhibits one of the conditions mentioned above, you need to enlighten him. Over time, I've come to favor another form of this ancient medicine: aquapuncture, or the injection of a liquid into the prime acupuncture points, which I've found has a more prolonged stimulatory effect than just the insertion of dry needles. The liquids of choice in typical cases are homeopathics, along with the "cocktail" discussed earlier. Generally, I've found that the combination of the three—the two liquids, plus the effect of injecting them at acupuncture points—is greater, to borrow a phrase, than the sum of its parts.

Another advantage of aquapuncture is that it takes a fraction of the time to perform that acupuncture does. Earlier this year, a well-known Hollywood agent, Andrea Eastman, began bringing in her old terrier Oliver for acupuncture treatments to relieve his arthritis. Smith Ridge clinic has a full-time acupuncturist, so after an initial consultation to confirm that acupuncture was advisable, Oliver began coming in for weekly treatments and responded favorably. A month or so later, the acupuncturist was away on the day Oliver was to be treated, so I filled in. Partly out of curiosity, partly because it was a busy day and I didn't really have the time to spend doing a full acupuncture treatment on Oliver, I went with aquapuncture. Instead of at least thirty minutes, the procedure took about two minutes. Days later, Andrea reported that the dog was jumping like a puppy. Now he gets aquapuncture every two weeks and, from time to time, a full acupuncture treatment to enhance total alignment.

A note on acupuncture: I've heard too much controversy about its use in treating cancer to want to risk trying it with cancer myself. If a cancer patient has other symptoms that are causing more distress than the disease, typically arthritis, I will do aquapuncture to bring clinical relief, but I address the cancer in the ways described in Chapter Eight.

Within the realm of acupuncture, by the way, lies the practice of magnetic therapy. The coursing of the chi—a quasi-electrical energy—will create magnetic polarities in the body. As a result, I've seen magnets used on animals with startling results, from pain relief, lameness, and even solitary tumor regression. I offer these two sources, two dear friends highly versed in the use of magnets: on the West Coast, and especially for horses, Joanne Nor of Norfield Inc. in Los Angeles, and, on the East Coast, Suzen Ellis of "Spoiled, LLC" in Weston, Connecticut (see source guide).

Ozone Therapy

By now, you may have discerned a pattern in many of the approaches I use. New as they seem, they turn out to have come to light decades or even centuries ago. Some, like acupuncture and homeopathy, enjoy wide acceptance in the countries where they were developed, but have met until recently with strong resistance here. Others, like Ehretism, met initial success but were eventually seen as passing trends. And a few, like glandulars, were pretty much dismissed when they appeared, and soon forgotten, until a future generation turned them over like so many mysterious rocks to see what lay beneath. In so many cases, when innovation met convention, innovation lost out. The status quo, when its vested interests are threatened, is like the Great Wall of China: hard to overcome. But sooner or later, a curious thing happens. Innovation, if it works, gets through, and the wall comes crumbling down. So it is now with ozone therapy.

Although ozone was discovered in 1840, its therapeutic possibilities were not noted until 1915, by a German physician named Albert Wolff, who treated skin ulcers with it. Later, other doctors noted that if blood drawn from a sick patient was exposed to ozone, the ozone appeared to energize it; injected back into the patient, the energized blood appeared to strengthen the immune system. Or perhaps the ozone itself killed infections in the body; certainly it did so when infectious agents were exposed to it in the laboratory. Promising stuff, yet what is the principal use of ozone today? To purify water.

In that, ozone does an impressive job, killing organisms in water as it does in blood. As a result, I have a list of twenty-five countries—most of the world's major ones—that purify their water with ozone. Unfortunately, the U.S. is not on the list. We choose instead to *chlorinate* our water, using a toxic chemical. (Why go the natural, inexpensive route when there's a buck to be made from creating a market for another man-made chemical?) In some of the countries where those plants are operating, ozone *has* been used in medical treatment, with fascinating implications. In Germany, a woman with a gangrenous leg so infected it was about to be amputated was subjected to ozone therapy, as a next to last resort, just as Wolff contrived it. Substantial quantities of her blood were tubed out of her body and passed through an ozone generator under ultraviolet light, then pumped back in— a process called hypertrophic oxygenation therapy (or autohemotherapy). Within twenty-four hours her leg was almost normal.

As reported in a reference mainstay called *Alternative Therapies*, by the Burton Goldberg group, the treatment of animals with ozone began, ironically, with animal tests to prove how *hazardous* ozone was to humans! The results were so positive that veterinarians in Europe began going back to Wolff's original work and applying it to their patients. The FDA remains unpersuaded, so ozone therapy is neither recognized nor sanctioned in any official way. On the other hand, it's not illegal, at least not in New York and four other states. What that means is that at Smith Ridge, we can use it. I'm grateful for that, because ozone therapy so often produces amazing turnarounds when conventional therapy fails—as it did, for example, with a shih tzu named Lucky.

By the time Lucky was brought in, all four of his legs were paralyzed, the result of a spinal tumor in his neck that clearly showed on a myelogram performed by a board-certified neurologist. The tumor, unfortunately, was too large and embedded to be removed by surgery. The couple who owned Lucky were ready to give up and have him put to sleep, but as a last resort posted a description of Lucky's condition on the Internet. When a client named Carol Marangoni urged them to come to Smith Ridge, they hesitated: both husband and wife are computer scientists to whom the very idea of holistic medicine sent up big red warning flags. And when they heard me suggest that the only hope I saw for Lucky was initially ozone therapy, they looked at me as if I were a snake-oil salesman. But then they viewed the videotape we have of Snoopy, a white terrier whose *malignant* spinal tumor and subsequent paralysis we'd reversed with a combination of treatments (and whose story appears in Chapter Nine). The videotape left them almost in tears. "Okay," they said wearily, "let's give it a try."

I took a blood sample for a BNA, the results of which would be a road map for detailed treatment. I also put Lucky on intravenous vitamin C and ozone. At the least, the fluids might make him feel better. Then I laid him gently in one of the boarding cages we have in back for overnight "guests," and sent the blood sample off to the lab.

The next morning, I came into the clinic and went back to check on Lucky. *He was standing.* When I called the owners, I could tell they didn't believe me. I got off the phone and looked in on Lucky an hour later. *He was walking.* I called the owners again. This time the owner actually asked if I was pulling his leg. Two days later, he and his wife drove down from Albany and Lucky walked over to greet them. We sent the dog home on a full therapeutic regimen. Several weeks later, the paralysis returned. That was a Friday. When the owners called, we talked about the possibility that Lucky had embarked on a healing crisis (see Chapter Six). We also considered whether to bring Lucky in for another "jump start" of intravenous C and ozone, since he'd responded so quickly to the first one. The owners decided to weigh the choices over the weekend. They called back on Monday morning: Lucky was walking again.

That was about two years ago. Recently, I spoke to the owners again, to see how Lucky was doing and ask for a blood sample to run more blood tests. Lucky was playing with his toys for the first time in eight years, the owners told me. Amazing. When the blood results came back, they showed protein values that indicated that Lucky's immune system was actively handling his condition, so that the cancer had ceased to be a factor in his clinical health.

Currently, we're using ozone therapy to help relieve other spinal problems and paralysis. We also use it topically, by infusing it into olive oil, to ease chronic ear problems not responsive to other therapies. By far the greatest success we're having with it, however, is in treating cancer, especially bone tumors. For that, see Chapter Eight.

Chiropractic

Imagine again you're that dachshund coming in to Smith Ridge. I'm hardly a mindreader when I say I know what you need before you trot in the door. Over time, dachshunds have been elongated by breeding, the better to live up to their name—literally, "badger dogs" in German—as terriers who can dig their way to the end of a badger hole and attack their sharp-clawed prey with surprising ferocity. "Many a zealous dog has been known to plunge into a tunnel after quarry—only to get stuck inside," blithely reports the Reader's Digest *Book of Dogs*. That in itself seems a cruel and unusual fate for any dog, but the genetic legacy of the dachshund's breeding is worse: a spine inexorably pulled out of alignment as a dachshund ages by the too great length between his fore- and rear legs, and by the weight of his abdomen in between. Chiropractic, the practice of manually manipulating the spinal column and other joints of the body to realign them, is a godsend for dachshunds. It has survived decades of scornful dismissal by the AMA to be recognized by all but the most conservative doctors as a useful tool in easing human back pain and restoring mobility. Along with many other holistic veterinarians, I've found it even more helpful with pets, especially dogs bred over generations to look cuter, win more prizes, or hunt better at the expense of their bone structure.

When I first examine a dog or a cat, whatever its breed or mix, I'll apply pressure to the back of his neck, shiatsu-style, and work my way down his spinal column. If I feel a back muscle jump, I'll suspect an imbalance and press more sharply with the palm of my right hand or thumb and forefinger in smaller pets. At times, that produces a distinct and sometimes audible clicking sound as the vertebrae realign. Occasionally, the results are more dramatic. A King Charles spaniel was referred to me by a board-certified surgeon who assumed I'd just do acupuncture to relieve the dog's spinal distress. The dog had severe arthritis of the spine and rear legs, had trouble walking, and hadn't jumped up on even a low chair in years. I examined the dog, took a blood sample, then performed a chiropractic manipulation of his back. Crack! The sound was so loud I was startled—and a bit worried, to tell the truth, especially when a colleague who was visiting for a day of observation took me aside and only half jokingly asked, "Did you break that dog's back?" The next day, when I got a call from the lady's husband, a prominent attorney, I really began to sweat. "What did you do to my dog?" the lawyer demanded. Great, I thought: lawsuit, charges of malpractice, the end of life as I know it. "Nothing much," I said cautiously. "Why?" "Because," said the lawyer, "he just jumped on the bed last night for the first time in years!"

The theory behind chiropractic is that such misalignments are not merely painful in and of themselves. They also disrupt the passage of nerve energy along the spinal column. This causes what chiropractors call a subluxation, which inflames the spinal nerves and in turn affects the organs and functions associated with that part of the nervous system. If you choose to believe the Chinese, it also blocks the flow of chi along the involved acupuncture meridians. Almost every cat and dog I treat is subjected to my spinal "once-over." Most turn out to have at least a minor imbalance or two that a judicious push of the palm or aquapuncture can address.

A note of caution on chiropractic, however. Practiced in its bluntest form, with aggressive manual manipulations, it may disrupt a bodily process of natural healing. A holistic veterinarian I know, Mark Haverkos, practices a gentler variation called network chiropractic, which involves subtle adjustments of the spine and main nerve trunks over a period of time. According to Haverkos, the body sometimes "pushes" a vertebra out to compensate for some internal pressure, and a chiropractor who abruptly cracks it back into alignment may subvert the body's own more gradual way of dealing with the disruption. Although I don't as yet practice network chiropractic myself, I do use the occasional chiropractic manipulation to relieve outward symptoms, keeping in mind the need always to address deeper problems.

Cryosurgery

Here's another practice that isn't new, but was merely rediscovered after its initial rejection by conventional veterinary medicine. The difference with cryosurgery, I'm proud to say, is that my brother Robert played a seminal role in its reintroduction.

In the early 1970s, when Robert began his own veterinary practice, the notion that diseased tissue might be "frozen" by liquid nitrogen, so that it might simply die and be rejected from the body, was discredited in veterinary medicine. Cryosurgery (*cryo* means "cold" or "to freeze") sounded arcane. It also appeared not to work, since various tumors and other diseased tissue, when frozen, grew back. To my brother, the theory seemed sensible; perhaps the problem was one of procedure. He began experimenting on animals who had rectal fistulas (internal tracts of pus that surface around the anus), and hard-to-get-at rectal and oral tumors. It was easy enough to persuade owners to let him try, since his efforts would be relatively benign: if cryosurgery failed, the fistulas or tumors would simply return and he would be back where he started. But also, these diseases were basically inoperable, because in cutting the tumor out, a surgeon would likely destroy the integrity of the rectum or the mouth itself. In that sense, too, the owners had nothing to lose.

With the first cases my brother took on, the tumors, as expected, grew back. That was when he had his epiphany. What if he froze the tumors a second time in the initial procedure and slightly widened the scope of this controlled form of frostbite to include a narrow border of skin around the tumor? Now the procedure worked as hoped. The body's immune system rejected the tumor as dead foreign material, and the area adjacent to it turned to healthy scar tissue, which kept the tumor from returning. With the liquid nitrogen clouding around him like dry ice, my brother looked a bit like Boris Karloff in his laboratory. Fortunately, instead of Frankenstein, he produced tumor-free dogs.

Even with two-phase cryosurgery, the tumors didn't fall off immediately. Days might pass. And as my brother began using cryosurgery on other kinds of cases, the unexpected sometimes occurred. One day he treated a cocker spaniel that had a tumor right in front of his ear. The two-phase cryosurgery seemed to do the trick. Ten days later, the dog's owner called up very irate. "Why did you charge me all this money for freezing the tumor when it's still there and looks terrible?" Glumly, my brother agreed to see the dog the next day. That morning, the owner called sheepishly to cancel the appointment: the tumor was lying on the kitchen floor. And where it had been on the dog's head, the skin was pink and healthy-looking.

What we've come to understand with cryosurgery is that every case is different. Sometimes the tumor dissolves, sometimes it falls out. In many cases, the surgical area appears unsightly and smells rotten for several days. Touch-ups of the affected area may be required weeks or even months later. But when the second "freeze" is done (followed, occasionally, by a third "freeze" with very resistant tumors), and if it includes a slightly wider area than the tumor itself, cryosurgery does work, sooner or later, almost every time. Its practice has been taken up in human medicine, too. One common application now is in treating ovarian cysts; another is in freezing tumors in human livers; and for years it's been used very effectively to remove cataracts.

In my practice, with many of the cancerous tumors I see, cryosurgery has become an absolutely essential tool. And unlike some of the other therapies I use, there's no leap of faith needed to appreciate its use. With cryosurgery, seeing is believing, time after time after time.

CHAPTER SIX

The Healing Crisis

O ccasionally, in cases of extreme toxicity, the body initiates its own dramatic confrontation with disease. Then even alternative remedies may be superfluous. This confrontation, when it does occur, may even seem life-threatening, but tends to produce a recovery so radical as to seem a miracle of nature. To those holistic veterinarians who recognize it as a valid process—and not all do—the phenomenon I refer to is known as the healing crisis.

Of all the dramas of natural healing I've witnessed, the healing crises are the most spectacular, and the most awe-inspiring. I've seen animals develop horrible rashes overnight, become paralyzed, or grow feverish enough perhaps to die, only to stage their own recoveries at the same breathtaking speed with which the crises began.

To anyone unaccustomed to it, a healing crisis *appears* to be the final stage of a terminal disease. It's not. Generally, a pet in ill health—but not in a healing crisis—will exhibit a steady decline of energy, a continuing lack of appetite, emaciation, and persistent or gradually worsening symptoms. A healing crisis, ironically, usually follows a period of seemingly renewed health. A pet's symptoms have eased, his energy has rebounded, and his owner has concluded that all will be well. Suddenly the disease seems to reappear. Various signs of increased elimination may occur: mucousy diarrhea and darker, more concentrated urine, mucus from the nose, excessive salivation, and all manner of inflammations and flakiness of the skin. The pet's fever spikes up, perhaps as high as 106 degrees. Yet the pet, though likely in pain, seems oddly *engaged* by the process, as if he knows something his caretakers do not.

At that point, the animal can lose his appetite and curl up in a corner, off by himself. This is no more than an extreme case of what animals in the wild do when they isolate themselves to gather strength and get well. Indeed, it's different only in degree from what we do when we refuse food when we're sick, and let our bodies focus on elimination: through sweating, expectoration, and intestinal release. Unfortunately, a domesticated animal exhibiting such behavior is force-fed almost immediately, which is antithetical to the fasting that is one of nature's prime methods of healing. He's also put on drugs. If the symptoms persist, the therapy intensifies. If all treatment fails, the pet is typically declared a lost cause and is euthanized. In some of these cases, the veterinarian is missing out on an extraordinary force to help restore health. As are, of course, the pets he treats.

Unfortunately, there isn't any certain way to tell, in the midst of a full-blown crisis, when to let nature take its course and when to intervene. A healing crisis is too profound, and too mysterious, to gauge as one does a fever with a thermometer. For owner and veterinarian alike, that makes the process an agonizing and alarming one, and the temptation to go for the quick fix—to administer the drugs that may not cure the disease but will at least relieve the symptoms—is always keen. That, to me, is the hardest part, even after presiding over as many crises as I have. A pet's life, and an owner's trust, are in my hands, and when I suggest holding off on drugs, letting a pet weather the crisis on his own, what I've advocated defies the entire canon of contemporary veterinary medicine.

That's a lonely place to be.

As with so many of the alternative therapies I practice, I came upon the healing crisis in dealing with my own health. I'd been working hard—too hard, I suppose, because I hadn't taken a vacation in three years. Finally, I was scheduled to go to St. John, in the U.S. Virgin Islands. Just before leaving, I went to my chiropractor, who made it part of his practice to test his patients' urine for various values. I had the highest level of one value and the lowest of another he'd ever seen. "You're passing so much nitrogen waste out of your body right now that you're *going* to get sick," he told me. By now, I was on a macrobiotic diet and felt healthier than I'd felt in years. I told him he was crazy.

I flew down with a friend to rent one of the tent cabins at Maho Bay, and at first I felt fine. My friend kept to a macrobiotic diet, too, so basically all we ate was brown rice and vegetables; all we drank was herbal tea. Yet four days into the trip I fell violently ill. My temperature skyrocketed, I had severe sweats and chills; I couldn't even drag myself from my cot in the tent to the central bathroom facilities, two hundred yards away. At one point, I turned my head while lying in bed to see who was coming into my tent, and literally blacked out for several moments. Three days later, I felt better than I'd ever felt in my life. It was a true healing crisis, the first of three I've had in my life. I was thrilled to feel so well, but also quite shaken and, while it was happening, scared: they don't call it a crisis for nothing. Had I not known intellectually what was going on, and had I not been forewarned by my chiropractor, I may well have checked myself into a St. John medical clinic—and who *knows* what would have happened.

My healing crisis, though it produced abrupt symptoms, was actually the outcome of my vigorous attempts over a period of at least two years to improve my health. It came not because I was sick or weak, but because my body was strong enough to stage an assault on the deeper level of the toxins within me, to eliminate them in one big push.

It's important to distinguish between a true crisis and the more immediate, crisis-like process a body experiences with any radical change of physical habit. A heavy smoker who quits his habit abruptly will have pangs of withdrawal that signal the body's first efforts to break the nicotine addiction and return to health; he'll probably expectorate a lot of nicotine- and tar-laced phlegm. (You do *not* want to suppress this cough with a cough suppressant!) Though his body's full recovery—and the end of his pangs—will take months if not years, he'll probably experience sharply aggravated symptoms somewhere along the way as the process of detoxification reaches the next level. Someone who switches diets in a radical way, especially from one of dairy foods and meat to one of grains and vegetables, will experience a modest healing crisis, too, as the body manages at last to expel food-related toxins. Switching from conventional drugs to holistic preparations or supplements often triggers healing symptoms that worsen before they improve.

And then there's the healing process that a heroin addict incurs when he quits cold turkey. For several days, he endures terrible recurring withdrawal symptoms, often growing so sick he appears to be dying, and if under medical care he may have to be confined by a straitjacket in a padded room. If the addict chooses to go cold turkey on his own and gets a "fix" of heroin by someone who panics and thinks he is dying, the addict will rapidly feel "better." But his addiction, of course, will not be reversed. (This, by the way, is not unlike what happens to a patient with skin disease who is on high levels of anti-inflammatory drugs. You try to wean him from them; his skin gets dramatically worse, and if you revert to the drugs, it appears to improve, but this is "improvement" of a most pernicious kind.) If, however, the addict gets through this private hell without reverting to heroin, he starts to get better for real. His body has purged its poisons and is on the way back to health. In time, a true healing crisis may occur if he continues the hard work needed to achieve it.

Heroin addiction, thankfully, is one problem I don't see in my practice. But whenever I'm confronted by a chronically ill patient on drugs, especially cortisone, I know that getting him off drugs while at the same time keeping his symptoms stable is more than half the battle. You can't truly heal a patient while he's on drugs.

Whatever brings it on, a healing crisis in pets unfolds in clear stages recognized as Hering's Law of Cures, after the American homeopathic doctor Constantine Hering. As the body initiates a major expulsion of toxins, pain appears in the neck, then moves down through the trunk and out the extremities—from the inside out, both in the sense of moving from the inside of the body to outside it, and from the neurological center of the body out the pathways of the arms and legs. At the same time, pain moves *up* and out, from the neck into the head, usually accompanied by a discharge of mucus from the nose. As a corollary, healing occurs in the reverse order in which symptoms have appeared. In order to get well, Hering says, a patient must go through a crisis. Expect it, look for it, and work toward it, he declares. In pets, Hering's law is harder to discern, because pets can't tell us what they're feeling. But the course of the crisis is identical to what it is in human beings. In pets, as in people, vomiting may also occur, along with diarrhea, pustules or a rash, and excessive thirst and urination.

Unfortunately, as clear as its course is, the *arrival* of a healing crisis is as unpredictable as its results. No doctor, no patient, no food or medicine can bring it on. I'm forever being asked by anxious owners, "When's the crisis going to come?" I have no idea. The body provokes its own crisis; it does so when it's ready, and not before. In some instinctive way we don't begin to understand, it tends to wait until it has enough strength to handle the force of the pain and eliminations associated with a crisis—thus the calm before the storm, that period of improved health after the body has been at its weakest—and to match the severity and pace of the crisis to what its own constitution can stand.

At the same time, the body is not a Swiss clock, and nature, which can shape one snowflake after another to have six points, can be as mysterious as it is precise. When owners whose pets are in the throes of a healing crisis call me for greater reassurance than that, I read them one of my favorite passages from Arnold Ehret:

"Nature wants to save you!" Ehret proclaimed nearly a century ago. "Disease is merely Nature's effort to start performing the process of healing—the elimination of wastes and disease matters that clog up your tissue system. Listen to the instinctive advice of Nature unfailingly given to both man and animals! 'Give me a chance to eliminate; to repair your bodily mechanism!' Take time to be 'sick' for a few days or even weeks, and I will help you! 'Remain still, quiet, rest, sleep and DON'T EAT!' "

And then I tell them the story of Ginger.

When I first saw Ginger, she was an eight-and-a-half-year-old boxer, and like many boxers of her age, she was in terrible shape. She had a couple of tumors, a condition all too common among boxers. She was also severely arthritic and had a low thyroid condition, both of which required synthetic medications that eased her pain but further damaged her immune system. Gently, we weaned her from the steroids and synthetic thyroid onto homeopathic remedies and multiple supplements; the tumors remained, but did not progress, and Ginger's arthritis subsided enough to let her live drug- and pain-free for another three years. Ginger's owner, a physical therapist named Pat, was thrilled—and so was I.

One April day, Ginger came in for a checkup and routine blood analysis. When the blood results came back from the lab, I was stunned. The normal white blood cell count in a healthy dog is between 6,000 and 16,000. Of those, about 70 percent should be bacterial infection fighters, called polys (a form of neutrophil), while 20 percent should be virus fighters, or lymphocytes. (The remaining 10 percent address various other conditions.) Ginger's white blood cell count was 38,000! Worse, the ratio of infection fighters to virus fighters was reversed. Typically with viral infections, the white blood count drops and the patient gets ill. This blood picture was more in line with a form of cancer called lymphocytic leukemia.

I told Ginger's owner not to panic. Perhaps the lab had made a mistake. A few days later, we repeated the test. Now Ginger's white blood cell count was up to 61,000! And immature lymphocytes were appearing—the equivalent of underage soldiers being sent off to war because the draft had taken everyone else, and another good indication that what we were seeing was lymphocytic leukemia. A consulting veterinary pathologist agreed with the presumptive diagnosis but advised drilling into Ginger's bone to extract marrow that would make the diagnosis definitive. I rejected the recommendation (as did Ginger's owner). She was doing so well *clinically*—which is to say that despite the dire blood count, she was exhibiting no symptoms of discomfort or disease. And why drill to confirm a diagnosis of a disease that we were already responsibly treating with specific supplements to support her immune system? Within a month, the count was up to 75,000, with an even more unbalanced distribution pattern between polys and lymphocytes. Now we knew for sure—without an invasive procedure—that Ginger had leukemia.

Rather than subject Ginger to chemotherapy, however, I decided to monitor the situation. Still symptom-free, Ginger appeared to be leading in all outward respects a normal life. By September, the count remained about the same. That was great! Ginger still had lymphocytic leukemia, but if it grew no worse and she could lead a symptom-free life, why send in the heavy artillery?

The call came one day in November while I was in California: Ginger had become severely ill with a temperature of 105. She'd been brought in to a clinic near her hometown, where an X ray revealed full-blown pneumonia. I was asked almost timidly if I agreed that Ginger should be put on antibiotics. Absolutely, I said. There *is* a place for medicine in our society. In an emergency like this, where the first priority is to keep the patient alive, antibiotics are an essential tool—and a great blessing.

By the time I got home and was able to see Ginger, she'd been on amoxicillin for three days, but still looked terrible. The pneumonia was in full force, and if that along with the underlying leukemia wasn't enough, she apparently now had lymph cancer, with palpably enlarged lymph nodes all over her body. At this point, I put her on Keflex, an even stronger antibiotic that fights nonresponsive pneumonia. Perhaps at least it would knock her fever down. Privately, I had very little hope.

Ginger's owner called the next day to report that Ginger's temperature was up to 106.5. What should we do? I wasn't sure, but a little voice in the back of my mind had begun to wonder if something powerful and unusual might not be going on here. It takes strength to run a fever that high; more often when the body begins to fail as a consequence of a terminal illness, its temperature drops. Why was Ginger's temperature rising?

I had Ginger's owner bring her in for a blood sample. If her internal organs had been damaged, that would be another indication that her illness was terminal, and cause to consider euthanasia. In the office, Ginger's temperature was over 107. I almost put her to sleep right there. Instead, I took a routine blood sample, stopped the antibiotics (since they seemed to be doing no good), and put her on a general homeopathic remedy for fevers. I told the owner I wasn't sure she'd make it through the night, but we'd hope for the best. The owner's preference, too, was natural passage rather than euthanasia.

The next morning, Ginger's owner called to say that Ginger seemed marginally better. She asked about the blood results. I looked at the results I'd just received, and was astounded: Ginger's white blood cell count was down to 9,400. That was normal! "What do you make of it?" the owner asked me. I told her it was obviously a mistake at the lab, and asked the lab to verify the results.

The results were verified. I remained incredulous. Surely the lab had mixed up Ginger's blood sample with another pet's. Meanwhile, Ginger's temperature was dropping down to 102.5. The swelling of her lymph nodes was starting to go down. Another blood sample was taken five days later: Ginger's white blood cell count was down to 7,100. One year later, the white blood count was still normal, with a normal distribution. And Ginger was normal, too.

This was a true healing crisis. Ginger had reversed three life-threatening illnesses. Moreover, the course of her recovery perfectly illustrated Hering's Law of Cures. The cancer was Ginger's core illness, the one that should have killed her but didn't because she worked so hard, over two and a half years, to cure herself of it and build strength to expel the last of it during her healing crisis. Her leukemia, lymph cancer, pneumonia, and nasal discharge were afflictions, in that order, from within Ginger's body to without; they were part of the recovery process from the cancer and, as a result of the healing crisis, were resolved in that same order. In all my years of practice, I've seen many minor-league healing crises, but only about a handful as wrenching and extreme as Ginger's. To me, they're nothing less than natural miracles.

At fourteen, still healthy, Ginger was in her owner's car when the brakes were slammed on at a traffic light. Ginger slid off the seat, hit her back, and was paralyzed. She came in, I gave her two acupuncture treatments, and she was outside running around in a week! In the end, she died of old age—an amazing achievement.

Ever since Ginger's extraordinary experience, I've welcomed high fevers. I've had a couple of cancer patients with temperatures of 107 and told their owners, "Terrific! We might have something to celebrate!" Because along with the calm before the storm, I've come to realize that high fevers are the surest sign that a healing crisis is in process. And both those pets, unhindered by antibiotics, did embark on crises from which they emerged in better health. But this is tough stuff, not only for a pet but for his owner and veterinarian alike. You tell the owner of an animal with full-blown pneumonia and a 107-degree temperature that you recommend discontinuing or not using antibiotics because a healing crisis appears to have begun, and you're risking your reputation and veterinary license. It helps—a lot—to have an owner who understands the risks, and who appreciates the potential benefits of holistic medicine enough to take those risks with you. The surprise, to me, is not how many owners do, but how many become as optimistic as I am!

So it was with the owner of Blake, the white terrier mentioned in the introduction to this book, whose skin inflammations had grown so severe and persistent that his previous veterinarian recommended putting him to sleep. The truth is that when I first saw Blake, I thought he was pretty hopeless, too. But homeopathic remedies and supplements would do no harm, and since every other measure of conventional medicine tried had failed, why not give them a try? After warning his owner that Blake's chances were slim to none, so as not to raise false hopes, I curtailed Blake's intense medical therapy and began to wean him off cortisone, putting him on alternatives as I did so. The owner, who was initially calling with progress reports every few days, stopped doing so, and when other cases rose up to engulf me, weeks passed into a couple of months.

One Saturday morning at the clinic, everything just seemed to flow. People were in great moods, we were running right on time—quite a rare occurrence at Smith Ridge—and every one of my cases that day was a pet who had suffered a serious illness but who was now doing incredibly well. Just before noon, I looked out into the waiting room to see a sight like none I'd ever beheld.

Blake's owner I recognized: she was the one sitting on a chair by the door. But the creature at the end of the leash bore no resemblance to the dog I'd treated. He was this little black *thing*; he looked like a miniature rhinosaurus. He had no hair whatsoever, and his skin appeared to be charred. I couldn't hide my horror, especially since he was sitting in full view of several other disconcerted clients, but to my even greater surprise, Blake's owner smiled. "It's all right," she said. "For the first time in his life, he's not itching. And look more closely."

I did. What I saw were thousands of little white hairs sprouting amid the blackness. The owner had realized even before I could explain it to her that Blake had detoxified. Indeed, he had gone through a healing crisis as dramatic, in its way, as Ginger's, with severely abraded areas of raw skin, hair loss, and so forth. In a sense, his crisis was worse, since Ginger's illnesses had been internal, and invisible, while Blake's was of the skin. The owner, who was one very cool lady, also intuited that Blake was *young* enough to endure the trauma he was experiencing. His constitution was strong enough to take it. An old dog might not have survived—but then, an old dog's body probably would not have embarked on such a brutal healing crisis. Nature knows what it's doing and, once headed in a positive direction, tends to make the "right decisions" in the best interests of the body in question.

In a sense, the correlation between crisis and constitution is an obvious one. If an eighty-four-year-old man consumes a pepperoni pizza and four beers, he could be set back for a while. Give that same meal to a twenty-one-year-old marathoner, and he'll feel fine, especially the next day after he goes out to run his usual ten miles. The age and strength of a patient have everything to do with the level of toxins his body can absorb and expel. Which is also to say that they have everything to do with whether or not he can withstand a healing crisis, and the extent to which it can be brought about. In no case, however, is the crisis predictable. As Bernard Jensen has observed in his *Doctor-Patient Handbook*, "A crisis comes usually after you feel your best. It is the will of nature. No doctor, no patient, no food, can bring a crisis on. It comes when your body is ready; it does it in its own time. It goes through slow or fast, according to the patient's constitution. You *earn* this crisis through hard work. A crisis can come harsh, small, violently, softly. Some crises come in the form of backaches, skin rashes, diarrhea and joint pains, or fever."

Because a *minor* crisis is likely to be brought on in a person by some conscious action—quitting cigarettes, changing a diet—its potential effects, can, and should, be rationally gauged. The closer a crisis candidate is to being twenty-one rather than eighty-four, the better his health is in other respects, and the better he'll cope with the temporary aggravation of symptoms associated with the crisis. So it is with animals for minor crises brought on by the switch from a poor diet to a nutritious one, or those weaned from antibiotics to homeopathics. Is the pet too old or infirm to withstand the aggravated symptoms associated with even a minor crisis? This is a decision no owner should make without the counsel of a seasoned holistic veterinarian.

A major healing crisis is initiated mostly by a pet—but not completely. A pet still has to be taken off drugs by his owner and veterinarian for the crisis to have a chance to occur. And a crisis in progress can still be reversed, or at least kept from resolution, by symptom-suppressive drugs. I sometimes decide, with older cats and dogs, that their health is simply too fragile for a crisis of any proportion. Our ultimate goal, after all, is to help provide a pet with as much pain-free time and energy on this earth as we possibly can. If an old cat with a degenerative condition is pain-free and may live that way for another two years, why try to induce a major trauma to his system which might buy an extra year or two, but force him to spend most of that time detoxifying and enduring painful symptoms? Generally, though, I think that a chronically ill pet who seems on the verge of a healing crisis deserves the opportunity to go through it. As Hering observes, a sick patient must always go through a healing crisis in order to fully recover his health. If in fact a pet is simply growing more diseased, and not going through a crisis, the use of synthetic medications at this stage may save his life but keep him chronically ill. I would rather risk having him pass out of his misery than deny him the chance to get well.

Occasionally, a pet I'm treating takes matters into his own paws no matter what we do.

Such was the case with Kismet, an Airedale I'd been working with for most of her life. Kismet had first come to me as a young dog with terrible skin inflammations and the typical verdict, from a conventional clinic, of incurable allergies. I'd reversed her skin problems the usual way—off antibiotics, onto homeopathic remedies—and thoroughly enjoyed seeing her bounce back in for annual checkups as a happy and healthy dog. Then, as she approached old age, Kismet developed a tumor in her left thigh. She was still vigorous enough for me to conclude that an X ray would do no harm, and might help us decide how to treat her, as it would make a tremendous difference if the tumor had invaded her bone.* The X ray showed a soft-tissue, intramuscular tumor the size of an orange, a finding I confirmed by drawing out a sample painlessly with a needle and sending it out for diagnosis.

At a conventional clinic, Kismet would have been operated on immediately. Either her tumor would have been removed, or her leg would have been amputated. Once the tumor had proved cancerous, she might have been subjected to an extensive regimen of chemotherapy. All this would have been painful for Kismet, traumatizing to her immune system, and terribly expensive for her owner. Given her age, Kismet probably would have died as a result; if she had lived, her remaining time would likely have been brief and unhappy. I chose instead to monitor the situation, hoping the tumor would grow slowly and cause Kismet no pain. Over the next several months, Kismet appeared pain-free but grew increasingly enfeebled, shuffling with the gait of a very old creature. Sadly, she also started growing another lump on the side of her body. When acupuncture treatments failed to produce more freedom of movement, I started talking to the owner about having Kismet put to sleep. We still had the choice of trying a program of intravenous fluids to flush out her system, but I thought the benefits would be at best temporary, and agreed with the owners that euthanasia was the sensible course at this point.

I went home that weekend feeling pretty depressed. The decision to put a pet to sleep is never an easy or unemotional one, and Kismet was one of my favorite dogs. Euthanasia has its place in veterinary care (see Chapter Ten), and when it's the only humane option left, I can administer the life-ending injection with the knowledge that life as the pet knew it and enjoyed it is over already; all I'm ending is the misery that remains. But even then, it's a trying experience, one magnified by the grief of the owners for whom this pet was a member of the family.

On Monday morning, I came in to work expecting to start my week by putting Kismet to sleep. In came Kismet's owners—with a dog who bore almost no resemblance to the one I'd seen the week before. On Saturday, her owners reported, Kismet's temperature had shot up.

---

*I may advise *against* X rays for older dogs when the nature of the affliction is clear enough and x-raying is only likely to confirm the obvious course of therapy. Too often, an X ray is performed needlessly—a routine procedure to be ticked off a conventional checklist; why in those cases expose the pet to unnecessary radiation?

Then, on Sunday, the mass on her side, which by then had grown nearly to the size of a melon, had broken open. Out had oozed more than a quart of slimy, clear liquid, deflating the lump altogether. The older, chronic tumor, as I felt it, was half the size it had been on Friday. With no external draining, it had rapidly shrunk, and Kismet appeared far less frail than before. Delighted, I put her on an intravenous vitamin C drip: if Kismet had undergone a healing crisis, the vitamin C would further support her immune system to finish the job.

The next day, Kismet's tumor was a marble-sized, hairless bubble. A second growth she'd developed on her spine was gone. And this dog who I'd assumed would never regain her youthful energy was romping around my office, barking to demand her dinner!

Here then was a healing crisis I hadn't anticipated or in any way tried to provoke, a healing crisis that I might have tried to avert had I known it was coming, given Kismet's seeming enfeeblement. Perhaps she'd understood from the sorrowful tone of my conversation with her owner that we were giving up on her, and that if she wanted more time on this planet, she would have to save herself. But whether she did or not, she'd healed herself.

More recently, I treated a Rottweiler named Whiskey whose referring veterinarian had predicted he had no more than a week to live. By then, Whiskey had been subjected to $3,800 worth of conventional therapy, and was only the worse for it. He was suffering from inflammatory bowel disease, an all-too-common condition among dogs and cats alike. Though in itself not necessarily fatal, it was compounded, in Whiskey's case, by significant lymphangiectasia, an associated disease of the lymph tissue in the intestines. Among many veterinarians, that combination in its advanced stages is felt to be 100 percent fatal among Rottweilers. When their own veterinarian had declared the case hopeless, Whiskey's owners had contacted nearly a dozen other sources, including two in Canada. They received the same grim verdict from all of them. Based on what I heard on the phone from the owners, and then their veterinarians, I had to say that Whiskey's chances seemed slim. But why not try to confound the odds?

Whiskey arrived on a stretcher, too weak to walk. A healthy male Rottweiler, powerfully built with considerable muscle mass, weighs about 125 pounds; Whiskey weighed 57 pounds. With the owners' permission, I cold-turkeyed him on all the drugs he'd been getting on a daily basis for so long (including cortisone, daily, for months). This was unusual, even in my practice: going "cold turkey" can do more harm than good. But in this case we had nothing to lose, since the drugs were obviously not working and Whiskey was about to die. At the same time, I hospitalized him and began a program of intravenous fluids, including high doses of vitamin C. Over the four days that Whiskey remained at Smith Ridge, his condition improved to the point where I felt comfortable sending him home on a full program of alternative therapy. I told the owners to administer the program meticulously, to stay in close touch—and to pray.

Within four weeks, Whiskey was much improved—walking, though still with considerable effort. Then one day after five weeks, one of the owners called in a panic. Whiskey's head had swollen to nearly twice its normal size, and blood was coming from his nose. "What should I do?" the owner pleaded.

"Go to the movies," I suggested.

When the owner was sure he'd heard me correctly, I added that this seeming turn for the worse, after weeks of slow but steady improvement from a dire state, struck me as a textbook case of a healing crisis in the offing (a textbook case, that is, if there *were* any textbooks on the healing crisis, which there aren't). And what was our choice but to hope that it was? We knew what would happen if Whiskey was put back on cortisone and other drugs: we'd be right back where we started. The owners chose to forego the movies, but they set Whiskey up in a bedroom and tried to go to sleep. The next morning, after several anxious check-ups on his condition, the owners noticed that Whiskey's nasal discharge was now half blood, half mucus. In two days, the swelling of his head began to subside. In five days, the swelling was gone altogether. The healing crisis—and it had been that—was over. Since then, Whiskey has returned to full and robust health. He weighs in at a svelte 140 pounds. Not only that: he's handsome enough, and game enough, to have appeared in a jeans commercial on television! From basket case to TV star: now *that's* a healing crisis with happy results.

If that weren't satisfaction enough, Whiskey's recovery was so inspiring as to persuade a human observer to dedicate his life to alternative medicine. At the time, Gary Nestler was a floor manager for the computer business run by Whiskey's owner. Gary happened to come from a family of five physicians; he was as allopathically oriented as a person can be. Yet he was so struck by Whiskey's healing that he began delving into alternative practices. Now he's the director of the department of alternative medicine (for humans), nationally board-certified in acupuncture and herbal medicine, at the University of South Carolina's medical school.

Even for holistic veterinarians, the decision to believe that a healing crisis is under way is an arduous one. I've often seen a holistic veterinarian do great things for an animal initially and then decide, nine months later when the pet comes back with a seeming turn for the worse, that that approach has failed. And so out come the drugs, or the euthanasia solution—just when the pet may be about to slough off his most deeply ingrained toxins.

What I say to those veterinarians at those times is what I say to the owners: Don't be afraid! Fear is such a terribly destructive force in medical care. So often, it inhibits us from letting the patient help himself. But also: Recognize the whole picture. How was the patient in the days preceding this apparent decline? A pet on the eve of a healing crisis will have seemed energetic, even frisky. "This feeling of strength is probably the most distinguishing feature that characterizes a healing crisis from a disease crisis," observes John Sherman, a doctor of naturopathy from Washington State who has studied the phenomenon. "The vital force is on the 'ascendency' in a healing crisis, whereas there is a lack of vitality in a disease crisis. . . . When the vital force intrinsic to the body has finally worked up to this acutely reactive event, taking any suppressive medication, even an aspirin, could damage the immunity and vitality of an individual."

If holistic veterinarians hesitate, what of conventional ones? The fact is that most seem incapable of accepting, even as a remote possibility, the notion that drugs might not always be the best approach to severe ill health, let alone that without them, a healing crisis might occur—as the case of Bristol Hill makes clear.

By the time I saw Bristol Hill, he was a three-and-a-half-month-old kitten with bone infections who'd been subjected to so many intravenous injections that his veterinarian had run out of veins to hit with a needle. The veterinarian simply hadn't known to consider any other course of treatment besides drugs. And now euthanasia was the logical and humane choice. When I saw Bristol, I felt we had a truly hopeless case, and the blood analysis seemed to confirm that opinion: his white blood cell count after two months of constant intravenous antibiotics was over 50,000, when it should have been between 6,000 and

16,000. Because the infections had spread to his joints, all four of Bristol's legs were crippled. Moreover, the chronic drug therapy had overwhelmed his immune system, and Bristol had become quite anemic. Though I was tempted to go along with the recommendation of euthanasia, I decided there was nothing to lose in putting him on injectable vitamin C and giving him a couple of homeopathic remedies for chronic and acute infections. Five days later, I couldn't believe my eyes. Bristol was sloughing off toxins from everywhere, but at the same time he appeared so much stronger. Alarming as the process appeared, I knew it was a healthy one. I also sensed that Bristol was feeling resolute. So I did nothing to try to stop it.

Over the next weeks, Bristol would improve; then another abscess would pop up and he would just slough it off. Here was a healing crisis in perfect stages, with Bristol marshaling strength for each approaching expulsion of toxins en route to glowing good health. Today, two years after I first saw him, Bristol's infections are completely gone. So is his anemia. And his owner reports that despite some vestiges of joint stiffness, Bristol just zooms around the house.

Consider, finally, the story of Scramble, as told by her owner in a letter written to serve as a testimonial to her own healing crisis.

"My dog Scramble has been treated for liver cancer for the last six months," Ken Davidson wrote of his fourteen-year-old mixed-breed shepherd in October 1995. "All that time, I'd had Scramble on the Immuno-Augmentative Therapy program (see Chapter Eight). For a while, she had appeared to improve. Then she'd gone into a steep decline that seemed the end. For two weeks Scramble could not stand up, let alone walk on her own," Davidson explained. "Her legs had been oozing blood and fluid that Dr. Goldstein called 'toxic cleansing.' . . . I was willing to do whatever I needed to do to help my dog live a long and healthier life. But we seemed at the end of the road. I was afraid that Dr. Goldstein's 'healing crisis' was his way of trying to keep me positive, but I could see that my dog was nearing death."

At 2:30 a.m. one dark morning, Scramble began breathing heavily. Her eyes seemed vacant, as if she'd died already. Knowing that the emergency-room veterinarians would sternly advise euthanasia, Davidson decided, as he put it, "to let her die in her own environment. Eventually I went to sleep expecting to wake up to a dead longtime friend and companion.

"Upon waking the next morning, afraid of what I would find, I went to the kitchen where I had left her the night before. What I found will be with me the rest of my life. Scramble was standing up, wagging her tail, and licking her lips for breakfast.

"Three months later, Scramble is still as healthy and vital as she has ever been," Davidson concluded. "She is still battling cancer, but she is playful and alive."

Understand: Not every seriously ill pet is lucky enough to incur a healing crisis. Too often, a sharp decline in health is just what it appears to be—a decline—and should be treated with antibiotics or any other measure at hand to keep a pet alive. But when a healing crisis does occur—and they *do* occur—the results that come from letting well enough alone, from letting the body heal itself, are more complete, and more enduring, than those that can come from anything we have to offer. I've seen those results. I hope, if your pet is ever so sick, that you see them, too.

CHAPTER SEVEN

An Alphabet of Ailments

T he list of ailments that constitute this chapter is hardly intended to be complete. Books can be written (and have been) on each of the conditions addressed below; a number of other conditions are not included at all. Rather, this chapter represents a synthesis of the problems I see most often in my own practice, and which I have treated, usually successfully, in the ways I describe. My hope is that an owner, having determined the problem his pet has, will be led toward effective treatment. With a relatively mild problem—fleas, for example, he may treat his pet himself. Many of these conditions, however, aren't mild at all, and initially should not be treated at home. My goal in describing these more serious problems is to make an owner aware of the gravity of them, and so to persuade him to get professional help for his pet sooner rather than later. If in reading these pages he's persuaded to seek out a holistic veterinarian, all the better. Trained though I am in conventional medicine, I've based most of my career on holistic practices; I've seen them work every day, and I truly think they work better than conventional medicine in most circumstances. (When conventional means *are* preferable for a condition described in the pages that follow, they're gratefully noted; holistic medicine, in my opinion, embraces the *whole* range of therapies needed for the pet's well-being— including conventional medicine when necessary.) If an owner finds himself at a traditional veterinary clinic instead, he will have an awareness, at least, of the holistic approach to the problem from this book, and can engage his veterinarian in meaningful dialogue about it. Not enough veterinarians are practicing the approaches outlined below, but a growing number are aware of and intrigued by them, and are often willing, with an owner's encouragement, to give them a try.

Understand, too, that this is a *reference* chapter. Don't feel you have to read it all now! Of course, if you have a deep, abiding fascination with fleas or anal gland problems, be my guest. Otherwise, make a mental note that this guide is here for when you and your pet need it, and skip to Chapter Eight.

Allergies

In dogs especially, but also in cats, allergies are an all-too-common problem. That doesn't make them easy to treat. Not only do they appear in a bewildering number of forms, their origins remain obscure. It's never easy to deal with a condition you can't define.

The conventional wisdom is that allergies are caused by a strong reaction of the immune system to some foreign protein: pollen, various molds, and grasses, to name a few. Fleas can cause allergic reactions as the immune system reacts to the protein in flea saliva. Bees and mosquitoes can precipitate allergic reactions, too. And the four food allergies most common in people affect pets just as keenly: red meat or meat by-products (in pet food); dairy; wheat (a common ingredient in pet foods); and yeast (often as brewer's yeast). Why do some people and pets react to these proteins while others do not? The conventional wisdom holds that an unlucky few have a genetic predisposition to react to those proteins. Though this is partly true, why do allergies often appear at one point in our lives and disappear at another?

My own approach to allergies begins with the premise that an allergy isn't the root cause of the symptoms it manifests. It's the symptom itself, which flares up when a body's immune system has become sensitized to an allergen. This is usually secondary to a buildup over time of toxicity that has affected the immune system. Genetics may be involved: a pet with a family history of allergies is definitely likelier to have them. An acquired weakness may also be a factor in allowing any symptom to manifest more easily, especially in a weaker part of the body. But either way, whatever leads to the toxic buildup forms the basis of the allergy complex. So the goal is to get the body detoxified and the immune system healthy again, not just to treat the symptoms.

In all allergic reactions, the common denominator is *inflammation*, usually external but sometimes internal, as the immune system reacts to the unwanted protein. In a healthy immune system, the inflammation will be brief, with healing through detoxification the happy result.

In an unhealthy body, the inflammation just grows into allergic symptoms. Most pets that manifest allergies do so in the skin, exhibiting rashes, hot spots, conditions like miliary dermatitis—little lumps all over the body—and other symptoms too various to list here. In pets as in people, allergies may inflame the ears and eyes, the respiratory and digestive systems. Problems such as asthma, bronchitis, conjunctivitis, and colitis with diarrhea may result.

The conventional treatment of choice for allergic reactions is usually cortisone. I've discussed cortisone elsewhere in these pages; in brief, it treats the external *and* internal symptoms of inflammation without addressing their causes, and so is rarely a cure. In conventional medicine, pets are also subjected to a battery of tests to identify the particular allergen that's plaguing them. They then receive shots on a regular basis to "desensitize" their immune systems to that allergen. The process involves administering high doses of the allergen to which there's an allergy in order to exhaust the appropriate antibody's ability to react to it. My question is: Would you rather have your immune system be sensitive . . . or desensitive? Golden retrievers, to take just one example, are famously allergic (especially plagued by painfully itchy "hot spots"). I suspect that because they've been so "desensitized" for their allergies, they're more prone as a breed to cancer. I've seen other animals with cancer, especially dogs, who have a medical history of "successful desensitization" for allergies. I'm convinced, though I can't prove it, that this process may be very contributory.

In my own practice, I avoid cortisone whenever possible. If a pet is really suffering, I'll administer a low dose of it just to rein in the symptoms and get the pet to stop exacerbating them by scratching or licking—but most of this injection will contain *natural* adrenal cortex. Also to address the symptoms, I'll inject a dose of Cutis, a homeopathic skin remedy made by the German company Heel (see source guide). Recently, I've gotten dramatic results using a new, oral product called natural hydrocortisone, which appears in a product line for animals called Pet Health Pharmacy. Derived from soy, the natural cortisone acts like the synthetic version, but without the side effects, and without leading to elevations in the adrenal and liver blood values. Orally, I also use Betathyme (Doctors Mutual), a supplement that contains a plant-derived form of cortisone, and a Chinese herb called Kai Yeung, both labeled for people and available in tablet form through holistic veterinarians, or perhaps by order from health food stores. (I'll give a thirty-pound dog one Betathyme twice a day, and two Kai Yeungs once a day; for cats, I'll halve these doses.) I'll also give the antioxidant enzymes AOX/PLX by Biovet. (Four tablets of AOX have the same anti-inflammatory effect as 2.5 milligrams of prednisone, currently the most commonly used form of cortisone.) The comparable brand for cats from Biovet is Feline Support. I use several topical solutions as well. Calendula (marigold) is one of homeopathy's most effect responses to allergy-related skin problems; I use a spray called Eco-VM (made by Imhotep). Traumeel (Heel) is a good ointment for marked red spots, and aloe vera in any form is always helpful.

Depending on a pet's symptoms, I'll prescribe an appropriate homeopathic remedy to alleviate the chronic allergic response. For skin-related allergies, I'll use BHI's "Allergy" because one of its ingredients is homeopathic histamine. (BHI's "Skin" and "Hair and Skin" are also useful.) The company Dr. Goodpet has two good products relevant to allergies: Scratch Free, and Flea Relief (when fleas are the allergy instigators). Echinacea in capsule form is worth including. Although we try to use the fewest number of products to achieve the reaction we want, I have no problem putting a pet on several of these preparations, simply because the chances are greater that one of them will work. (Remember: As rational and scientific as Western medicine presumes to be, it can't tell you exactly what causes or cures allergies any more than I can. Nature does work in mysterious—and unpredictable—ways. Why not hedge your bets?) For a pet who's suffering, I'll administer combined homeopathic remedies as often as every fifteen minutes until the cycle of inflammation and scratching is broken. Be sure, too, for all allergic skin problems, especially those that appear to be caused by fleas, to avoid chemical shampoos. So many effective herbal brands are on the market now that owners should just make straight for the nearest health food store and scan the shelves.

You'll notice that all of the above remedies address allergic problems of the skin. Allergies may provoke all manner of systemic reactions, however. For inflammations of the ear, I give BHI's "Ear and Inflammation" orally, and Dr. Goodpet's Ear Relief topically; sometimes I add Seven Forests' Forsythia herbal tablets. For conjunctivitis or gummy secretions of the eye, I give Similasan "Eye" drops. For coughs, we have remedies from ProV Line and BHI (both called "Cough"), as well as three homeopathic formulas from Similasan. BHI also has an "Asthma" homeopathic remedy, and one for bronchitis.

The best way to tell if a food allergy is responsible for a pet's digestive problems is to put him on an elimination diet. Feed him a strict diet of chicken, rice, carrots, and distilled water. Each week, add one of the foods that might be the problem, and see if a reaction occurs. If it does, just eliminate that food from his diet while you continue to work on getting him allergy-free.

Cats incur allergic conditions of the skin, too, and should be treated the same way dogs are (though typically given smaller doses). If the allergen is a food, the cat should also be put on a homeopathic remedy, as recommended for dogs, and at the same time put on an elimination diet. In cats (and in dogs), if a food allergy causes intestinal inflammation leading to diarrhea or other digestive problems, take the steps outlined below, under "Diarrhea."

I should mention that many holistic veterinarians have touted bee pollen as working miracles with allergies—especially those apparently provoked by pollen and bee stings. I'm not persuaded. It's true that bee pollen contains high concentrations of protein and will dramatically affect an allergy's protein-protein reaction, but the result may be more inflammation, not less. You can try it if you like, but if you do, start with very low doses and build up gradually.

With allergies as with all illness, my goal is to restore the body's metabolic balance. Because of the inflammatory nature of allergies, the adrenal gland, the producer of natural cortisone, is almost always one that needs support. Adrenal supplements are the answer. Health food stores carry a number of them; one I use frequently is Drenatrophin, from Standard Process Labs; Miladrene, from Miller, is another. But there are so many more.

Anal Gland Problems

A dog has a small, sac-like gland on either side of the anus which secretes a particular scent. The anal glands are probably what dogs are smelling when they sniff one another's behinds. They are what dogs use, along with urine, to mark territory. Designed to empty naturally during defecation, the anal glands sometimes become impacted or abscessed, painful conditions that lead the dog to drag his behind across the floor, in an attempt to alleviate them. Cats can incur similar anal problems, but do so more rarely.

In most cases, the sacs can be manually squeezed to release the fluid and ease the blockage. Given that this is just about the most foul-smelling liquid in the world, I try to minimize the chances of a recurrence by placing a small amount of Panalog into the anal sac when I empty it. Panalog is actually an allopathic ointment for the ear, but it's effective with the anal sacs, and a little goes a long way. It does contain an antibiotic and cortisone, but because the body absorbs the medicine minimally if at all, it has no systemic side effects. I also use a homeopathic remedy for hemorrhoids in people, because hemorrhoids are also rectal inflammations, and the remedy seems to address both conditions. It's produced by BHI and called, poetically enough, "Hemorrhoid." I mix it with BHI's "Infection." To alleviate the problem chronically, I suggest adding more fiber or whole grain to a dog's diet to bulk up his bowel. A bulkier bowel increases pressure on the sacs to allow them to empty naturally.

A common misperception about the anal sacs is that they should be emptied frequently, so veterinarians squeeze them empty as a routine matter. In my experience, that only increases the prospects of inflammation and impactions. Since these sacs are lined with secretory cells, the natural state of the glands, in fact, is not to be empty.

Anemia

In pets, as in people, the overriding symptom of anemia is weakness, exacerbated by loss of appetite. Pets tend to have pale gums; the color inside their ears may be pale, too, rather than pink. Because anemia is a generalized condition, it also exaggerates other symptoms: a lame dog, for example, will appear lamer if he becomes anemic.

Anemia occurs, in essence, when the body's red blood cell count drops. Since iron is needed to produce these cells, an iron-poor diet, especially when accompanied by general malnutrition, can lead to anemia. Another obvious cause is chronic loss of blood; a pet with a serious open wound will almost certainly become anemic if the bleeding is not stanched. Kittens can die of anemia when attacked by enough blood-drawing fleas. Worms, especially hookworms in severe infestations, can also absorb enough blood to cause anemia. And certain blood parasites, such as hemobartonella in cats, destroy red blood cells, leading to anemia. Internal bleeding from ulcers or tumors can cause anemia, which may become life-threatening. The kidney can be involved more subtly. It secretes a hormonal substance called erythropoietin that stimulates the production of red blood cells in the bone marrow, so that chronic kidney disease often causes a marked anemia. Cancer involving the bone marrow usually causes anemia. So does leukemia, which, while a cancer of the white blood cells, wreaks havoc on the red blood cells, too. (A commonly seen form in cats is due to FeLV.) Finally, anemia can be an autoimmune disease—autoimmune hemolytic anemia—in which the body attacks its own red blood cells, in my experience a result of vaccination.

Because the causes are so varied, the first step in treating anemia is to determine just what the cause is. Anemia is *not* a condition to be treated by the layman acting on his own creative initiative. Diagnosis by a veterinarian is critical—especially if, for example, the cause turns out to be autoimmune hemolytic anemia, from which a dog can die within twenty-four hours. Emergency cortisone and a lifesaving transfusion are typically required. If parasites are the cause, they must be handled appropriately (see "Fleas" and "Worms" below). Internal tumors and cancer are, of course, also conditions to be treated professionally.

At times, a severely anemic pet will require a blood transfusion. Pets, like people, have different blood types, but the differences are much more muted than ours are. My experience with hundreds of pets needing blood transfusions is that almost all are universal donors. So grab whatever blood you can get from a donor—using dog blood only for dogs, cat blood only for cats, etc.—and administer it to the recipient. Although rejections have been reported, I haven't had one yet. (Often, in critical cases you don't even have time to obtain the blood type results from a laboratory.) A recent godsend is Hemopet, a line of blood components available through Jean Dodds, the veterinarian whose vaccine work is so fascinating and important. Hemopet, located in Irvine, California (see source guide), supplies purified, properly typed red blood cells, plasma, and other components available by Federal Express.

For less severe cases of external or internal bleeding, I use an herbal remedy called Yunnan Paiyao, the very powerful Chinese herb discussed in Chapter Six. It comes as a powder in capsules and can be sprinkled on an open wound, or ingested orally for any kind of bleeding disorder. For anemia secondary to chronic kidney disease, injectable erythropoietin (Epogen) is available through all veterinarians (conventional and holistic). I've had a lot of success using it.

Inevitably with anemia, whatever the cause, enriching the diet with iron is important. I recommend eggs, raw beef, or calf's liver, and green vegetables. Vitamin B_{12} is also very helpful as a supplement, as is apple cider vinegar, liquid chlorophyll, and kelp—all available at health food stores. I now use a product called Hemaplex (Progressive Labs), which contains red-blood-cell-building components: beets, raw liver, chlorophyll, and iron, among others.

Arthritis

The condition we think of as arthritis in pets actually has several different manifestations: spinal arthritis, hip dysplasia, degenerative joint disease. Some involve a genetic predisposition, especially in large breeds of dogs that experience rapid long-bone growth but also disproportionate weight gain (Great Danes, for example) and those bred to have long spines (dachshunds, for example). At the same time, poor diet is a factor, especially with the pregnant mother, as a fetus's bones and joints are being formed. I also believe that arthritis is exacerbated, if not sometimes actually caused, by the whole gamut of environmental toxins that afflict people and pets alike, as well as by the autoimmune reactions caused by vaccines. The inflammation that characterizes all kinds of arthritis may occur as the body struggles, unsuccessfully, to remove toxins that have settled in the joints. Inflammation, remember, is simply the body responding to foreign invaders, external or internal, by concentrating blood cells around them in an effort to expel them. Secondary to the inflammation process that occurs in the joints, I often see either a diminishing volume or leakage of the natural joint lubricator called synovial fluid, which in turn causes the joint surfaces to rub against one another and grow further inflamed. In my experience, arthritis is seen more often in dogs than in cats.

The standard medical response is to "drug" the symptoms. Cortisone, aspirin, ibuprofen, and phenylbutazone were, until recently, the drugs of choice. Now a much touted drug called Rimadyl has reached the market. Though classified as one of the NSAIDS—nonsteroidal anti-inflammatory drugs—that are considered to have milder side effects than steroids, Rimadyl in my experience has produced disturbing side effects, particularly liver anomalies. A recent newsletter from Tufts University's School of Veterinary Medicine notes as much, with the qualification that these anomalies have only been seen in a "few" dogs. In fact, Rimadyl's manufacturer, the Pfizer corporation, sent a letter to veterinarians on July 30, 1997, stating the risks in more dramatic terms. "Currently about 150,000 dogs take Rimadyl each day. . . . We have received approximately 750 reports of side effects of any kind during the first six months of marketing. This represents 14 reports of a side effect of any kind for every 10,000 dogs treated. The most frequently reported effects have been mild gastrointestinal signs, and we have also received reports involving suspected renal, hematologic, neurologic, dermatologic, and hepatic effects. Some of these cases include an acute hepatic syndrome 16 to 21 days after initiation of Rimadyl therapy. The affected dogs [are] all Labrador retrievers." That was meant as reassurance, though I consider the percentage high. (Also, whenever I see a claim of that sort, I wonder: How many other incidences of side effects *weren't* reported?) The reported side effects include severe vomiting, nausea, and liver toxicity—proof to me that dogs on it are trying desperately to rid themselves of its toxicity. In sum: Give Rimadyl a miss.

The first step I take in treating arthritis is to put a pet on the natural diet outlined in Chapter Three. At the least, a good diet may help prevent a worsening of his condition. I'll also try to wean the pet from whatever arthritis drug he's been on. As I do so, I'll dispense a new natural supplement, Cosequin, which contains primarily glucosamine and chondroitin sulfates. There are many products on the market with similar formulations, but I've had my best responses using Cosequin. It enhances the production of the lubricating fluid in the joints and therefore appears to actually help the joint repair itself. Now widely sold by veterinarians (and available at health food stores as Cosamin), Cosequin has proved immensely helpful.* For a more rapid response in severe cases, I'll start by using Adequan—injectable glycosaminoglycans—which I give initially twice a week for four weeks. A good second line of defense is the herbal supplement Ar-Ease (Crystal Star), which contains the herbs yucca, alfalfa, and devil's-claw.

With all arthritics, I use an antioxidant enzyme called superoxide dismutase that comes in liquid, tablet, or injectable form. SOD, as it's called, is produced naturally in the body to help destroy harmful free radicals that contribute to degenerative diseases such as arthritis, but the body's natural stores become depleted. The supplemental form

---

*A product similar in its effects to Cosequin, but less expensive, is Glycoflex. It contains perna canaliculus, an extract from the green-lipped mussel, which I believe to be nearly as effective as Cosequin for improving symptoms of arthritis.

is available at health food stores (and from many veterinarians) under various brand names. Also available for cases of more serious degeneration is AOX/PLX, which has SOD as its primary ingredient, but that includes three other antioxidant enzymes. Two other antioxidants I use are Pycnogenol and any of the proanthocyanidin complexes (I use Anti-Ox, by Vetri-Science); both are derived from grape seeds.

Another effective treatment for arthritis is, of course, acupuncture. Traditional acupuncture is almost always helpful. Because it's more effective, I now prefer the procedure called aquapuncture. I inject the Smith Ridge "cocktail" of B_{12} and adrenal cortex, and also homeopathic Zeel, or Traumeel, at the acupuncture points relevant to the patient's condition. In minutes, a pet's pain can ease, and the effects can last several weeks. The effects are also cumulative, so if needed, I'll do several more treatments weekly or bimonthly. Usually, I'll send an arthritic pet home from his acupuncture sessions with an oral form of Zeel or BHI's "Arthritis."

As soon as I get blood results back from the lab, I'll act on them, too. An arthritic pet almost inevitably will show a high level of alkaline phosphatase, the telltale sign of an overtaxed adrenal gland. (The adrenal is the gland that controls inflammation in an effort to eliminate damage and toxins, and thus has a close relation with arthritic joints.) A body's pH factor is its balance of alkalinity and acidity; to reduce a high alkaline count, I'll give substantial doses of vitamin C in the ascorbic acid form.

Ultimately, the best approach to arthritis is preventative. If a pregnant mother is kept on a good-nutrition diet, her fetus will develop strong bones and joints and not be programmed to get arthritis. If a newborn is put on that same diet, vaccinated minimally, and subjected to few or no medications, including antiflea and antiheartworm drugs, his chances of developing arthritis should be virtually nil.

Bladder Problems

Cystitis/feline lower urinary tract disease (FLUTD) Because the bladder is merely a container for urine, the problems it develops are usually not its own, but rather the result of toxicity passing into it as part of the urine and inflaming its walls. Hence cystitis: literally, inflammation (*itis*) of the bladder (*cysto*). In cats, cystitis is also known as feline lower urinary tract disease, and formerly known as feline urological syndrome (FUS).

As the inflammation spreads from the bladder down the urethra, a cat feels pain and irritation that make him think he has to urinate even after he's voided. He makes frequent efforts to do so, but only manages a few drops. If the condition worsens, the urethra will swell until the passage is constricted, preventing the animal from urinating completely when he *does* have to go. For male cats, this is a painful and potentially very serious condition, because their urethras are smaller in circumference than those of females, and the inflammation that forms, along with a mucousy, gritty "plug," can prevent any urination at all, backing up their systems and causing fatal uremia. *A male cat with a blocked urethra is in need of emergency care. If not tended by a veterinarian, he will die in twenty-four hours or less.* Of all the conditions listed in these pages, this is among the most dire. Yet it's relatively easy for a layman to diagnose. A male cat with severe FLUTD will strain noticeably to urinate often and spend a lot of time in and around the litter box, or try to urinate in odd places like a sink or bathtub. His bladder will soon be as swollen and hard as a plum (or larger) and be able to void little, any, or no urine. (If he does pass urine, it will likely be bloody.) He will also appear sensitive to the touch, especially in the abdomen, and may feel cold and clammy. When in doubt, don't deliberate: bring your cat in immediately for treatment, calling first to warn your veterinarian as to what the problem may be. (After hours, use an emergency facility; don't wait until your regular veterinarian is open the next morning. You may be too late.) A veterinarian will need to catheterize the cat to alleviate the blockage. If the problem reappears, he may ultimately decide to do a surgical procedure called a urethrostomy, in which the penis of the male cat is removed and the urethra reconstructed so as to be wider and act, in effect, like the urethra of a female. Severe as it sounds, a urethrostomy can be a lifesaver for a cat prone to urinary blockage; when the situation merits it, I strongly recommend it.

This blockage problem also occurs in male dogs, but less frequently, in my experience, than in cats. When it does, it's almost always due to the formation of bladder stones that slide into the urethra. Blockage is aggravated, however, by a bone that male dogs have in their penis (appropriately called the os penis). Female dogs will incur bladder problems, to be sure, but the width of their urethras, as with female cats, minimizes the chances of an emergency-condition blockage. However, I have seen female urethras blocked by just the right-sized stones.

Since most of the wastes the bladder passes are from food and drink, it's hardly surprising that cystitis tends to be the result of a poor diet. In pets, a history of low-grade commercial food, especially of the dry kibble variety, often seems to be the cause. Switching the pet to a good natural diet can help clear up many cases over time. The emphasis with cystitis should be on foods that have a high-quality protein, as poorer-quality proteins—found, for example, in meat by-products—tend to be less digestible and pass as waste, exacerbating the inflammation. If you're choosing among commercial pet foods, especially for cats, look for one that indicates low ash and low magnesium content.

Cystitis many times responds dramatically to vitamin C. The bacteria in the urine that causes inflammation tends to increase the urine's alkalinity; the acidity in the ascorbic acid form of vitamin C brings the pH factor back into the proper acid range, thus killing the bacteria, and so is indicated for the most common forms of cystitis. (Note that vitamin C in its *ascorbate* form may *raise* the urine pH factor, and so is indicated in certain less common urinary problems. Obviously, a veterinarian should be consulted to make an accurate diagnosis.) During an episode, I give a cat 500 milligrams, three times a day, crushing the tablets and mixing them with food. For a dog much heavier than thirty pounds, I double the dosage. I also use a cranberry supplement called Cran Actin, an acidifier especially effective with cystitis. (A layman can determine the amount of acidifier needed by using a "dipstick" for pH factor available at a pharmacy or swimming pool supply store.) At the same time, I put a pet on homeopathic remedies: "Bladder" (BHI), mixed with "Inflammation" (BHI) or "Bladder Irritation" (BioForce or Natra Bio), using one-third to one-half the dosage recommended for people. One other product I've had tremendous success with for all forms of urinary problems is the herbal combination called Tinkle Caps (Crystal Star). If I suspect a stubborn infection, I'll include the bee hive medication called propolis, at half the human dose.

This is how I treat all routine bladder infections, and in 90 percent of the cases, these treatments suffice—without antibiotics. In the other 10 percent, I *will* use antibiotics, the choice of which will be based on culture and sensitivity testing of the affected urine. But it is better in all cases to insist on vitamin C and homeopathics at least as a first measure, because a pet with a history of cystitis put on chronic antibiotic therapy is, in my experience, likely to have ever-worsening bladder problems, up to and including bladder cancer.

Bladder stones   Blood in the urine may indicate the presence of bladder stones (calculi). Stones are an indication of chronic urinary problems and must be taken seriously. Small stones tend to pass from the bladder into the urethra, where they can impede the flow of urine, especially in male dogs. The first measure is to establish a proper diagnosis, then put the pet on a natural diet, which should emphasize high-quality protein sources. This helps restore metabolic function of the liver, which in turn will minimize the production of wastes. For many of the common stones, the diet should be supplemented by 500 milligrams of vitamin C in its ascorbic acid form three times a day for cats, and double that dosage for larger dogs; these measures alone may be enough to dissolve tiny stones. (A pet who's had bladder stones once should be kept on low levels of vitamin C until a metabolic analysis makes clear that he's producing enough C to maintain proper acid-base balance.) Larger stones which remain in the bladder irritate the walls and cause bleeding, leading to secondary bacterial infections. Often these stones need to be removed surgically. However, I've also seen results from a food called S/D, manufactured by the Hill's company. I hesitate to recommend it because it's composed mostly of cornstarch. It's certainly not for a healthy pet, but the absence of minerals encourages the body to reabsorb the minerals that form certain kinds of stones. I've also had success using a Chinese herb called Akebia 14 that's indicated for stones, or the herbal product Tinkle Caps (Crystal Star).*

A final note: For all pets suffering with stones, use only steam-distilled water, as it's devoid of minerals that help form the stones. Ordinary tap water is loaded with such minerals; but so is spring or well water. All should be avoided.

Cushing's Disease

The symptoms of this canine illness are a bloated abdomen, thinning hair coat, and drinking and urinating to excess. If ignored, this condition can ultimately lead to liver, lung, or kidney disease. The symptoms of Cushing's can be traced to the immediate problem of an overactive

*Some less frequently occurring types of bladder stones, i.e., cystine or oxalate stones (seen particularly in the dalmation), form in very different ways, so that the above recommendations do not apply. Each one has its own, very specific therapeutic and dietary requirement. How to distinguish among the types? Don't try! The only sensible course of action is to seek a veterinarian's advice.

adrenal cortex that produces too much natural cortisone, known as cortisol. (Medically speaking, Cushing's is known as hyperadrenocorticism.) In the majority of Cushing's cases, the adrenal cortex is overproducing because of another gland: the pituitary, which controls the adrenal from its location at the base of the brain. In these cases, a benign but functioning tumor in the pituitary is the underlying problem. For treatment, conventional medicine focuses on the adrenal gland, and so prescribes a drug called Lysodren, structurally related to DDT (that's right, DDT) that selectively destroys the cells of the adrenal cortex to curtail its production of cortisol. To me, that's just another case of killing the messenger who brings the bad news. A relatively new therapeutic drug called Anipryl (or L-deprenyl) is recommended, and is reputed to work indirectly by making the dog feel better—a psychological effect that may produce physical improvement. Anipryl is also supposed to be less toxic than Lysodren. However, the only three cases I treated with Anipryl suffered unfortunate side effects, so I've stopped using it.*

At Smith Ridge, we've had considerable success with Cushing's dogs by focusing instead on metabolic balance. We put patients on homeopathic pituitary and adrenal supplements ("Pituitary" and "Adrenal" drops from Professional Health Products), along with a nutritional supplement called phosphatidyl-serine, the active ingredient in lecithin. In human alternative medicine, this supplement is reported to alleviate the symptoms of multiple sclerosis in some cases, and is remarkable in enhancing mental acuity. In dogs, it naturally suppresses cortisol output. I've seen it bring about clinical improvement in some Cushing's patients for whom other supplements were of little help. It also imparts a tremendous luster to their hair.

Dental Problems

Animals in the wild usually have pearly white teeth. Why are our pets so often plagued with rotting teeth, abscesses of the mouth, and gum disease? The difference is: *us*. To begin with, for generations we've bred many kinds of dogs to hunt or show better, or merely to look cuter. In so doing, we've distorted the natural shape of their jaws. Most

---

*The antithesis of Cushing's disease is Addisons: an *under*functioning adrenal cortex. Patients typically need a form of synthetic cortisone called mineralocorticoids. This is one condition that holistic therapies usually cannot help without conventional treatment.

toy breeds have jaws too small to accommodate all their teeth. The crowding leads to impactions and misalignment, which fosters gum disease. Many Yorkshire terriers, in my experience, lose half their teeth by the age of two. Cats have also been malformed by breeding. The heads of Siamese cats are getting longer and narrower for aesthetic reasons; as a result, the incidences of chronic gum disease among Siamese and other inbred lines are skyrocketing. Whether the increase is due directly to head shape or genetic immunodeficiency is hard to say, but these factors do appear to be linked.

Man's other contribution is commercial pet food. Animals are meant to eat food in the raw: chelated, rich in vitamins, minerals, and enzymes, a bounty of nutrition as it's found in nature. Cooking of any sort breaks down some of those values, rendering the food less vital, and more congestive, to the body. Commercial pet food, as outlined in Chapter Three, takes ingredients that have almost no nutrition to start with and heats that little bit into oblivion. Even the texture detracts. Canine teeth especially are meant to gnaw raw bones and other hard structures; the incisors are actually meant to rip flesh. The process helps keep them healthy, as exercise does for the rest of the body, and helps prevent the buildup of tartar. The soft, almost predigested texture of "wet" commercial foods, and even of dry kibbles (which are really just compressed powders), provides no workout at all for a pet's teeth. They form a kind of glue that adheres to the teeth, contributing to dental decay. Poor food also leads to foul breath, as it festers in the intestines and the stink of it backs up.

For both dogs and cats, dental problems pose a painful, chronic threat to health. They also tend to suppress the immune system, rendering a pet vulnerable to other degenerative diseases. For dogs with congenital tooth problems, surgery is often the only answer: misaligned or "extra" teeth may just have to be removed. For other pets, prevention, as they say in the Crest commercials, is the best way to fight both tooth and gum disease. People can use toothpaste on a daily basis to address their problems topically; for a pet, the changes must come, for the most part, from within. Fortunately, the healthy diet outlined in Chapter Three will keep most puppies and kittens free of dental problems.

That—and regular maintenance. Pets' teeth do require professional cleaning, by a veterinarian, as often as needed. (The frequency varies from as much as four times a year to once every four years, depending on the breed and particular pet.) I try to clean the teeth of every pet I treat. I'll chip off chunks of tartar from even the healthiest patients and flush out deposits of food and bacteria from the gums. In more severe cases, I'll use ultrasonic scaling, especially under the gum line. Most veterinarians anesthetize pets in order to clean their teeth and gums. I find that by working gently, with a soothing attitude, I can usually clean a pet's teeth while he's conscious, and so avoid anesthesia's assault on the system. At Smith Ridge, ultrasonic scaling may require a mild tranquilizer, but rarely general anesthesia. At the same time, I'm amazed by how often veterinarians fail to clean a pet's mouth when he's under anesthesia for removal of a tumor or some other surgery. Some don't seem to realize how important clean teeth and gums are, especially with pets who have severe degenerative diseases and need all the help they can get in boosting their immune systems. I do—because I've seen it make all the difference in a pet's struggle to regain his health. All too often, unfortunately, pets are brought to me for a second opinion soon after surgery, so I get to see how festering their mouths are, packed with years-old tartar—a revolting sight that could easily have been addressed while they were under anesthesia. Cleaning is the best treatment even when a pet's dental problems have gone unattended long enough to produce bleeding gums, substantial buildups of tartar, excessive salivation or chewing, and, sometimes, a loss of appetite.

There are many topical products available at health food stores. One I've used is Oxyfresh, a gel that contains a peroxide to help oxygenate the teeth and gums. Two products I use to fight dental disease are the homeopathic "Teeth and Gums" (Natra Bio) and Biodent tablets (Standard Process).

Afterward, a change in diet is crucial if the mouth is to heal itself. For dogs, include raw large soup bones from the butcher (ones that are not splinterable), at least one every few days. You may not be able to duplicate the healthful environment his ancestors enjoyed in the wild, but raw bones will make him *feel* as if he's a predator again—and strengthen his teeth in the process. Keep in mind, too, that a lot of tartar comes not from food in the mouth but from the backup of a congested digestive system, up through the salivary glands. We brush our teeth before going to sleep, only to wake up in the morning with foul breath and a film on our teeth. We don't get that way from eating in our sleep! And neither do our pets.

Diabetes

In pets, as in people, diabetes is a deficiency of the pancreatic hormone called insulin. The purpose of insulin is to transport sugar out of the blood into the cells, where it's used as energy. When the pancreas fails to make enough of it, sugar in the form of glucose accumulates in the blood. When it reaches a certain threshold, it passes into the urine. And since the chemistry of sugar attracts water, a diabetic begins to urinate (and drink) excessively—often a first sign to an owner of what his pet's condition may be.

Other symptoms include lethargy, weakness (leading to anemia), inordinate appetite yet increasing weight loss (due to the inability to use food energy properly), and vomiting. Frequently, diabetes provokes complications: urinary infections, liver and kidney disease, eye problems (principally cataracts).

Usually in emergencies, when a patient's blood sugar has risen rapidly, there's no question of what treatment should be: insulin, administered immediately and at the proper level, under a veterinarian's care. When the blood sugar level returns to normal and the patient is properly regulated with the correct dose and schedule, conventional medicine prescribes continuing insulin administration on a regular basis, for the rest of a pet's life.* That's not a cure. It's a treatment in which external insulin compensates for the deficiency caused by improper pancreas function. I show owners how to administer insulin, and counsel them on how to regulate it. But as a holistic veterinarian, I also try to get the pancreas back in balance with its associated metabolic organs so that it can again make its own insulin. The standard protocol of supplements includes injectable homeopathic pancreas in dilution, pancreatic enzymes (NESS) (see source guide), "Pancreas Drops" (Professional Health Products), raw pancreas glandular (Pancreatrophin from Standard Process Labs), and a Chinese herb called Rehmannia 16 (Seven Forests) known in the Orient to help in diabetes treatment. I also use goldenseal (an herb) and chromium (a mineral known as the glucose tolerance factor), both of which help regulate blood sugar levels. I administer one capsule of goldenseal to a medium-sized dog one or two times a day, and half as much to a cat; with chromium, which is packaged for people, I give 100 micrograms

---

*In an infrequent condition called transient diabetes, the pancreas is only temporarily shut down, so insulin in those cases is administered only during those periods.

to a medium-sized dog, and 50 micrograms to a cat. Diet, not surprisingly, is an especially important factor with diabetes, too. I put a diabetic pet on 50 percent complex carbohydrates (brown rice, millet, buckwheat, and rye, for example); 25 percent chopped and steamed vegetables; and 25 percent protein, such as egg yolks, organic beef, steamed fish, and organic chicken.

When I send an owner home with this regimen, I also show him how to test his pet's urine to determine the glucose level on a daily basis, as this is a gauge of his level of blood sugar. A sudden increase in blood sugar demands an increase in the insulin dosage (and a call to the veterinarian). Even if a diabetic pet appears to be doing well on insulin and supplements, frequent monitoring is imperative. Why? Because if a pet's pancreas suddenly "kicks in" and starts to produce its own insulin as it grows healthier in response to the supplements, giving insulin could dramatically reduce his blood sugar level to a critically low level. (If you give insulin to a healthy pet or person, you can bring on convulsions or even death, which actually made insulin the murderer's drug of choice until forensic scientists learned to detect an insulin overdose.) For emergencies, always have honey or even Karo syrup on hand. Either should be administered orally as soon as possible if he starts becoming shaky or begins to experience a seizure. Then rush him to an emergency clinic to be evaluated unless you're confident that he's stabilized.

Despite these dangers, the blood sugar in many cases will decline to a normal and stable level as the pancreas repairs itself. To a culture taught to view diabetes as a chronic, incurable disease, that may seem little short of miraculous. But given that we have nearly a total turnover of virtually every single cell in our bodies every seven years—and in dogs and cats, probably every three years—why *shouldn't* the pancreas heal itself? In fact, we've had considerable success with diabetic cats, dramatically lowering the insulin requirement in every two out of four cases and eliminating it in one out of three. Dogs are more of a challenge, but the odds of improving canine diabetes holistically are certainly better than just using conventional medicine, which basically gives them no chance for reversal at all and doesn't address the original degenerative condition that led to the diabetes in the first place.

Diarrhea

The key to understanding and treating diarrhea is to realize that it's not really an illness. It's a symptom: the outward sign of any number of problems that interrupt the large intestine's regular work of resorbing water from the wastes passing through it. Basically, the intestines recognize that some very unwanted toxins are passing through them, and react by hurrying them out as quickly as possible, while the wastes are still soft or liquid. Bad food (or something else eaten by your undiscerning pet) is the most common provocation, but diarrhea may also result from bacteria or parasites absorbed by licking one source or another (including, yes, other dogs' behinds). Separately, it may be the result of various internal organ malfunctions, especially of the kidney and liver, which can get overwhelmed by toxins they're supposed to process. These will back up through the liver and then get jettisoned to the intestines. Toxicity, in short, is what leads to diarrhea, though that's not always a bad thing. With cancer or other degenerative diseases, the purging of toxicity as diarrhea *may* signal a healing crisis.

The standard approach to diarrhea is to treat the symptom, usually by administering Kaopectate (in liquid or tablet form) or Imodium, along with antibiotics, often in conjunction with good old cortisone. I'll use Kaopectate when the symptoms are dire enough or chronically nonresponsive, though I'm not nearly as happy with the new kind, which has various chemical flavorings and colorings, as I was with the old, which was composed more purely of kaolin and pectin, ingredients borrowed directly from herbal medicine. But Kaopectate merely addresses the symptoms of diarrhea, not the cause, unless it happens to help bind some of the toxins involved.

Different root causes may require different treatments. Intestinal worms, for example, must be dealt with on their own (see "Worms"). If diarrhea results from a failure of the pancreas to produce enzymes properly, or of the liver to metabolize, those organs must be addressed (for starters, with supplements and homeopathics). The essential step with all diarrhea, however, is to put the pet on a liquid fast. This may seem contraindicated: after all, a diarrhetic pet has been depleted of nutrients, is likely very hungry, and ought, by logic, to be fed so he can rebuild his strength. Not so. The digestive system has what's called a gastrocolic reflex. Its own logic is to empty the colon as the stomach fills. To stop the colon from emptying and thus to break the diarrhea cycle, there's a simple strategy: don't eat! Or at least, eat as little as possible.

I've seen great success (with people as well as pets) with an old remedy called the potato diet: 50 percent white potatoes, 50 percent sweet potatoes, a slice of turnip, and a slice of leek, all boiled and then mixed with boiled chicken or lamb for flavor. I've seen the potato diet stop chronic diarrhea almost overnight (even in a ferret!). I also put the pet on homeopathic remedies: BHI's "Diarrhea" and Dr. Goodpet's "Diar-Relief" are both good. Instead of killing the bacteria, they enhance enzymatic function, which helps end the diarrhea naturally. And for chronic diarrhea, I'm a big advocate of a supplement called Acetylator (Vetri-Science), which contains lactobacillus, enzymes, and glucosamine sulfates, all of which help natural intestinal function. I've had pets with severe diarrhea on the potato diet, along with these supplements and homeopathic remedies for months, gradually easing them back onto a regular diet. Chronic diarrhea takes time to treat. Eventually, though, it does succumb to holistic measures—without antibiotics.

One final note on chronic diarrhea. In recent years, I've seen an increasing incidence of it, both in cats and dogs, as a symptom of inflammatory bowel disease. Dr. Deva Khalsa, one of my holistic colleagues, feels strongly that the condition is caused by vaccines, more specifically by the meat extracts in which certain vaccines are grown. In absorbing these vaccines, puppies and kittens become sensitized to meat protein—which is to say, *too* sensitive to it. Later on, after ingesting meats with similar proteins, the proteins may trigger an immuno-mediated allergic reaction. When this cause and reaction become chronic, the result is inflammatory bowel disease.

Distemper, Canine

The acute, culminating stage of this disease, which resembles pneumonia and often results in fatal encephalitis with paralysis and seizures, is the one for which dogs are vaccinated repeatedly in their first several months of life and annually thereafter. It's a viral disease so rare now that I can count on one hand my last several cases of it over the last decade, though I'm including it here because who knows? It might reappear in your part of the country. The rarity of the disease is a situation for which the vaccine may be credited, though also one that has led to overvaccination (see Chapter Four). In its milder, chronic form—itself the result of the distemper vaccine, as Dr. Richard Pitcairn among other holistic veterinarians believes—canine distemper incubates without symptoms, manifests as a fever that quickly recedes, then reappears in more potent disease form, often with loss of appetite, conjunctivitis (with a pus-like discharge from the eyes), diarrhea, and skin eruptions on the stomach or the hind legs.

The best course of action for acute canine distemper is to have a veterinarian administer high levels of intravenous vitamin C, carried into the body by one of the two standard intravenous fluids, sodium chloride or lactated Ringer's solution. If available, intravenous ozone (which kills bacteria, fungi, and viruses on contact) should also be administered. At the same time, I'll address the symptoms with specific homeopathic remedies. If the dog is still failing, I'll use a distemper nosode—a homeopathic preparation, with its minute quantity of distemper virus "succussed" to a high potency. (Though often effective as a preventative, a nosode can also be used for treatment of an existing condition. I'll start with low potencies; if there's no response, I'll work up to higher potencies.) I'll also put the dog on a liquid fast of vegetable broth. If in its acute phase a dog exhibits seizures—the result of the disease affecting his central nervous system—I'll use acupuncture, herbs, and specific homeopathics to address them.

The fact is, though, that a dog is far likelier to contract a chronic form of distemper from the distemper vaccine—the condition called vaccinosis—than he is to get the full-blown disease without the vaccine. Just to be safe, I give an eleven-week-old puppy one distemper vaccine, making sure not to overdose a puppy or small dog. If no more distemper vaccines are given and the dog is raised on a healthy diet, in my experience that's the last time a pet or his owner need worry about distemper ever again.

Distemper, Feline

Its name suggests that this terrible illness is the feline counterpart of canine distemper, with pneumonia-like symptoms. In fact, it's an intestinal virus, better known by another name: feline infectious enteritis (*enter* denotes the intestines; *itis* means inflammation). Often, too, it's referred to as feline panleukopenia because of the rapid lowering of the white blood cell count, secondary to the virus (*pan* means all; *leuko* means white blood cells; and *penia* means deficiency). Whatever you call it, it's a swift, usually unstoppable killer that begins with a cat's shunning of the food bowl, progresses quickly to high fever, vomiting (first a clear fluid, later yellow bile), and severe bloody diarrhea. In kittens especially, it tends to end rapidly in death. The course is for the virus to devastate the white blood cells of the immune system, rendering the body vulnerable to fatal secondary infection. If caught in the early stages, it *may* be arrested with a liquid diet and high levels of intravenous vitamin C. Administered, that is, at a hospital: this is a medical emergency, not a disease to be treated at home.

Though it can quickly rise to epidemic levels, feline distemper today appears to be almost wiped out. This may be due to the feline distemper vaccine, though at not inconsiderable cost, as described in Chapter Four. The vaccine appears to produce a low-lying, chronic form of the disease, and I have discerned a disturbing correlation, based on experience, between the vaccine and increased incidences of hyperthyroidism in cats. (A similar case could be made with the vaccine for feline leukemia.) The best course is to vaccinate a young cat once for feline distemper when the immune system is mature enough for the vaccine's effects to be permanent, and not again. Of course, give your cat good nutrition to support his health. His chances of getting the disease later in life will be about as great as yours of winning the lottery.

It's worth noting, too, that just because a cat is vomiting or experiencing diarrhea doesn't mean an owner should assume the worst. Most of the time, vomiting and diarrhea denote far more mundane conditions. Though it's by no means a clear indication itself, one clue that your cat's condition may be feline distemper is if he hovers over his water bowl without drinking, while appearing gaunt and debilitated. If he does that consistently, call a veterinarian right away.

Ear Problems

Both dogs and cats often incur irritating or painful ear problems of a chronic, hard-to-treat nature, from inflammation and infections to buildups of wax. In fact, I have a higher success rate in reversing cancer than chronic ear problems. The likeliest cause is allergies (especially if the symptoms appear during pollen or hay fever season, or in association with a certain kind of food). For many dogs, unfortunately, the problem may be genetic. Spaniels, retrievers, poodles, and pointers, among other breeds, all have floppy ears that inhibit air circulation, trap water when they're swimming, and generally help foster what I think of as a "swampy" environment that promotes bacterial growth. In unhealthy or metabolically unbalanced pets, the discharge is thickened as their bodies struggle to eliminate toxins via the ears, among other channels, leading to waxy buildups. The wax becomes another medium fostering the growth of bacteria and fungi. (From personal experience, I know that fasting can lead to a marked increase in earwax production as the body eliminates residual toxicity.) In dogs, excess wax exacerbates the already less than ideal design of the ear, with a canal that begins horizontally and then takes a sharp turn *upward*, creating a bend in which wax and other material are apt to collect even with dogs whose earflaps stick up straight.

Many veterinarians, and especially groomers, conduct routine cleanings of the ear in an effort to keep the "swamp" from forming. It seems logical, but in my experience, such frequent intrusions only provoke the ears to produce *more* wax in response to the irritation created by the cleaning. Another common practice is to pluck ear hairs in those breeds that tend to have a lot of ear fur, on the assumption that the hairs help trap material. Also wrong, in my opinion; I've seen severe inflammations occur as a result. Members of a few breeds of floppy-eared dogs—poodles and bichons, for example—may benefit from an *occasional* pruning of ear hair. Most don't, unless the ear is already a mess and the wax and hairs are adding to the problem. Use common sense: if no problem exists, leave well enough alone. Or as the pun has it, play it by ear.

Often a cleansing wash, conducted gently, will help. A classic natural acidifier is apple cider vinegar; apply a dropperful of it in a dilute solution (a teaspoon of vinegar to a half cup of distilled water) to the affected ear, massage gently from outside so that the fluid circulates through the ear canal, then let the pet shake it out. I'm partial to an herbal ear wash called Halo, which contains several soothing oils, including sage and clove, and several herbal extracts, among them chamomile. I've also had success with the brand Noah's Kingdom, which along with the ingredients above contains mullein oil and liquid garlic; the garlic helps kill bacteria. (Kyolic garlic liquid, also diluted fifty-fifty with water, is particularly helpful.) Seven Forests, the line of Chinese herbal remedies (Institute of Traditional Medicine), has Forsythia for chronic ear infections and Picrorrhiza 11 for ear problems caused by yeast infections. (Both remedies are taken orally.)

In severe or nonresponsive cases, I'll start by taking a culture of the ear, have a lab identify the bacteria in it, and test various antibiotics on the sample. If one works well, I'll use it topically—not systemically—

to get short-term results. Meanwhile, I'll try to judge from a metabolic analysis which imbalances or allergy may be linked indirectly to the problem and treat them with supplements accordingly. The ear, remember, is also an eliminative channel, providing the body with yet another pathway (two pathways!) through which to jettison toxicity. More often than not, when the metabolic organs are restored to balance and the pet is on a good diet, the chronic ear problems get better or go away. If, as balance is being restored, the "swamp" needs a bit more encouragement to clear up, I'll sometimes take olive oil and infuse it with ozone to create what's called medical olive oil. Then I'll flush the ears with it in the manner described above. The ozone is especially helpful because it kills bacteria and fungus on contact; the only catch is that it soon defuses out of the oil, which must then be reinfused. Unfortunately, ozone is commercially hard to come by and not even legal in most states for medical purposes. I use it in my own practice, and I know of a few other holistic veterinarians who use it in theirs, but the field remains pretty limited.

Occasionally, I'll see a pet whose ear problems have become so severe that the entire canal is scarred and shut. In those cases, I'll recommend opening the canal surgically and removing that part of the exterior wall where the canal bends upward. Obviously, this should be performed by a good surgeon. It's not an ideal cure, in that it fails to consider what the source of toxicity may be, but the surgery does alleviate the physical condition contributing to the buildup. If a metabolic analysis is then done, and the pet is put on the appropriate supplements, the problem ought not to recur. Such was the case with Dottie, a three-year-old cocker spaniel referred to me by Dr. Martin DeAngelis after he'd opened up both ear canals surgically, which unfortunately did nothing to alleviate the problem. Dr. DeAngelis referred Dottie to Smith Ridge, as a last resort, to have cryosurgery performed for the many benign growths and thickened folds she had in her ears, the canals of which were darkened with waxy buildup. Instead, I started by putting her on supplements as indicated by a BNA, along with a three-day intravenous vitamin C flush. I also gave her ozone intravenously and topically. Rapidly the buildup vanished, the canals turned pink, the folds and growths dissipated. Now, years later, her ears are still fine, subject only to occasional flare-ups that we treat as before, though more mildly. Cryosurgery, as a result, was never performed.

Ear cropping   Some breeders and veterinarians still endorse the practice of cropping the ears of certain breeds of dogs for show purposes or just aesthetics. Besides being cruel and painful, this practice ignores a crucial fact: there are eighty-eight acupuncture points in the ear flap which correspond to every major function of the body. Imagine what happens to the balance of the rest of the body when a significant number of these points are suddenly sheared off! It's an awful, awful practice, completely unjustifiable.

Ear mites   Unlike the nuisances described above, ear mites are parasites, invisible to the naked eye but for the brown granules of their discharge. They usually dwell first in cats, though if a dog is in the house, they'll soon take up residence in his ears, too. In either case, a pet's misery, in shaking his head and scratching his ears, will be all too apparent. (A foul odor is the other telltale sign.) Use one of the washes described above, and shampoo the head and ears with an herbal formula specifically for killing parasites (any health food store ought to carry one). Recognize, too, that like all parasites, ear mites prey on pets with weak or underdeveloped immune systems. Strengthen the immune system to prevent the mites' return. If, however, the mites persist despite these measures, I do recommend using a conventional topical preparation just long enough to kill the mites and put an end to your pet's suffering. As soon as they're gone, focus on health, starting with a good diet, and they ought not return.

Epilepsy

By definition, epilepsy is seizures of unknown origin. A heartbreaking, historically incurable condition among people, it appears in both dogs and cats, though most often in the young dog. Western medicine's best guess is that epilepsy is caused by a neurological dysfunction in the brain, but after years of research, no one has found anything organically wrong with the brain of an epileptic. I believe, as do a growing number of holistic veterinarians, that the likelier cause is vaccines. As Richard and Susan Pitcairn observe in *Dr. Pitcairn's Complete Guide to Natural Health for Dogs and Cats*, experiments with laboratory animals have clearly shown that vaccines can cause allergic encephalitis, a low-grade inflammation of the brain that may result in attacks; and the Pitcairns are not alone among holistic veterinarians in having seen dogs exhibit initial epileptic attacks shortly after their annual vaccines.

The conventional approach to epilepsy, both with people and pets, is to use drugs to lessen the likelihood of attacks. Phenobarbital is a standard choice; Dilantin is another; a third, newer option is potassium bromide. These drugs are often used in combination with one another. The problem with them is that they're toxic, especially to the liver. Also, like most drugs, those for epilepsy become less effective over time, and so must be given in ever greater quantities. This is because they're actually fostering the condition while suppressing its symptoms—what I call the catch-22 of conventional medicine. Fortunately, there is another way. If I'm treating a dog who's having multiple severe seizures and not responding to alternatives, I have to use a drug, too: intravenous Valium, the only means powerful enough to break the seizure cycle. And if the dog is in a continuous seizure, a condition called "status epilepticus," the dog must also be anesthetized to help ease it out of the attack.

Usually, though, I'll see the animal between seizures. Typically, I'll hear that when the attacks began, they occurred just once or a few times a year. Now, I'll hear, they're becoming more frequent: perhaps every three or four weeks. What I do is take a blood sample, then send the dog home with one or more of these preparations: an herbal compound containing black cohosh, valerian, and skullcap (several brands are available at health food stores; the one I use most is Relax Caps [Crystal Star]); a homeopathic product called "Epilepsy" drops (Professional Health Products, distributed by Nutritional Specialties); Neurotrophin (Standard Process Labs), to support normal brain function; and a supplement, also readily available, called phosphatidyl-serine, which enhances food and oxygen uptake by the brain and nervous system. As I add these, I'll also wean the pet from the conventional drugs he's on—slowly enough to be sure the changeover doesn't bring on an attack.

These supplements alleviate the symptoms and often postpone attacks. But each one also has the potential to reverse the seizure disorders. When the metabolic analysis of the blood sample comes back, I focus on the imbalances. Inevitably, with epilepsy, the liver is implicated. Since the gallbladder is part of the liver complex and stores bile produced by the liver for the initial breakdown of fats, one of the supplements I give is Lipocomplex (Progressive Labs, distributed by Nu Biologics), which helps the gallbladder do its job (it actually contains ox bile). To that end, I also use a magnesium supplement, especially if the analysis reveals a paucity of magnesium in the blood. Both magnesium and vitamin B_6 are integral to fat metabolism, and also to the proper functioning of the brain's pituitary gland.

Acupuncture can be very useful in keeping an epileptic in balance. Along with the association point on a dog's spine and other indicated points, there's one on the top of the head (called GV20) that's the point of general sedation for the body. Typically, if you feel there, you'll detect a slight depression. I've taught owners to find it on their own epileptic dogs, and told them to rub it during a seizure: many times, they've reported back to me that the rubbing stops the seizure.

My own theory about epilepsy comes from the acupuncture master with whom I first studied some two decades ago. He reported that he'd never seen an epileptic or any seizure-disorder patient without an imbalance in the gallbladder energy meridian. This meridian courses up the back of the neck and traverses the top of the head and temples, ending at the eyes. Personally, I have never had a dog with epilepsy who didn't have a gallbladder meridian imbalance, either. Consider, too, that among the acupuncture points on a dog's spine which correspond to various organs and glands in the body, there's one for the gallbladder. Invariably, with an epileptic dog, it's out of alignment. Press it and you'll provoke an immediate reaction among the nearest muscles.

In the intriguing-if-unproven department, a breeder of corgis told me not long ago that she'd read that epilepsy might be caused by a migration of parasites through the brain. She had a dog named Racer who was severely epileptic; she had tried treatments both conventional and holistic without success, so she decided to try the herb black walnut, which kills parasites. The dog's seizures were dramatically reduced for years. I should add that I've since tried black walnut on dogs and not found it as successful. But who knows? Perhaps corgis are especially affected by it; perhaps another variable was involved, which in time, with more experimentation, will come to light.

Eye Problems

When a pet's eyes grow irritated—reddish or swollen, teary or gummy at the ducts—the most obvious possible cause is a foreign intruder: dust, a bug, perhaps an airborne insecticide. A drop of cod-liver oil applied to the eyes three or four times a day makes a good wash for all irritations. The herb eyebright, so called for its tonic effect on any eye problem, can also be applied directly to the eyes in an infusion (a half dozen drops of the extract, or a capsule of the powdered herb, should be mixed with a cup of distilled water; several drops of the mixture should be applied three or four times daily). Although there is controversy over the use of eyebright, especially topical use, I've used it many times with no side effects, and sometimes with remarkable positive results. Probably the best and easiest choice now is an herbal eyewash kit called Anitra's Herbal Eyewash (Halo), which contains eyebright as its chief, but not only, ingredient. On their own or in conjunction with any of the above, I'll use Similasan #1 homeopathic eyedrops to alleviate dry, reddened eyes.

When a larger, more abrasive object is the cause—a splinter, for example—a pet's cornea may be ulcerated, or scratched. (With dogs, a common cause is the swipe of a cat's claw.) A good clue, of course, is that only one of the eyes is likely to be irritated. If you can see the irritant, make no effort to remove it yourself; bring your pet right into a veterinary clinic. Any sign of blood is also reason to bring the pet in for treatment immediately. Only if the pet appears to have worked the irritant out already through his tears should you try to facilitate the healing process with an eyewash. One preparation I've found that's particularly good for chronic corneal ulcers is Adequan (injectable chondroitin sulfate) diluted with sterile water* and used topically as an eyedrop.

A less obvious—but no less common—cause of eye irritations is allergies. Many dogs suffer during pollen or hay fever season just as people do. One course of action, to be sure, is medical suppression of the inflammatory symptoms. I much prefer the holistic route, for reasons discussed above (see "Allergies"). Similasan makes a particularly good homeopathic eyedrop called Similasan #2 for burning and itching brought on by allergies. And eyebright, in any of the mixtures noted above, is helpful for allergic reactions, too. If the reaction is severe enough, emergency medical assistance may be necessary.

In pets, as in people, one of the most common degenerative conditions of the eye is cataracts. Environmental pollutants and ingested toxins are at least partly to blame, for cataracts are nothing more than the accumulation of toxins in the lens of the eyes. But the aging process

---

*The ratio I use is one part Adequan to three parts sterile water, although stronger concentrations may be used for severe ulcerations.

plays a role, too, as free radicals, in their generalized attack on healthy cells, accelerate degeneration of the eyes. And among diabetics, cataracts are an all-too-frequent side effect, as high blood sugar affects the eyes. Whatever their origin and kind, the toxins crystallize in the lens, clouding vision and occasionally bringing on blindness if unchecked. Surgery is the standard treatment for cataracts, and certainly in people it's become a highly sophisticated, painless, and effective solution. For pets, it can seem an expensive course of action; in my opinion, it's often unnecessary.

Diabetic cataracts, it's true, come on suddenly and are so dense that nothing helps but surgical removal. The more typical cataract progresses slowly enough that a regimen of homeopathic and herbal remedies, along with overall health improvement and metabolic balancing, can usually keep it from getting much worse—thus saving an animal's vision—or even reverse the disease. Eyebright and bilberry are the two herbs integral to holistic cataract treatment. They're the primary ingredients in a supplement I use called Visioplex (Progressive Labs), which also contains vitamin A and raw eye concentrate and comes in capsule form, to be given orally as directed. Another useful measure is the herb succus sineraria. It comes as an eye preparation to be applied topically, a drop in each eye once a day. It's also contained in a homeopathic combination called "Cataract Drops" (Professional Health Products), which is taken orally and has been reported to have positive effects with cataracts. I've used two other topical products with some success. One is a homeopathic drop that a dear friend and holistic veterinary associate of mine, Joanne Stefanatos of Las Vegas, Nevada, formulates (see source guide); the other, if you can find them, is vitamin B_{15} drops. Because cataracts *are* a degenerative condition, a logical corollary is that they occur in a body that is itself degenerating. The inverse is also true: get a body healthy, and its cataracts will improve. So along with these remedies, I put a pet with cataracts on the diet outlined in Chapter Three, and supplements indicated by the BNA. You'd be surprised at the difference it makes.

Another chronic and disturbing condition of the eyes is progressive retinal atrophy, a shrinking of the main functioning section of the eye—the vision screen, so to speak. It too responds to good diet (and the aforementioned remedies). With cats in particular, the condition is often linked to a lack of taurine, an amino acid that is part of a cat's natural diet but is often not present in commercial foods. Change the cat's diet accordingly, and add a capsule of taurine to each meal

(500 milligrams per day) as a supplement; it's available at health food stores. Also, the enzyme supplement VetZimes V2 contains taurine.

Less frequent but of no less concern is a chronic condition called indolent ulcers. The superficial layer of the cornea keeps sloughing off and fails to heal. The conventional treatment is to constantly cauterize the eye, or to undertake a surgical procedure called a keratectomy. I've found that the eyebright infusion, applied topically three or four times a day, can heal indolent ulcers completely in less than a week. I believe that Adequan also works on indolent ulcers, but I haven't yet had the chance to try it on this condition, as this use is relatively new.

A final thought: In Chinese philosophy, the eye and the liver are linked. When I do a metabolic analysis of a pet with chronic eye problems, almost inevitably I find a liver imbalance. Along with putting him on a good diet, I'll start him on liver supplements. The combination tends to produce strong results. The link also explains why vitamin A and carrots have been so celebrated for aiding vision. Vitamin A supports proper liver function by acting as a "lubricant" for its cells.

Feline Immunodeficiency Virus (FIV)

The first thing to be said about so-called feline AIDS is that it's cat-specific. Which is to say that it doesn't spread to people, dogs, or any other species. It is, however, a virus in the AIDS family which, like human AIDS (though not as severe), weakens the immune system, leaving the patient open to secondary infections that, while harmless or mild in healthy cats, can further debilitate a cat with FIV. (Like AIDS, FIV is also a new plague; the first case was discovered in 1986 in a California cattery.) The second thing to be said is that in my opinion, FIV and the other feline viral disease described below are spread not so much because of the virus as because of a compromised immune system's vulnerability to the virus. Wherein lies the clue to treatment.

With FIV, the number one symptom, along with a run-down appearance, is severe gingivitis: gums that are inflamed and painful. A fever and swollen lymph glands may follow. Often the condition subsides for months or even years, then flares up again when the immune system is stressed or deteriorates and is rendered vulnerable to infection.

Although FIV can be spread by contact at birth, the most common route of viral transmission is through bite wounds, so that "outside" cats, especially unneutered males who tend to get into fights, have a disproportionate chance of contracting it. (Unlike AIDS in humans, FIV is *not* transmitted sexually.) My own feeling is that any kitten put on the diet outlined in Chapter Three and subjected to a minimum of vaccines is unlikely to catch the FIV virus. It goes *almost* without saying that males should be neutered as a matter of course, not just to curb FIV but to help contain the cat population. If he does get the virus, his immune system is highly unlikely to succumb to the acute stage of the disease, so that he can lead, in effect, a normal life. A surprisingly high percentage of cats do carry the virus, but far fewer get full-blown FIV, an indication that diet—and the broader state of good health—plays a pivotal role. (A cat that does have the low-grade, chronic form of FIV should *not* be given any vaccines, no matter what your local veterinarian says.) Indeed, FIV offers a perfect illustration of the principle that disease is an excuse to get healthy.

Along with a good diet, I'll put all FIV cats on supplements initially. Then, when I get back their BNA reports, I'll add whatever specific supplements are needed to help each individual case. Chances are, they'll include Feline Support (Biovet), a thymus supplement or a homeopathic like "Thymus Drops" (Professional Health Products); and Co-Enzyme Q10 (Vetri-Science), which supports heart function and also acts as a catalyst for enzymatic action throughout the body. Co-Enzyme Q10 also has reported beneficial effects in pets with gum disease, which makes it even more useful with FIV. If I see an associated suppressed bone marrow, I'll use Millettia 9 (Seven Forests), which contains astragalus, salvia, and cnidium, and nourishes the blood. Also useful from Seven Forests is Viola 12, generally for immune deficiency. And as a last resort, I'll use the homeopathic nosode for FIV (one is from Washington Homeopathics; the Hahnemann company also makes one). Most cats do well without it, and occasionally a nosode will produce an exacerbation of symptoms, but for most cats who've failed to respond to other treatment, it can sometimes bring impressive results.

I've treated a lot of cats successfully for FIV with this support program. Does that mean the cats are cured? No. FIV is a stubborn organism; once in the host, it tends to stay there. But if a cat with FIV can be rendered symptom-free for the duration of a normal life span, the question of whether or not he carries the virus becomes, as far as I can see, academic—especially if you responsibly don't expose the cat to other felines. I've seen multiple-cat households where one cat is positive for FIV and others remain negative for years.

Feline Infectious Peritonitis (FIP)

Like FIV, this is a viral disease that compromises the immune system. Like FIV, it cannot be passed to humans. Unlike FIV, unfortunately, FIP is nearly 100 percent fatal.

FIP is one of the coronaviruses, the most insidious of the bunch because in its initial stage, it appears to be a routine cold or mild fever (if it manifests any symptoms at all). Tragically, that is when the virus can be "shed" to other cats; I've seen whole catteries wiped out by FIP. The coronavirus vaccine is of limited efficacy because it isn't designed specifically for FIP. In fact, there's considerable anecdotal evidence to suggest that one or another of the standard vaccines brings on FIP by compromising the immune system and rendering it vulnerable to the virus. In a cattery or a home containing more than one cat where FIP has appeared, the best preventative measure is to keep cats apart and apply rigorous standards of sanitation. This is because the virus is spread through feces and bodily fluids, including saliva. Cat-to-cat transfer via the licking of the fecal area, or a shared litter box, is the most common route.

By the time more pronounced symptoms start to appear, the cat is no longer "shedding" the virus. Unfortunately, his own prospects of recovery have diminished considerably. Along with a higher fever and loss of appetite, FIP manifests symptoms of two sorts, the "wet" and the "dry." The abdomens of cats with "wet" FIP swell dramatically with a thick, high-protein fluid. Their fevers respond neither to antibiotics nor to holistic measures. Over the next two to four weeks, they grow progressively debilitated, then die. "Dry" FIP affects the eyes and the nervous system. The eyes acquire a white filminess (which feline leukemia can produce as well), while the neurological effects can vary: pain, paralysis, seizures. The fever is not as pronounced, and the course of the illness is more prolonged—stretching over months, rather than weeks—but the end, in my experience, is likely death.

That said, I *have* heard encouraging reports from Dr. Deva Khalsa, one of the holistic veterinarians I most admire, whose practice is in Yardley, Pennsylvania. Apparently, she's been able to arrest, even reverse, cases of FIP, using homeopathic remedies. I've also found grounds for optimism in situations where more than one cat is involved. Carlyn Clayton, a dear client and adopter of exotic cats, had a newly introduced kitten die of FIP; by then, the rest of her cats all tested strongly positive for it. "They're all going to die," she told me, disconsolate. I urged her to change her perspective. "Think of it as: They were all exposed, and they have high titers [high concentrations of the antibodies to the virus in their bodies], which shows they're all strong and healthy enough to fight off the full-blown disease." She did. Not one of the other cats died.

Feline Leukemia (FeLV)

Of the three main feline viral scourges, leukemia sounds like the worst but actually is much less likely than FIP to result in death. About one in five cats carries the virus, but far fewer will contract the full-blown disease, and fewer still will die of it. Unlike FIP, it's also a viral disease that with the right diet and remedies *can* be reversed clinically.

Like FIV (and human AIDS), feline leukemia compromises the immune system, leaving the body vulnerable to secondary infection. The telltale symptom is a lack of energy, often coupled with anemia (which, if it becomes severe enough, requires blood transfusions to keep the cat alive). Often the chest and lungs become filled with fluid. The kidneys can also become infiltrated by the disease. From my experience treating an inordinate number of cancer patients, I've often seen leukemia as an associated disease. My hunch is that it sometimes appears first, ravaging the immune system and, in so doing, enabling the cancer to form.

FeLV is spread mostly through saliva and blood (and, like FIV, cannot be spread to humans). A common route of infection is mutual grooming; another is blood transfusions.* Sadly, a third route for the virus is from a pregnant mother to her litter in utero or, to newborns, via nursing. If the disease progresses, it will usually spread from the mouth to the lymph nodes into the blood and bone marrow. Some cats, however, ward it off before it gets that far, which offers the obvious clue to treatment.

With a logic that seems willfully perverse, conventional medicine has tended to treat feline leukemia by killing the cat. Really! By putting the cat to sleep. It's true that a dead cat whose leukemia was detected early enough cannot infect other cats. But even if the leukemia progresses, a cat can be treated in such a way that it can lead a largely symptom-free life and, if kept inside, away from other cats, will pose

---

*FeLV is often said to be passed via shared water or food bowls, but this is unlikely, since the virus quickly dies in open air.

no threat of infection. Remember the household of cats I discussed in Chapter Two: three related cats came down with leukemia; three others, not related but in constant contact with the first three, never did.

If I see a cat that has the virus but not the full-blown disease, I'll put him on immunosupportive supplements and a healthy diet. If the cat is clinically ill, infusions of vitamin C solution can be extremely helpful. So can a special "leukemia" diet developed by Dr. Ihor Basko (see source guide), who reports having reversed leukemia with it. Along with raw calf's liver, Basko recommends carrot juice, vitamin E, brewer's yeast, and aloe vera, among other ingredients. With FeLV, more so even than with most illnesses, the stronger a cat's immune system is, the likelier he is to keep leukemia at bay.

Conventional medicine does believe leukemia can be prevented— with the feline leukemia vaccine. That may be true, but at what cost? In my experience, cats vaccinated for feline leukemia have a greater chance of becoming immune-suppressed after the vaccine than before, and have a higher death rate from other diseases than nonvaccinated cats. Although they remain FeLV-negative, I've seen so many cats ravaged by bizarre immune-suppressed conditions. Almost inevitably, these cats' records reveal a history of recent leukemia vaccination. As noted in Chapter Four, I've also seen a correlation between the increase in hyperthyroidism among cats and the introduction of the feline leukemia vaccine. Does the vaccine work for some cats? Perhaps. But I can't imagine playing the odds unless a cat were being brought into an area of high leukemia incidence—which in itself would be irresponsible. And even then I'd never advise inoculating the cat on an annual basis, as conventional medicine does. Or vaccinating the cat for half a dozen other diseases at the same time on the assumption that his leukemia might render him that much more vulnerable to them. Enough with the vaccines! Go for health, and let the body do the rest.

Fleas

For both cats and dogs, fleas are an almost inevitable irritant. Scarcely a pet owner in America hasn't had to confront the sight of his animal companion miserably scratching at the little pests in summer or fall (or through the winter and spring as well, especially in year-round warm climates). By the time that happens, chances are the house or apartment is infested, too, as innumerable fleas propagate in the carpeting, cushions, bedding, towels, and other inviting fabrics. So maddening is the problem, and so overwhelming, that even an herbal-tea-drinking, yoga-calm vegetarian is tempted to say: No more! Give me the chemicals! Bombs away!

An entire industry is dedicated to easing you into that choice. Racks of chemical flea products at your local pet store and in veterinary waiting rooms are packaged with soothing assurances (if you read only the big type). Pesticide services stand ready to dispatch workers to your home with canisters of odorless spray to bomb it clean. Many of the products appear to work: the fleas do vanish, at least temporarily. So why not use them? Let's take a closer look—because only when you appreciate what these products contain will you do the harder work of keeping your pet flea-free without them.

Since the 1970s, when attention began to be paid to commercial flea collars, and the phrase "necklaces of poison" came to be used, the pet product industry purports to have made flea products safer. It's true, for example, that collars no longer contain diclorvos, a chemical used in nerve gas. However, most commercial flea products contain one insecticide or another, ranging in toxicity up to the organophosphates, which act like nerve gas in that they paralyze the nervous systems of fleas—at doses low enough, ostensibly, to do no harm to pets. Members of that family, including fenthion and Vapona, can cause tremors and heart and respiratory complications in pets, and even leukemia and death. Another highly toxic group called the carbamates includes propoxur, the principal ingredient in Vet-Kem, the brand of flea collar most prominently displayed at my local pet store. The "precautionary statement" on the back of Vet-Kem advises the user not to get the dust that coats the collar in his mouth or eyes; if swallowed, he should call a poison control center. Is a poison that might kill you a substance you want around your pet's neck twenty-four hours a day, month after month?

As a supposed improvement on collars, the industry began to offer new kinds of protection a few yeas ago. With Proban, dogs ingested tablets whose main ingredient was the very toxic chemical cythoate. The idea was that the dogs would exude the chemical through their skin, killing the fleas in the process. "The dog acts as the drug delivery system to the flea," declared a university report titled "Perspectives on Systemic Flea Control" which provided an overview of the rationale for developing these products. Great! At the same time, Proban's warning label read: "If swallowed by a human, IMMEDIATELY call a physician, poison control center, or hospital emergency room." Soon, reports of side effects—vomiting, seizures, and acute liver toxicity—began to accumulate. A professor of mine at Cornell did numerous autopsies on dogs that had died after taking Proban for some time. He found a "jellification of the liver," meaning that the liver had been virtually destroyed. Proban has been superseded by Program, supposedly a more benign flea fighter. Active ingredient: lufenuron, a chemical that disrupts the flea's reproductive cycle. I treated a golden retriever who had been put on Program on a Friday and fallen into a coma by Monday. (There was nothing I could do to save him.) Over the next months, there were reports of side effects, brain damage in particular, in both Europe and the U.S., including a special report of its toxic effects by New York's WABC-TV Eyewitness News in September 1996. Currently on the FDA's internet chart of adverse drug reactions in animals (www.fda.gov//cvm; click "online library" and then "adverse drug reactions"), lufenuron is listed as causing an alarming incidence of reactions and deaths. Among 256 cats treated, there were 54 cases of vomiting, 39 of depression, and 31 of anorexia; in all, 22 cats died. Among 639 dogs treated, there were 189 cases of vomiting, 96 of depression, 92 of diarrhea, 84 of pruritis (intense itching), and 54 of anorexia; in all, 27 dogs died. Yet Program is still a dominant product in the commercial flea-control market and continues to be promoted as nontoxic.

Along with tablets, there's the "droplet" approach, in which a small plastic vial containing just a few ounces of highly concentrated chemical flea repellent is squeezed out between the shoulder blades—sort of like applying perfume. A prominent "droplet" product is Defend, whose active ingredient is pyrethrin. It's less toxic than the chemicals mentioned above, enough so that it's actually labeled nontoxic. But overuse can still lead to vomiting, headaches, and neurological dysfunctions, among other symptoms. And to other creatures, it can be lethal. I recommended it to a client whose two dogs were suffering intensely. He put a drop between each of their shoulder blades, as directed. That day, the dogs swam in his pond. The next day, numerous fish in the pond lay dead on the surface. How can a few drops of a chemical that kills fish not be harmful to dogs? Yet the trend continues. The latest "droplet" product, Bio Spot, contains a chemical called permethrin (making up 45 percent of its contents), which is in the same group of insecticides as Defend's pyrethrin, though more powerful. Along with the standard warnings about how it can poison humans, the label contains the following caution: "This product is extremely toxic to fish. Do not add directly to water." In fact, Bio Spot, which is made for dogs, is even harmful to cats. "DO NOT USE ON CATS," says the warning (their capital letters, not mine), "or animals other than dogs. Cats which actively groom or engage in close physical contact with recently treated dogs may be at risk of toxic exposure."

This is progress?

In one sense, I sympathize with the makers of these concoctions, and with the owners who buy them. For all the advances made in chemical flea treatment, pets in my experience seem plagued more today than they were a decade ago. Partly, that's the result of the warmer weather in most of the U.S.: fleas have more hatching cycles before the frost, if the frost comes at all. Also, though, it's a perfect example of how wrongheaded we can be in treating problems with chemicals and drugs. Fleas, like most parasites, seek out weak hosts on which to land, those whose immune systems won't repel them. They're like little vultures, circling overhead, eyeing the stragglers in the herd. When we douse our pets with chemicals to repel their fleas, we further weaken their immune systems, rendering them even more vulnerable to next year's hatch. When, at the same time, we call in the chemical sprayers to deflea our homes, we solve an immediate problem—but at the cost of having our pets, and our families, ingest particles of industry-grade insecticides (surely you don't believe the claims that a spray capable of killing trillions of fleas in your home vanishes without a trace in two hours?), further degrading their immune defenses. Given how awesomely adaptable fleas are to toxins, we also know that sooner or later they'll develop a tolerance to—and perhaps even thrive on—whatever chemical we hit them with next.

The first step to dealing with fleas is to recognize that *they aren't leaving*. Remember the movie *The Hellstrom Chronicles*? It started with an aerial view from a helicopter of a nuclear test site. Everything was dead and barren. As the camera moved downward, the ground was seen to be covered with swarming insects. Insects have survived the Ice Age; they've survived whatever wiped out the dinosaurs; if there's an apocalypse, they'll survive that, too. Fleas are particularly tough, and by God, they're plentiful. If a male and female flea are placed in a new home and provided with adequate food like a dog or cat, they'll propagate a flea population of literally millions in less than a month.

The right approach is not to address the symptom but to get to the cause of the allergic reaction that a flea bite stimulates in a vulnerable pet. It means getting your pet healthy enough that fleas will cause no reaction in him—and ultimately the fleas will have no interest in him. Some time ago, I went to Switzerland to research holistic pet remedies. Through my entire stay, I was struck by the radiant physical health of all the people I saw. When I got to Zurich, I learned just how healthy the country's animals were, too. I stopped in at a veterinary school and asked one of the professors what he used for flea problems. "Flea problem? What's a flea problem?" He had two golden retrievers who roamed free in woods thick with fleas and ticks. Yet when they came home, the few fleas and ticks they brought back with them just dropped off within minutes. The dogs were healthy enough not to be targets. For your own pet, that suggests the obvious: the good, nutritional diet outlined in Chapter Three, and no flea-fighting chemicals.

Fine, you say, but what about the flea infestation my pet has *right now*? I'm holistic, but not holier-than-thou: if a pet is really suffering, and one or more of the various available nontoxic products have not worked, I'll steer an owner to one of the over-the-counter chemical treatments just to break the cycle of more bites and scratching. If so, I'll recommend that an owner choose a product containing citrus-based d-limonene, the "herbal insecticide." One spray I keep around my own home is Quantum's "Flea & Tick" repellant. It contains the herb erigeron (flea bane). "Flea & Tick" also contains rose geranium, which is one of the effective tick repellants. In severe cases, I may recommend Front Line or Advantage, two of the more benign popular brands, though not without trepidation.

In all cases, I recommend two natural substances: garlic and brewer's yeast. Both exude odors or tastes that discourage fleas. And garlic is as close to a panacea as a natural product can get. Grate or chop a clove or two into each meal, both to combat fleas and for general health and longevity. Add a tablespoon of brewer's yeast (half a tablespoon for small dogs and for cats). Every day or two, also sprinkle brewer's yeast on your pet's coat, working it in with your hands. Be sure to get him out of the house at that point, since the fleas may desert him.

Among the many herbal flea preparations that can be useful, I'm partial to Earth Animal's Herbal Internal Powder, a powdered mix of natural ingredients which contains garlic as well as alfalfa, wormwood and yellowdock, and pennyroyal. Sprinkle the powder liberally into a pet's food; it smells so good you may want to sprinkle it into your own! (I do, especially when cooking pasta.) It will repel fleas without hurting your pet. Another product high in garlic and brewer's yeast is Internal Powder (Earth Animal), which my brother, veterinarian Robert Goldstein, makes another of his own chief recommendations. To round out the nontoxic approach to flea prevention, Earth Animal also offers everything from herbal collars to shampoos and rinses to nontoxic products for in and around the home. The most effective I've seen is a borax powder (originally put out by a company called Flea Busters) that helps eradicate fleas from the home nontoxically.

In theory, a pet redolent of garlic and brewer's yeast ought to repel all fleas and thus not bring any into the house. In fact, a few fleas may get inside anyway—and we know what happens when they do. To keep them from taking up residence, an owner must be absolutely vigilant. Rugs and carpeting should be steam-cleaned at the start of flea season. The home must be thoroughly vacuumed once a week. Also once a week, a pet's bedding must be put through the washer and dryer at high heat. These measures may seem time-consuming, but when coupled with herbal preparations and a good diet, an amazing thing will happen: trillions of fleas will head off in search of animals less healthy—and less odiferous!—than your own.

Another highly popular approach I endorse is herbal collars. Some come in the form of a standard flea collar—flexible plastic that an owner cuts to size—or as a rope-mesh collar that can be resupplied with the herbal oil it contains. Three common ingredients in these herbal flea oils are pennyroyal, eucalyptus, and citronella, preformulated in the bottle. I actually take this oil, put a few drops in a spray bottle filled with water, and use it to spray both the pets and the house.

As an aside, many owners are tempted to bomb their houses with powerful insecticides during Indian summer, when the flea population enters its final peak. Try to hold out for a couple of weeks. As the days get colder, let the house get colder, too, especially while you're out. (Make sure the plants are in a room with a heater.) This wipes out the fleas.

Gastric Bloat/Gastric Torsion

Large-breed, deep-chested dogs occasionally suffer a severe bloating of the stomach several hours after a meal. Almost always, the meal turns out to have been a commercial kibble that expanded with water in the stomach. The dog will grow visibly uncomfortable, try in vain to vomit, and often drool. The stomach, inflated and hard to the touch, will put pressure on the abdominal area around it, pushing liquids from the blood into it out, and precipitate dehydration and shock that will most likely result in death in a few hours if not treated as a medical emergency.

A not infrequent complication of bloat is gastric torsion. The stomach, filled with food and water, manages to twist at each axis where the esophagus and the small intestine rise to meet it respectively. The torsion prevents any food from being released into the small intestine, which makes the bloat that much worse. All too often, dogs afflicted with either of these conditions turn out to have been playing or engaging in some form of rigorous activity an hour or two before.

If dry commercial foods are one cause, I suspect that another contributing cause is overvaccination. One theory claims that vaccines appear to damage the nerve bodies in the central nervous system which innervate the stomach. A breeder of standard poodles witnessed such a high incidence of gastric bloat among her dogs that she conducted and published a study, vaccinating one-third of her dogs with the standard regimen of combination vaccines, one-third with vaccines on an individual basis, and one-third with no vaccines. The incidence of gastric bloat correlated exactly as she suspected it would; the combination group suffered the highest incidence of bloat, while the nonvaccinated dogs remained bloat free. (Interestingly, there were also correlations between the vaccine and stained teeth, as well as seizures.) Another contributing factor to gastric torsion may be too many generations of the easy life, with pets eating preprocessed foods that don't require the stomach to do its own processing, so that the stomach muscles grow slack and more likely to swing and twist.

The best prevention for bloat is a natural diet free of dry kibble, with no more food than necessary at each meal. Withholding water at least half an hour before and one full hour after mealtime can also be very helpful in prevention of this condition and to aid generally in proper digestion. Veterinarian Richard Pitcairn reports that a breeder of Great Danes swears by freshly made raw cabbage juice, given at the onset of bloat, as an effective means of easing the condition. I also recommend the use of a stomach glandular supplement and BHI's "Nausea" combined with BHI's "Stomach." Unfortunately, the situation tends to recur. If a late-night trip to the emergency clinic is repeated, the best course may be a surgical procedure that in effect "tacks" the stomach down internally.

Gastritis

Another, less threatening condition of the stomach that affects both dogs and cats occurs when some agent inflames the stomach walls. Symptoms include vomiting, loss of appetite, and fewer bowel movements. These are symptoms that can suggest a dozen other problems, so a professional diagnosis is needed. I usually treat gastritis by putting the pet on a fast, giving only small amounts of liquid, even just ice cubes to lick, then ease him onto a bland diet of chicken or turkey, white rice, and chicken broth. For good measure, I'll include the homeopathic remedies ipecac (from the South American plant ipecacuanha) or nux vomica, both of which stop vomiting. Another product I recommend is BHI's "Nausea," and in persistent cases, a suppository called "Vomitus Heel" (Heel), which I've found to be extremely effective.

Heart Disease

Unfortunately, many older pets tend to develop some degree of heart disease. The good news is that if attended to before it becomes severe, heart disease can usually be arrested, if not actually reversed.

Among cats, the most common kind of heart disease is cardiomyopathy, which takes one of two forms. The heart muscles can become weak and dilated, and so unable to maintain proper blood flow. Or they can thicken, constricting blood flow. A specific problem seen commonly in dogs (and people) is a mitral insufficiency. The heart's mitral valve (located on the left side of the heart, between the receiving and pumping chambers) may fail to shut perfectly, allowing blood to leak through and cause a murmur. Whatever the exact failing, heart disease in pets produces general symptoms: a cough, because blood backs up from the constricted muscles or valves of the heart into the lungs; labored breathing, for the same reason; gums that become cyanotic, or blue, from lack of oxygen; and also a bloated belly if fluid backs up into the abdomen. When a pet begins having trouble going the distance of his usual walk, climbing a flight of stairs, or jumping onto a bed he's jumped on for years, all in combination with respiratory symptoms, especially a choking cough, the possibility of heart disease is very likely and should be investigated.

I say this to encourage owners to bring their pets in for proper diagnosis, and to refrain from reaching their own conclusions and thinking they can treat heart disease themselves. The conditions of heart disease are various and complex, and so is their treatment. In fact, this is a realm where the most advanced drugs and techniques of conventional medicine are often needed (and much appreciated by holistic veterinarians). Electrocardiograms, echograms, and X rays leading to specific diagnosis and treatment by heart medication all form the likely course for a pet with serious heart disease and can prolong his life. Holistic measures, however, can be a wonderful adjunct even in serious cases and, once the disease symptoms are under control, help a veterinarian to ease the pet completely off conventional drugs and onto alternatives exclusively. I've even seen holistic therapies reverse serious heart disease *without* conventional medicine.

Generally for heart disease, I use a supplement called Heartsease/Hawthorn Caps (Crystal Star). The herb hawthorn berry is known for its therapeutic effects on the heart, and although not as specific as so many drugs are for diagnosed heart diseases, I've seen it be very helpful with a broad range of heart patients. It's soothing and sedative, so that it also reduces stress, and in so doing eases high blood pressure. At the same time, I'll use Co-Enzyme Q10 (distributed by many suppliers), because besides helping enzyme functions in the body, its number one indication is to aid with proper heart function and support. Vitamin E is helpful, because it helps strengthen the heart muscles (and the rest of the musculature). Since heart disease leads to an accumulation of fluids in other parts of the body, a diuretic is often prescribed; the most commonly used in medicine is Lasix. I'll use Lasix, too, though I'll try to put a pet onto an herbal diuretic instead. If I have to keep using Lasix—which *is* stronger—it may deplete the body of potassium. In that case I'll use Vital K, an herbal preparation high in potassium that is available in health food stores. Better, though, just to go with an herbal diuretic if it does the trick.

Heartworm

To judge by your local veterinarian's stern insistence on regular heartworm pills for your dog, you'd think we're in the midst of a brutal epidemic, leaving piles of the dead in its wake. I think there's an epidemic, too, but of a different sort: of disease-causing toxicity instilled in our pets by heartworm preventative pills.

Granted, heartworm is a serious condition. An infected mosquito bites your dog (cats are rarely affected), injecting microscopic worms that first hibernate, then gain access to his bloodstream. The worms find their way to the heart, where they grow to as long as twelve inches, constricting the heart's passages and causing symptoms that range from coughing to labored breathing to heart failure. If the image of giant worms literally blocking the life blood of your dog isn't horrifying enough—and it can seem more so when viewing a real heart preserved in a jar of formalin, on display in a veterinarian's office as a sales tactic for heartworm preventative—the fact that they spawn hundreds of thousands of baby larvae, called "microfilaria," which circulate through the bloodstream, is nothing short of grotesque.

A few caveats are in order, however. Only a small percentage of dogs who get heartworm die of it, especially if they're routinely tested twice yearly for early detection. Even in untreated dogs, after a period of uncomfortable symptoms, the adult worms die. The microfilaria do *not* grow into adult worms on their own. To reach the next stage in their life cycle, they have to be sucked back *out* of the body by another mosquito, and go through the other stages of their maturation process within the mosquito. Only when that mosquito alights again on a dog and bites it can the microfilaria reenter the bloodstream with the ability to grow into adults. The chances of a microfilaria-infected mosquito biting your dog the first time are slim. Of it happening to the same dog twice? *Very* slim. And after two decades of pervasive administration of heartworm pills in the U.S., the chances of your dog contracting heartworm in most parts of this country even a first time are slimmer still. Early in my career, I saw and treated hundreds of cases of heartworm disease, most with routine medication, yet witnessed only three deaths (the last was in 1979). By comparison, we're seeing cancer kill dogs on a daily basis. To my mind, the likelihood that toxicity from heartworm pills is contributing to the tremendous amount of immune suppression now occurring, especially in cases of liver disease and cancer, is far greater and more immediate than the threat of the disease they're meant to prevent.

The most common form of heartworm prevention is a monthly pill taken just before and during mosquito season. (Many veterinarians recommend giving it year-round, even in areas of the country that experience winter.) Its toxins—ivermectin, for example—sweep through the body, killing any microfilaria that have been introduced by mosquito bites in the previous month, and thus preventing the growth of adult worms. Some brands also contain other toxins to kill intestinal parasites. The other approach to treatment is with a daily dose of the drug diethylcarbamazine, starting several weeks before mosquito season. The drugs called for in either course of treatment are, simply put, poisons. Unfortunately, while they kill off microfilaria, they have the toxic effects of poisons, and can be especially damaging to the liver. I've saved a 1987 product evaluation for diethylcarbamazine mixed with oxibendazole, a preventative also used for hookworm. The evaluation, published by the company itself in a medical journal, reported that of 2.5 million dogs given the stuff, the company received only 176 reports of problems, including cases of liver toxicity and fatalities. To me, 176 is too many. But also, how many more went unreported? The evaluation concludes, "Of course, not all incidences are reported to the manufacturer, so the true magnitude of occurrence is really unknown." The manufacturer would argue, no doubt, that many of the symptoms I've seen cannot be linked in any provable way to any of the heart-worm preventatives. Perhaps—though the anecdotal evidence has long since persuaded me not to put dogs on the stuff. But I have seen one obvious, immediate effect of these once-a-month preventatives in case after case: when you give a dog that pill, over the next few days, wherever he urinates outside, his urine burns the grass. Permanently! In some cases, you can't grow grass there until you change the soil. What, I wonder, can it be doing internally to your dog in that time?

When the first daily preventatives came out, my brother and I witnessed evidence of hemorrhaging in the urine of several dogs put on them. We stopped the medication; the bleeding stopped. We started it up again; the bleeding resumed. When we reported this to the manufacturer, we were informed that the company was aware of the problem from other complaints. Aware—but not about to pull its product from the shelves. All we could do was to stop giving the medication ourselves to the dogs we treated. Since then, the company has changed the product, diminishing this side effect and bringing it into the realm of acceptability for use in areas of high heartworm incidence.

The dogs I treat from puppyhood receive no heartworm preventative pills. It may be said, of course, that I practice in an area where cases of heartworm are pretty infrequent. But while my clinic is in Westchester County, just north of New York City, my practice encompasses patients from around the country. In the last decade, 98 percent of my patients, on my recommendation, have not been given heartworm preventative. In that time, I've seen less than a handful of clinical cases. Two of them I treated herbally, starting with heart support supplements (a heart glandular, vitamin E, Co-Enzyme Q10) and regular doses of black walnut, an herb known to kill parasites. (It comes in a liquid extract form; I recommend putting a dropperful in the food or mouth at each meal.) The third I treated medically, with a new drug (Immiticide) reported to be a lot less toxic than intravenous arsenic, at a lower-than-recommended dosage. All three are clinically normal—no evidence of heartworm recurrence—years after treatment.

As a precaution, I recommend that all dogs be tested twice a year for heartworm. For clients who insist on a more active form of prevention, I suggest doses of black walnut given two to three times a week, as I've actually reversed clinical heartworm with it. (For a thirty-pound dog, one capsule three times weekly during mosquito season in areas that have reported any incidence of heartworm.) We also use a homeopathic nosode. In areas where the chances of heartworm exposure appear greater than those in my own—like southern Florida and the Bahamas, where the chances of contracting it are high—I recommend adding to this regimen the conventional daily heartworm pill, given three times weekly. Veterinarians trained in homeopathy can get your pet on a good nosode program for heartworm prevention.

Hip Dysplasia

This is a hereditary joint disease that affects as many as 50 percent of some large and giant breeds of dogs. The bone and socket in the hip grow misaligned with each other, creating an abnormal fit that over time creates a proliferation of excess tissue in and around the joint. Bony spurs, deformation, degeneration, and inflammation result. Sometimes the joints even partially dislocate due to poor integrity. (The word "dysplasia" means "bad development.") Though usually not present clinically at birth, the propensity may first appear in puppyhood. By the time a dog has reached adulthood, the entire structure of his hip (or hips) may be terribly misshapen, causing pain and lameness. The symptoms seem obvious—a reluctance to walk up stairs; difficulty standing up; apparent discomfort while walking or running; even crying and outright pain—but they can be deceptive, perhaps indicating some other degenerative disease (or even a disease like Lyme). A radiographic diagnosis is therefore crucial. However, an owner who observes his dog limping is certainly doing no harm by administering the supplements detailed below in the meantime.

Conventional medicine generally holds the view that hip dysplasia can't be prevented, or its degeneration halted, and takes its usual tack of drugs and surgery: the former to treat the symptoms of inflammation and pain, the latter to change the angular dynamics of the joint itself, or to replace the hip or socket altogether with a prosthesis. Though effective, these procedures are extensive and require a very experienced surgeon. Years ago, I had limited success with a surgical procedure to relieve the pressure on the hip by cutting a small muscle bundle inside the thigh called the pectineus. Though not clinically cured, the dog would be more stable and in less pain for a while. But I've come to feel that surgery is usually not necessary in order to provide a dog with a good, pain-free quality of life.

First comes the Bio Nutritional Analysis, which allows me to work up a regimen of supplements to redress all of the dog's imbalances, not just his hip condition. In almost every hip dysplastic dog I see, there's an imbalance in the pituitary gland in the brain, which controls growth factors in the body. In most, there's also a need for adrenal support (because the adrenal is being called upon to deal with stress and inflammation). Along with putting the dog on supplements for those two problems, I'll give him AR-Ease (Crystal Star) for the arthritic symptoms that arise when extra mineralization forms like barnacles around the ball end of the femur bone and socket of the pelvis. The nutritional supplement Cosequin (Nutramax) in capsule form helps rebuild cartilage and promote lubrication lost in the hip joint; it is relatively new, though I've been recommending glucosamine sulfate, its main component, for years. First developed to help injured racehorses, Cosequin is now used widely by holistic veterinarians to address not only canine hip dysplasia but other joint disorders that animals incur, such as any type of arthritis. Another supplement to consider in less severe cases is Glycoflex, which contains an extract of green-lipped mussels; some holistic veterinarians use both at the same time. In more severe cases, I'll start with injectable chondroitin sulfate, called Adequan, which rapidly helps increase joint fluid production and in so doing can lead to dramatically greater mobility and diminished pain. A veterinarian administers it by intramuscular injection, usually in an eight-injection series over the course of four weeks, and follows it up with oral administration of Cosequin. There are many Cosequin-like formulas on the market; I've just had such success with Cosequin that it's the one I prefer to use.

Additionally, when I first see a young dog with hip dysplasia, I'll put him on high doses of vitamin C. This is because the blood results of these patients typically show an elevated level of the enzyme called alkaline phosphatase. As its name suggests, this enzyme is an indicator of alkalinity in the blood. We therefore use vitamin C in the ascorbic acid form to help counterbalance the alkalinity and restore the body to a more stable acid-base balance. I try to ease off the C eventually, though, so that a dog receiving an external source of C doesn't lose the capacity to produce his own. Also with young dogs, I'll include collagen supplements; a brand of choice is Collagen Complex (Professional Health Products). Collagen is a matrix of all the connective tissues in the body, and does wonders, especially in treating these dysplastic dogs that are still developing new tissue.

If a pregnant mother with a genetic history of hip dysplasia is put on a proper nutritional program, usually with vitamin C, the disease can be prevented in her puppies. It's important not to overfeed the puppies or let them overexert, as both have been shown to contribute to the disease once the propensity to develop it is there.

Hyperthyroidism/Hypothyroidism

The thyroid gland, which is located in the throat area and controls the body's metabolism, often becomes hyperactive in cats. So often, indeed, that hyperthyroidism has come to be considered an epidemic. It's a serious development, since the hyperthyroid cat has a very fast heartbeat and can be especially susceptible to heart disease. Yet no one knows exactly what causes the condition, or why a condition that's neither viral nor bacterial should have reached epidemic proportions. Is it, as they say, something in the water? I'm not the only holistic veterinarian who's intrigued by the correlation between the distribution of the feline leukemia vaccine and the increased incidence of hyperthyroidism. I can't prove the link, but many times I see a cat with the condition—which happens now at least once a week on average—I find a full battery of vaccines, including one for leukemia, in her recent medical history.

The drug typically used to treat hyperthyroidism is Tapazole, which can produce dramatic results. A hyperthyroid cat will show high levels of the hormone thyroxine (with which it regulates metabolism), sometimes *twenty times* the amount it should have. After the cat has been on Tapazole for three days, the thyroxine can plummet down to normal or below. Unfortunately, Tapazole is also toxic, especially to the liver and kidneys. Another established and toxic treatment is radioactive iodine. Iodine has an affinity for the thyroid gland; when radioactive iodine is administered to the cat, it acts rather like a heat-seeking missile, making its way toward the overproducing thyroid and destroying it. Though the procedure is said not to be toxic, the cat has to be kept in quarantine (from pets and people both) for a couple of weeks in a lead-lined room!

Alternatively, I've had considerable success in treating hyper-thyroidism metabolically. Most cats with the condition have elevated levels of liver and adrenal enzymes, so a first step is to redress those imbalances with the standard liver and adrenal supplements. The home-opathic remedy flor-de-piedra at low potencies is also helpful. (Manu-factured in France, flor-de-piedra is sometimes hard to find; a more widely available homeopathic substitute is lophophytum leandri.) Sometimes I'll add Thyrodrops (Professional Health Products), which is homeopathic thyroid. If the condition is persistent, I may add a little Tapazole into the program, but at one-quarter to one-eighth the rec-ommended dose, and monitor well. If the condition remains out of control, chances are the thyroid has developed a tumor on one or the other of its sides. Here's a situation where conventional surgery can be successful in complementing holistic alternatives. When the tumor is removed, I've seen the hyperthyroid cat make a fast and complete recovery.

Hypothyroidism is, as it sounds, the reverse of hyperthyroidism. It's a condition more commonly seen in dogs than in cats. Since the thyroid is underperforming, the standard symptoms are sluggishness and weight gain, and also hair loss on both sides of the body in a symmetri-cal fashion. But I've also seen many dogs with low-thyroid function who exhibit none of these classic symptoms. Standard treatment is to give a synthetic thyroid drug that can do the thyroid's work for it and speed up the sluggish metabolism. I prefer a more natural thyroid sup-plement called Armour, or a similar, less expensive version called USP thyroid; both come as tablets to be given orally, and both should be supported with a thyroid glandular such as Thytrophin (Standard Process) or Thyrocomplex (Progressive Labs). It's important to note that sometimes the thyroid may seem imbalanced but is actually just fine; the problem gland is either the pituitary in the brain or the hypo-thalamus, both of which coordinate thyroid activity. When our stan-dard supplements for the pituitary or hypothalamus redress those imbalances, the hypothyroidism subsides. Many times, I can establish normal thyroid function just by means of metabolic balancing, even without the use of a thyroid replacement like USP thyroid.*

Jaundice

Though we think of it more as a human condition, with its telltale sign of yellowish skin which is symptomatic of an obstructed liver and the subsequent overabundance of bile in the blood, jaundice appears commonly in both dogs and cats. In fact, it's becoming more common. In pets as in people, the exposed skin gets visibly yellow (over the eyes, inside the ears, and across the abdomen). But so do the whites of the eyes and the gums, and sometimes even the nails.

The principal—but not the only—cause of jaundice is liver disease, and more specifically liver cancer. Obstructed, the liver releases bile it should be directing into the gallbladder's system of bile ducts to emulsify fats from food. The bile, actually yellow, produces the characteristic color of jaundice as it gains access to the bloodstream. Another distinct cause is a rapid breakdown of the red blood cells, perhaps from a blood parasite, perhaps from autoimmune hemolytic anemia, perhaps from a poison. Whatever the cause, the breakdown releases bile pigments from the red blood cells which leads to jaundice as well.

As a warning sign of real trouble in the liver or the red blood cells, jaundice constitutes an emergency and should be treated immediately. Bringing those conditions under control is the main priority. With chronic jaundice, this is cause for concern, though not as critical. It causes no pain, and is itself just a condition, not a disease; I've seen cats live happily enough for years with it. At the same time, I want to determine the cause and then address it. If the liver is to blame, I'll keep a pet on liver supplements (see "Liver Problems," below); the healthier the liver is, the less the degree of the jaundice. Hepatitis very often responds well to intravenous vitamin C, a rapid agent of cellular detoxification, along with intravenous ozone (see Chapter Five). The

---

*In her own work, Dr. Jean Dodds has demonstrated the important role that the thyroid plays as a mediator of environmental stress factors, particularly vaccinations. She believes that an overstressed thyroid leads to a condition called autoimmune thyroiditis, in which the immune system, through a sensitivity, actually attacks its very own thyroid gland. Young dogs with aggression problems, for example, may be suffering from this condition. By correcting the thyroid balance, Dodds has actually reversed such aggressive tendencies and saved dogs from unnecessary euthanasia. If left unchecked, autoimmune thyroiditis can lead to a hypothyroid condition.

ozone quickly breaks down into oxygen, which helps promote cell activity, a key indication of an improving liver. If the condition is the result of red blood cell breakdown, I'll control the crisis medically, if necessary, but also inject adrenal cortex and, if indicated, bone marrow ("Medulla Ossis" from Heel). I'll also administer natural hydrocortisone orally, and a product called Hemaplex (Progressive Labs), whose ingredients support the production of new red blood cells.

Kidney Problems

In older dogs and cats, the symptoms of kidney disease can seem hard to distinguish from the general slowing down associated with age, but with diligence they can be spotted early on. They must, for by the time symptoms appear, the kidneys have probably sustained some degree of irreversible damage, and symptoms usually don't appear until a good percentage of normal kidney function is compromised. Beyond a certain point, if the damage is not contained, no measures will be able to keep your pet from failing rapidly.

In both dogs and cats, increased thirst and urination are the classic symptoms. The kidneys fail to reabsorb water back into the blood as they're eliminating wastes, so excess water is excreted in urine, and the body grows dehydrated as a result. The increased urination may also lead to incontinence, and so a pet may leak urine in the house. Because the kidneys are working improperly, wastes also back up into the blood. Often I've seen this excess toxicity settle in the mouth, which leads to inflamed or ulcerating gums and foul-smelling breath, and also causes frequent vomiting.

If the situation deteriorates, it will lead to the general poisoning of the blood, called uremia. In such cases, intravenous fluids are administered to help flush poisons out of the body and enhance kidney function. In the most extreme circumstances, the only way to keep a patient alive is by dialysis: passing the blood through an outside dialysis unit that does the job of the kidneys. But dialysis is simply not a viable option in general veterinary practice. Kidney transplants are another extreme measure. Although they are being done at a few facilities, they don't always succeed and are prohibitively expensive, and the drugs needed to prevent tissue rejection, if the operation is successful, take a severe toll on the pet's overall health and immune system.

In manageable cases, every effort must be made to lighten the kidneys' load. As few toxins as possible must be ingested, which is to say that no vaccines, and in most cases no drugs, should be administered. Since the kidneys also process out unused phosphorus and proteins from the food your pet eats, a special diet containing high-quality meat in relatively low-quantity servings is recommended. (A few good choices: rice, turkey, chicken, and all the steamed greens you can get your pet to eat.) Vitamins A and C should be part of the diet, since the body's own stores may have been sluiced out of the kidneys along with everything else. Vitamin A acts as a lubricant for the kidney tissue. C helps because there's a tendency in kidney disease for the urine to become alkaline, so the C acidifies it, which also helps destroy any bacteria present. Also, C is a natural diuretic, enhancing the flow of liquids through the kidneys, especially of wastes. I'll also put a pet on supplements to redress any other metabolic imbalances that may have been adding wastes to the kidneys' load, along with the injectable kidney solution Ren Suis (Heel) and herbal remedies such as Tinkle Caps (Crystal Star) or "Kidney Bladder" (Quantum). The main ingredients in these are parsley, juniper berries, and uva-ursi, all known to have a diuretic effect that enhances proper kidney function. Many times a pet with chronic kidney disease will need the continued support of subcutaneous (under the skin) fluids administered several times a week. This maintenance can be done by you at home, and your pet, as a result, can enjoy an extended, good-quality life.

Common sense might suggest that a condition as severe as kidney failure should be treated with as much medication as possible. However, having treated literally thousands of pets with kidney problems, I know how much better patients do without drugs. The only exception to this is a condition called pyelonephritis, which is a bacterial infection of the innermost region of the kidney. If a diagnosis of pyelonephritis is confirmed, I will use antibiotics chosen specifically from the results of a urine culture—in conjunction with all the alternatives listed above.

What causes kidney disease in the first place? The list of possible contributing factors is long, but in many cases I think a prime suspect is vaccines. Another is synthetic cortisone. Used indiscriminately and routinely for skin problems and arthritis, cortisone is known to stress the liver and kidneys, and over long periods may cause irreversible damage. To a lesser but not insignificant degree, all of the other environmental pollutants and poor diet detailed in Chapter Two contribute to kidney degradation as well. Though the kidneys are resilient enough to grow new tissue and reverse limited damage, they're also tiny organs not designed to withstand the modern world's onslaught of toxicity. If your pet is not yet afflicted with this dire condition, take these three simple measures: put him on the diet outlined in Chapter Three; forget annual booster vaccines but do bring him in for regular blood tests to track the three telltale values of the kidney (creatinine, phosphorus, and urea nitrogen); and administer supplements to redress even slight imbalances. By taking those easy steps, you'll have a far greater chance of saving him from the sad demise that kidney disease brings on in its final stages.

Liver Problems

The liver is the body's largest organ, and probably its most versatile, performing many distinct and crucial tasks. It metabolizes food for use in the body and passes the wastes on for elimination. It's the body's main detoxifier. It produces bile for the proper processing of dietary fats. Its reticuloendothelial system is a major component of the body's overall immune system. It serves as a storage depot for food reserves. And as if all this weren't enough, it manufactures factors necessary for blood clotting. Unfortunately, in its role as the great detoxifier, the liver bears the accumulated brunt of low-grade food, synthetic drugs, and environmental pollutants, which can leave it diseased.

The usual result is inflammation, which we call hepatitis. But pets, like people, can also incur cirrhosis. In humans it's associated with alcohol, but the link is not intrinsic. Cirrhosis is simply a fibrosis of the liver due to replacement of normal tissue by scar tissue. In animals, that can be the result of anything that chronically overworks and damages the liver: malnutrition, poisons and toxins, drugs (such as heartworm preventative pills), and more. A classic sign of liver disease is jaundice (see "Jaundice"), which occurs when the malfunctioning liver loses its bile to the bloodstream. Other warnings: loss of appetite and vomiting, an abdomen distended by fluid; and diarrhea or light-colored stools. Unfortunately, symptoms in a pet often don't appear until the liver has sustained significant damage. Fortunately, the liver has extraordinary recuperative powers.

Conventional medicine usually focuses on treating the symptoms of the disease by prescribing a battery of antibiotics and steroids. My own treatment begins, once again, with nutritional analysis and a program of supplements not just for the liver but for other organs that may be contributing, by their own malfunctions, to the liver's woes.

Initially for the liver, I'll administer a liver glandular in capsule form, tablet, or liquid. (Doctors Mutual Service is one supplier, and Miller Pharmacal is another. Both are listed in the source guide.) I'll also use vitamin A in modest doses—for general liver support I recommend 10,000 IU for a fifty-pound dog and 1,500 IU for a cat, once a day. Be careful, as too much vitamin A can actually be harmful to the liver by causing a disease called hypervitaminosis A. The homeopathic combination remedy called Hepaticol (Professional Health Products) has proved helpful. Initially, too, I'll use the Chinese herb Tang Kuei 18 (Seven Forests), alone or in combination with the herb milk thistle, or silymarin, both powerful promoters of liver health. Tang Kuei 18 comes in tablet form, milk thistle in several different forms; all are available at health food stores. Often I'll give a dog one Tang Kuei tablet in the morning, and a milk thistle tablet at night (large dogs may be given two tablets for each dose, cats generally one-third to one-half of a tablet). Milk thistle also appears as an ingredient in several products for liver disease. One such is Lipotrope (Progressive Labs), which in addition to milk thistle contains inositol and choline, factors that help support liver function. Lipotrope is available in capsule form at most health food stores. Finally, I always advise owners to get their pets out into the sun on a regular basis: sun-generated vitamin D helps support liver function.

In more severe or nonresponsive cases, I'll admit a dog into the hospital and use intravenous therapy (vitamin C, ozone, injectable homeopathics). I'll also inject the Smith Ridge "cocktail" (multi B vitamins, vitamin B_{12}, and injectable adrenal cortex) and injectable homeopathic liver (called Hepar Suis, from Heel) at acupuncture points that are indicated for liver malfunction (see Chapter Five).

Often, by the way, an initial nutritional analysis may indicate other organ imbalances and show normal or even depressed levels of liver enzymes. As supplements begin to bring the other organs back to health, the liver enzymes may rise to levels that seem alarming. In fact, that may indicate an inhibited liver "waking up" to do its work of detoxification. As the liver grows healthier, it replaces the diseased tissue with healthy tissue. That, in turn, enables it to work better, and thus show more enzyme activity. Soon enough, if the liver *is* healthy, its enzymes will finish their backlog of detoxification, and levels will go down to normal. Cirrhosis may actually produce depressed levels of liver enzymes at first, because the scar tissue no longer produces enzymes.

Lyme Disease

Since 1975, when the first human case of this tick-borne disease was diagnosed in Old Lyme, Connecticut, its debilitating symptoms have afflicted tens of thousands of Americans. It principally affects residents of eastern suburbs and exurbs, where populations of the white-tailed deer that carries the tick have exploded. Unfortunately, dogs have proved susceptible to Lyme disease, too. (I *have* seen cats test positive for Lyme, even indoor cats whose owners have probably brought the tick indoors—on themselves or the household dog—but this is less common.) Given how much romping dogs do through tick-infested fields and woods, it is no surprise that many dogs in the eastern U.S. have been exposed to the Lyme disease organism. But not all will develop symptoms of the disease itself.

In humans, the first telltale sign of Lyme is a solid red "bull's-eye" circle on the skin caused by the bite of the deer tick and the successful transfer of the Lyme disease organism—a "spirochete"—from the tick into the bloodstream. Dogs, in my experience, don't manifest the red spot, but may get some of the other symptoms humans do (headaches, fevers, chills, and chronic weakness, sometimes leading to dizziness). The most common symptom is a marked lameness, which may shift from one leg to another. Another indication of Lyme in dogs is kidney disease, with all its attendant symptoms (see "Kidney Problems"); for reasons that are unclear, the disease has an affinity for the kidneys. More rarely, Lyme may affect the heart and central nervous system; twice, I have seen it produce seizures that indicate encephalitis surrounding the brain.

At least three vaccines to prevent Lyme disease in dogs are now in wide use. Unfortunately, I'm not impressed by any of them, as all appear to produce side effects and, in some dogs, the symptoms of full-blown Lyme disease.* In any case, they seem to impair the immune

---

*Dr. Richard Jacobson of Cornell University's School of Veterinary Medicine has researched each of them more thoroughly than anyone else I know of in the field. His report: "Fort Dodge's vaccine is a whole-cell bacterin; all of the 100–200 different Lyme disease antigens are in this agent, or preparation." *So a pet has 200 different antigens infected in him, with the idea that he'll develop antibodies to all of them, and be ready for whichever one he happens to encounter!* "Solvays' vaccine is bivalent," Jacobson goes on, "which means that while it's a whole-cell bacterin, too, it contains only two antigens." *Better, but not great.* "Meriel's is a recombinant preparation," Jacobson says. "It only has the outer-surface protein, and not any antigen in its entirety, just enough protein to provoke the immune system to recognize it, and per-system unnecessarily, leaving a dog that much more vulnerable to the chronic symptoms of vaccinosis. I'd recommend not using them except in areas where the disease is epidemic. To date, I have not ordered one dose for my clients at Smith Ridge.

So what do I do when pets show symptoms of Lyme disease? First, test for it, though that's not as useful as it sounds. The test for Lyme disease in dogs is notoriously unreliable. Often the test will come back positive, suggesting that the dog has Lyme disease, when at worst he has a small, inactive number of spirochetes in his system, indicating an old but now controlled exposure.* However, if a strongly positive test is accompanied by the usual symptoms of the disease, I'll assume that the dog does have Lyme. In the deer-tick-infested exurb of Westchester, New York, where I live and practice, that's a pretty safe bet.

Though I never like to reach for antibiotics, the Lyme disease spirochete is a fiendishly stubborn organism often unresponsive to holistic measures. Besides, I'd rather deal with the aftereffects of antibiotics on the body than those of uncontrolled Lyme disease—especially irreversible kidney failure. My drug of choice these days is doxycycline, which is relatively mild but usually effective. Holistically, I'll add an impressively potent herbal preparation called Spirokete, put out by the renowned herbalist Hannah Kroeger; her combination of five herbs, including nettles and organic tobacco, will actually kill the organism in most cases. (It did for me—just five days after experiencing the bull's-eye redness of a severe tick bite I received in Old Lyme, Connecticut!) I'm also partial to a homeopathic remedy called Lym D (Bio-Active Nutritional) that contains the Lyme nosode and several others to help ameliorate the associated symptoms of the disease. In a real-life example of this product's potential effects, one of my clients used it as a preventative for her two dogs and called me to let me know that within ten minutes of administering it, she saw the ticks on her dogs literally drop off. The homeopathic remedy ledum, which in my experience works well for people, doesn't work as well with animals,

---

haps react to it." Safe enough? Not necessarily. "Although it seems logically better," says Jacobson, "I have nine dogs right now that are lame with a history of getting the Meriel vaccine while having no natural exposure to the disease."

*A newer test called the Western blot differentiates between the positive reaction caused by the vaccine and that caused by the active disease. But in my experience and from conversation with a close associate, Dr. Alan Schreier, who has done a tremendous amount of study and lecturing on Lyme disease, an old but now inactive exposure can still make this test appear positive, indicating a disease state that doesn't really exist, especially if the dog is free of symptoms.

though other holistic veterinarians report more success with it than I've had.

Mange

A very common mange mite is a tiny, crablike creature that descends on dogs, burrows into their skin, and causes terrible itching. Known medically as sarcoptic mange, the mite is invisible to the naked eye, and so the reaction it causes is often misdiagnosed as a severe allergic skin reaction. Even the recommended "skin scraping" method of diagnosis often fails to reveal this little creature.

Usually, sarcoptic mange begins on the ears and at the elbows, then spreads down the legs. The telltale sign is ferocious scratching at skin that seems to grow more inflamed and itchy with every scratch. As it progresses, it emits a characteristic, pungently foul odor. Another indication that these microscopic mites are at work is that cortisone—usually given to most dogs with symptoms of itching—will provide relief for at best a day (rather than weeks). Usually, an owner will find a scattering of red, itchy dots from the mange mites on his own arms, or in areas where clothing is tight against the body, such as belt lines. With a creature as microscopic as mange, this can be a critical clue. What I've found surprisingly helpful is Selsun shampoo—a prescription formula, not the milder, over-the-counter product Selsun Blue, although I've used the latter on younger and smaller dogs and cats with mange caused by differently named mites. If Selsun doesn't work, then I'll resort to medical treatment; a harsh dip, though toxic, is a onetime immersion that will eliminate the mites. But I will not use injectable ivermectin in treating this condition, as many conventional veterinarians will, because I feel that it is too toxic and immune-suppressive.

Much harder to treat in one of its two forms is demodectic mange. Considered a normal inhabitant of dogs' skin, the demodectic mite remains benign until an immune deficiency allows it to proliferate. One manifestion is "localized," involving several small patches of hair loss, usually around the head area of puppies; the patches become a little scaly, though generally not itchy. They tend to heal spontaneously as the animal matures, though treatment can be hastened with tea tree oil (or *Melaleuca alternifolia*); just apply the oil on the lesions. The other manifestation of demodectic mange, again due to an immune deficiency, is "generalized," which is to say that it involves any part of the body, and sometimes the whole body. This is one of the most difficult problems to cure in veterinary medicine. The medical treatments are very toxic: with one, the so-called Scotts dip (named after its creator, a former teacher of mine at Cornell), no more than one-third of the dog can be dipped at a time or he'll possibly die from the toxicity. A dip called Mitaban is also pretty toxic. It kills the mites but fails to address the immune deficiency that allowed the mites to take hold in the first place, and thus may not prevent their speedy return.

I treat demodectic mange by putting the dog on the nutritional diet outlined in Chapter Three, along with two herbal supplements: Viola 12 and Astragalus 10 Plus, both from Seven Forests. I've seen tea tree oil ameliorate mange spots. Also, I use supplements containing thymus extract, to add immune support. I've had tremendous success in several cases using the IAT program (see Chapter Eight) developed by Dr. Lawrence Burton. (Although he used his therapy almost exclusively for cancer patients, Dr. Burton designed for us a protocol to treat mange from his own personal research on AIDS.) In some cases, after giving a lot of support and still seeing symptoms, I'll recommend a Mitaban dip as a last resort to help kill those mites that have already proliferated.

Obesity/Fat Metabolism

Because nutrition is one of our specialties, Smith Ridge very commonly treats overweight pets, either as a primary concern, or as part of their illness. (A dog with chronic arthritis, for example, will often be overweight.) Within this category I also place pets with fatty tumors, or lipomas. Unless your pet is accustomed to eating hot fudge sundaes and banana splits, his excess weight is a matter of metabolic imbalance, so the primary goal is to establish proper metabolic function through specific supplements. The course for each individual pet is set by the BNA results, in combination with good-quality foods (see Chapter Three). Added to nearly all fat metabolism programs is L-Carnitine, found in any health food store (I advise 250 milligrams for a 20–30 pound dog, 125 milligrams for a cat); Chromium Picolinate, also found in health food stores (100 micrograms for a 30-pound dog, 50 micrograms for a cat); and a homeopathic preparation called Weight Off Drops (Professional Health Products). If a pet fails to respond in a few weeks, I'll add vitamin B_6 (50 milligrams for a 30–50 pound dog, 25 milligrams for a cat). Specifically for lipomas, I'll administer Chih-ko & Curcuma (Seven Forests). Here the recommendation is two tablets daily for a 30-pound dog. Lipomas are so much more common in dogs than in cats that cats hardly ever need to be addressed, though a tablet a day is appropriate if needed.

Pancreatitis

When the pancreas stops making insulin to convey blood sugar into the cells for energy, the result is diabetes (see "Diabetes"). If the pancreas become very inflamed, the result is pancreatitis, a common condition in dogs, especially overweight dogs. It also occurs in cats.

The trouble likely begins when a pet eats something too rich (like a whole birthday cake) or too foreign (a dead bird) for his digestive system to absorb. The pancreas, overburdened, becomes inflamed. Rather than sending its enzymes to the intestines, it starts to leach them into the abdomen and raises the digestive enzyme levels in the blood. The abdomen becomes distended; the pet also experiences severe nausea, loss of appetite, and pain in the belly. In its acute stage, pancreatitis can be life-threatening and must be treated immediately, likely with intravenous fluids. Serious cases can sometimes be relieved subsequently with surgery. As a lower-grade, chronic condition, it usually responds well to a few simple measures.*

For most veterinarians, a simple measure of choice is antibiotics. Until recently, they also used atropine. Although it stops the secretions of the pancreas, my problem with it is that it inhibits the parasympathetic nervous system. This is the *unconscious* nervous system that coordinates internal functions, among them the digestive organs. In so doing, atropine disarms the part of the nervous system which also happens to be the number one facilitator of holistic therapies. Acupuncture especially, but also herbal and homeopathics, all rely on it to help effect the process of healing. So atropine is the very antithesis of holistic medicine—and unnecessary, in my experience, for treating pancreatitis, unless nothing else is working. Now an increasing number of conventional veterinarians are choosing not to use atropine either.

Because it's a food-provoked condition and feeding stimulates pancreas function, the *really* simple measure for treating pancreatitis is NPO. That's medical shorthand for *non per os*, or "nothing through

---

*An interesting manifestation of this condition, usually in its chronic form, is that the pancreatic enzymes leaking into the abdomen start to work on the fat naturally located there, and actually turn it into soap, a process called saponification, as soap is simply the product of enzymatic degradation of fat.

the mouth," which is to say: No food! Given time off from its job in digestion, the pancreas usually heals itself. In examining the dog, I'll administer injectable homeopathic pancreas ("Pankreas," by Heel) and prescribe a program of homeopathic remedies: "Pancreas" and "Inflammation," both by BHI, or "Pancreas Drops" (Professional Health Products). Also, I'll use a pancreas glandular like Pancreatrophin (Standard Process Labs). The dog will then be put on a liquid fast for several days—on chicken or vegetable broth and all the distilled water he can drink, though in small amounts each time. Afterward, I'll ease him onto the natural diet outlined in Chapter Three, with a special emphasis on foods low in fats and oils: along with chicken and turkey, and grains such as brown rice and millet. So as to burden the pancreas as little as possible, I'll advise setting the food out in five or six "mini-meals" throughout the day. Vitamin E tends to enhance pancreas stability and will further help the pancreas heal itself.

Viewed holistically, by the way, pancreatitis is less often a distinct condition than it is a part of a larger disease complex. A dog with some systemic illness, especially one that induces chronic vomiting, will usually have elevated pancreatic enzyme values. You can diagnose pancreatitis at that point and start pumping in the drugs—or you can focus on the larger complex. In my experience, as that larger problem eases in response to holistic measures, so, in most cases, will the pancreatitis.

Occasionally, pancreatitis may even be part of a healing crisis. Though it's unproven as yet, one theory of pancreatic function, according to Dr. Donald Kelly, is that the digestive enzymes have a second job—moonlighting, in a sense, as "janitors" to digest diseased cells, especially cancerous ones. In a healing crisis, when the body is engaged in an all-out effort to repel disease, especially with cancer, the pancreatic enzymes may be called on to work overtime. To be sure, careful diagnosis by a veterinarian familiar with healing crises is crucial in these cases, and if the pancreatitis grows too acute, even a holistic veterinarian may have to administer intravenous fluids, or even antibiotics. But drugs really should be a last resort, not only because they're usually unneeded, but because in my experience, the freer the use of the drugs, the greater the odds that the condition will become chronic. (I've studied the background of my cancer patients and found that a number of them actually did have a history of pancreatitis treated medically.) Have the drugs impaired the immune system in a general way? Or in suppressing the production of pancreatic enzymes, have they thwarted a quite specific means by which the body curbs the proliferation of diseased cells that lead to cancer? I don't know, but the association is disturbing.

Parvovirus

Though largely eradicated over the last two decades, presumably by vaccine, parvovirus still crops up here and there among dogs, and can be devastating when it does. In just a few hours, it can progress from high fever and vomiting to bloody diarrhea to death. Through the epidemic years of the 1970s and early 1980s, since I knew relatively little of holistic measures, I used all of the antibiotics and fluids available—along with prayer—to try to break the fever. Some dogs I saved; all too many, unfortunately, died. By the time I saw the last of my epidemic parvo cases, I'd begun delving into alternative therapies. When I brought them to bear, I found that my success rate shot up to nearly 100 percent. I used homeopathic remedies like "Bleeding" (BHI) to address the bloody diarrhea; its principal ingredient is phosphorus, known in homeopathy to stop hemorrhaging. As before, to maintain hydration, I kept the dogs on intravenous fluids, including high doses of vitamin C—as much as a gram per pound of body weight per day. If needed, I also put them on high doses of Kaopectate to coat the intestinal walls, whose outermost layers had been sloughed off by the extreme diarrhea (exposing the body to rapid toxic uptake, which is how parvo actually kills). Recognizing how effective the Kaopectate was, I went so far as to give them Kaopectate enemas, which further speeded the intestines' recovery. In about two days, the disease receded and the dogs survived.

I haven't seen much parvo since then. When I did, I used the same homeopathic remedy for bleeding, probably mixed with "Diarrhea" or "Intestine" and "Inflammation" (all from BHI). I'd also add the herb slippery elm, and to help reestablish healthy intestinal bacteria, I'd add lactobacillus acidophilus (either in fat-free yogurt or as separate supplements). If there was liver involvement, I'd use two herbs I've come to rely on: milk thistle and Tang Kuei 18. And to prevent the postviral scarring of heart tissue which parvo can bring on, I'd include vitamin E in the program.

Perhaps thanks to the vaccine, few owners will have to worry about parvovirus. They should, however, worry about the vaccine (see the discussion of it in Chapter Four). One inoculation in a dog's life is plenty, as far as I'm concerned. The current emphasis on three or four parvo shots in a dog's first year of life, followed by annual boosters, is excessive by any measure, and renders the dog that much more vulnerable to the chronic symptoms of vaccinosis. When the disease was epidemic, Rottweilers, who were considered extremely susceptible to parvo, were given half a dozen or more vaccines for it by four months of age; they now have a shockingly high incidence of cancer, particularly of bone and lymph cancer, especially among young members of the breed. Coincidence? I don't think so.

Rabies

If you're reading this entry because your dog or cat has rabies, there's nothing that I or any other veterinarian can do: rabies is a hideous, lethal disease, and because it can be spread to humans by the bite of a rabid animal, either your pet must be put to sleep immediately or he will die shortly.

Now: *Does* your pet have rabies? I'll bet you my house and car that he doesn't. And this is where a sane discussion of this dementia-producing disease really ought to begin.

On the matter of rabies' horrors, there's no debate. When the saliva-borne virus infects an animal or person through a bite, it travels inexorably up to the brain—sometimes in a week, sometimes in up to a year—where it produces severe mood shifts, either to violent rage or, as often, to catatonia, followed by dementia and death. This is a matter of grave concern, as is the fact that rabies can be spread from animal to human. Taken together, they're clear justification for the rabies vaccine's status as a legal requirement throughout the U.S. How often that vaccine should be given is, however, a very different matter.

Administered annually by law in many states, and by veterinarians' recommendation in most others, the rabies vaccine bombards a pet's immune system with alarming amounts of foreign substances. In cats, the vaccine has been linked to fibrosarcomas. In both cats and dogs, it contributes to chronic vaccinosis, as well as the rabies miasm (see Chapter Four). If you live in a state that does require annual rabies vaccination by law, all you can do is protest—or move. If you don't, let moderation, not the fearful images of rabid dogs from the movies, be your guide.

The fact is that rabies is as rarely reported today as polio. In my twenty-five years of veterinary practice, I haven't observed or treated *a single case* of it. Does the vaccine get all the credit? I think not. My own suspicion is that in certain species of wild animals—skunks, for one, raccoons for another—rabies is a latent virus that lives naturally in the population, erupting only rarely as the disease. Indeed, a trigger for it to erupt in those species may be none other than the vaccine itself, administered to these wild animals when the domestication of them as pets became a fad starting in the 1960s. This may have added enough rabies-modified antigens to a skunk's or raccoon's system to push the latent virus into activity. (I learned this from an associate who worked in Albany, New York, where the rabies control center is located; he was told this by a veterinarian who worked for New York State.) Then all it takes is finding one of these animals for the rabies scare to be born, and a sudden push to vaccinate all dogs, cats, and wildlife follows—even if they've been vaccinated within the last year, as in the case of Maggie, whose startling story appears in Chapter Four. As for the rare case of a rabid bat, say, biting a person and infecting her with rabies, it's true: those cases occur. Do we all submit to annual rabies vaccines as a result? Of course not!

So why should our pets?

Reproductive Problems

There's an easy way, of course, to prevent reproductive problems in male and female pets alike: neuter the males, spay the females. Though a first-time pet owner may wince, the fact is that these procedures are painlessly performed under anesthesia, with little or no observable lingering discomfort, and in no way prevent a pet from leading a long and happy life. All they do is keep your pet from adding offspring to a world so overpopulated with dogs and cats that as many as 5 million homeless pets must be put to sleep each year in the U.S. alone. Because of those numbers, I always urge a prospective pet owner to adopt from an animal shelter, thus saving a life that very likely would be lost, rather than buying a full-breed puppy or kitten that just as likely will find another home. I recognize, however, that some owners either want show animals, and intend to breed them, or have their hearts set on a particular breed, as at times have I, so that spaying and neutering are not always options. For that matter, some owners of mixed breeds are adamantly opposed to altering; their rationale is that it's not intended by nature. But then, neither is cancer, and the fact is that altering significantly decreases the incidence of mammary cancer in females, and prostate problems and cancer in males.

Owners who still choose not to alter their pets may have to deal with problems of the reproductive system. One of the most common in female dogs and cats is pyometra, essentially a pus-filled uterus. A pet with pyometra will be visibly ill, with loss of appetite, vomiting, pained whimpering and fever, and excessive urination. Open pyometra is so called because the cervix opens and the pus drains out of the vagina. Closed pyometra is more dangerous because the cervix stays closed and the pus builds up, distending the abdomen and easily becoming a life-threatening situation. The best—and sometimes only—course of action is spaying (removal of both the uterus and the ovaries), though the procedure is more difficult than in a healthy pet.

With mild cases, we can afford to remember that in general, the body discharges vaginally for a purpose: to expel toxicity. And the toxicity initially comes from within. The discharge, in other words, is not provoked by bacteria in the vaginal region; the bacterial growth is secondary to the toxic condition. Once this cause-and-effect process begins, the bacteria themselves produce toxins, making the condition more serious. Whenever I can, I try not to suppress the discharge so much as to help the body complete it and return to health. Both "Menstrual" and "Feminine" are homeopathic remedies from BHI which help balance the female reproductive organs; I usually add "Infection" (BHI) to this mixture. Also, red raspberry leaf tea is very good for supporting the uterus, and the glandular "Uterus" (Allergy Research) is a good supportive measure. These may deter toxins from backing up in deeper internal organs, or even from precipitating cancer. (I've noticed that in some of my successful cancer patients, one of the last stages of recovery is a vaginal discharge, even if the patient has already been spayed, as if the toxicity, which has accumulated over the patient's lifetime, now gets expelled in the healing process. This is another reason not to suppress these discharges earlier in life with antibiotics.) In its mildest form, pyometra is known as endometritis, and treatment would be the same as described above, though I'll also add propolis, the natural antibiotic, in case any bacteria are festering. And, to be sure, I will use an antibiotic indicated by the results of a culture of the discharge, when accumulation becomes life-threatening, or to save a valuable breeding bitch when spaying is not an option.

Among nursing mothers, a not uncommon condition is agalactia, a lack of milk. I've seen mothers' milk restored literally in minutes after administering the homeopathic combination "Lymph, Inflammation, and Exhaustion" (BHI).

With males, the most common problems of the reproductive system concern the prostate. One condition is a noncancerous growth called hyperplasia. Another is prostatitis, an infection of the prostrate. A third is prostate cancer. The best way to prevent all of these, as implied above, is castration. The owner adamantly opposed to altering will be sorry to learn that the best treatment for these problems is also castration. The condition of hyperplasia almost invariably heals within two weeks of neutering, and is unlikely at best to recur. Castration also diminishes prostate infections, and helps in the battle against prostate cancer.

Besides castration, treatment of these conditions includes "Prostate" (BHI) and "Inflammation" (BHI). I add "Infection" (BHI) where appropriate. There is also a Natra-Bio product called "Prostate-Difficult Urination," which I've used with positive results. A prostate glandular called "Prostaglan" (Progressive Labs) is useful. Generally, the mineral zinc and the herb saw palmetto are well known to aid in prostate problems, and are contained in the above-mentioned products. For difficult or nonresponsive infections, I will resort to antibiotics, the choice of which will be determined by a culture. For prostate cancer, I have had success supplementing these treatments with Immuno-Augmentative Therapy (IAT), as discussed in Chapter Eight.

Respiratory Problems

Pets, like people, get respiratory problems that range from common colds to pneumonia. In all but the most extreme cases, I avoid the use of antibiotics, which can suppress the symptoms but do so by killing the bacteria that are actually helping digest the toxic, mucous buildup in the respiratory system. Holistic treatment starts with the recognition that most respiratory infections are really signs of the body's healthy effort to expel toxicity, via mucus from the nose, sneezing, puffy red eyes with mucousy secretions, and coughing with phlegm. I put a pet with a cold on vitamin C tablets (for a thirty-pound dog, 500 milligrams three times a day; and half that much for a cat); the homeopathic liquid Grippheel (Heel); or homeopathic Pneumo Drops (Professional Health Products) if there is lung involvement. Garlic, goldenseal, and propolis, all with natural antibiotic properties, are also useful.

Pneumonia is a trickier issue. It doesn't appear too often in dogs and cats, probably for the simple anatomical reason that both species walk on four legs, with their lungs horizontal to the ground, so that mucus and the toxicity it contains are more likely expelled through the mouth and nose than in human beings, who have gravity working more against them. It's serious, however, when it does occur. Usually classified as either viral or bacterial, it results in labored breathing, coughing, lethargy, high fever, and, if allowed to progress to advanced stages, especially in older pets, may lead to a fatal congestion in the lungs. I'll treat life-threatening cases with antibiotics as quickly as any conventional veterinarian, but if I see it at an earlier stage, I'll first try the program of vitamins and homeopathics I use for colds, along with vitamin A, which acts as a lubricant for the lungs (and kidney and liver); I'll also use a lung glandular like "Pneumotrate" (Progressive Labs) and an injectable body-part homeopathic like "Pulmo Suis" (Heel). As important, I'll try to understand the context of the condition: to see it as part of the whole, or holistic, picture. If an X ray reveals congestion in the lungs and the pet has a fever and elevated white blood cell levels, certainly that's pneumonia. But if I've been treating a pet for cancer, say, or some other degenerative disease, and if the pet has been working hard to regain his health, marshaling strength and boosting his immune system, pneumonia-like symptoms *may* signal the onset of a healing crisis. I treated a boxer named Ginger for leukemia for six months; over a weekend, the dog developed symptoms of pneumonia, with violent nasal discharges and a very high fever. When the fever broke, the leukemia was gone; a healing crisis had occurred (see Chapter Six).

For dogs, the most common respiratory infection—besides colds—is kennel cough; for cats, it's feline viral rhinotracheitis (FVR). Both are irksome but easily treated.

Kennel cough, often called bordetella bronchiseptica, is characterized by a dry, hacking cough with frequent gagging. Though it's not life-threatening and tends to run its course in a few days to a week, kennel cough is frustrating for pet and owner alike. Because of its high incidence in kennels and animal hospitals, where dogs are kept in close proximity and tend to infect one another once a concentration of the organism has reached unnatural levels in the immediate environment, a bordetella vaccine is commonly given to puppies at as young as six weeks. To my mind, this is unnecessary on three counts. First, the vaccine is probably useless and may even provoke symptoms of kennel cough. Second, it can be immunosuppressive (as in the case of Wilhelm the Great discussed in Chapter Four). Third, kennel cough can easily be treated by isolating the afflicted puppy and putting him on a program of homeopathic remedies like "Cough," "Bronchitis" (both from BHI), and "Cough" (Professional Health Products). These combination remedies all contain homeopathic ingredients such as bryonia and drosera, both excellent for cough-related conditions. The Swiss company Similasan has three different homeopathic cough preparations (called #1, #2, and #3), each for a slightly different kind of cough, labeled for humans but useful for pets. As a complement to these, herbal cough syrups can help; a brand I use a lot is Olbas, which is available at health food stores.

Coughing also characterizes feline viral rhinotracheitis, though the dominant symptom is sneezing, along with thick nasal discharge and gummy secretions from the eyes, and fever, as in a flu. If the symptoms are making the cat acutely miserable, antibiotics will alleviate them (antibiotics don't fight viruses but do address the secondary bacterial infections that viruses can provoke in immune-suppressed patients), but the only way to speed the virus on its course is to initiate a liquid fast of chicken or vegetable broth, supplemented by vitamins A (2,500 IU) and C (250 milligrams, three times daily), garlic and goldenseal, and the homeopathic Grippheel (Heel), "Cold and Flu" (BHI), and propolis. As with bordetella, a vaccine is available; its record of efficacy is no more impressive, however, and so best not used.

The worst respiratory problem is, of course, lung cancer. For treatment, I use all the supplements listed above, plus Immuno-Augmentative Therapy (see Chapter Eight).

Skin Problems

The three most common problems I see are, without question, cancer, arthritis, and conditions of the skin; and for years, skin problems topped the list. (Cancer, unfortunately, has superseded it.) That the skin should be disrupted so often, and in such various ways, is nothing if not logical. The skin is an eliminative organ as much as the liver, kidneys, and intestines; that's why it's sometimes nicknamed "the third kidney."

The most common skin conditions I see are allergic in nature. As the immune system's antibodies react to an unwanted allergen in the body, the skin often grows inflamed, red, and itchy, appearing as "hot spots" or rashes. A second kind of skin condition is pustules, usually diagnosed as a chronic staphylococcal infection. A third kind, more often seen in dogs than in cats, is flaky, smelly, or greasy skin, often accompanied by matted, foul-smelling hair or regions of hairlessness; usually this is the result of poor diet, vaccinosis, or both, and appears especially in overweight dogs.

The therapeutic approach I take for these different conditions is consistent, just tailored somewhat to each set of symptoms. With all, I'll do the Bio Nutritional Analysis to determine the internal cause of the problem, and address those imbalances accordingly. I'll also take a pet off commercial foods and put him on the natural diet outlined in Chapter Three; many skin problems respond quickly to a change in diet alone. For allergic inflammation, I'll use the remedies discussed above, under "Allergies." For pustules, I'll use BHI's "Skin" or "Sulfaheel" (Heel), mixed with BHI's "Infection." For smelly, thickened skin and greasy hair, I'll use BHI's "Hair and Skin," or "Psorinoheel" (Heel). Both a change in diet and vaccine schedule are also critical. To the natural diet I'll add cold-pressed safflower oil, available at health food stores, because the flaky skin is evidence of lost free fatty acids. Flaxseed and sesame oil are good, too, especially if the pet has an immune deficiency; both are immune-enhancing. One product I've had impressive success with, and which my pets love, is Animal Essentials (see source guide).

All skin problems benefit from regular use of an herbal shampoo. Oatmeal shampoos are generally soothing. Those that contain calendula, plantain, and aloe are all anti-inflammatory. I also favor the herbal-based shampoos containing tee tree oil, including ProCare (Melaleuca), because they work like medical shampoos without chemical ingredients.

Finally, a three-day liquid fast is wonderfully restorative for skin problems. Since any skin disruption is evidence of the body's efforts to eliminate toxins, a fast can speed up the process considerably, enhancing the flushing out of foreign bacteria and other unwanted agents. It takes a lot of energy to eat, digest, metabolize, and assimilate food—energy that during a fast can be expended entirely by the body on elimination. I don't do much fasting in my practice only because so many of the pets I see are in dire straits. At home, however, I put my own dogs and cats on one-day fasts every few weeks. Far from being enervated by the process, they're galvanized by it, and are jumping around with energy by the time it nears an end. Just be aware that because of the enhancement of the detoxification process as a result of the fast, your pet may experience a temporary worsening of symptoms which should shortly subside, either after more toxins have been expelled or with the resumption of feeding, which slows down the elimination process.

Spinal Problems

The most common spinal conditions I see are spondylosis and intervertebral disc disease (or slipped discs). Spondylosis is essentially an arthritic condition between two vertebrae, in which a mineral deposit eventually fuses the bones together by forming a bony bridge between them. Rigid when meant to be flexible, the spaces between the vertebrae grow inflamed, causing pain and usually impaired mobility of the legs, especially the hind legs. If severe enough, there can be an inflammatory response from them, leading to neurological deficit symptoms. Though considered a condition of aging dogs, I've seen it appear with depressing regularity among young dogs, apparently the result of toxic accumulations in the body, often from a bad diet, probably also from environmental pollutants, genetic predispositions, and vaccinations. The slipped disc syndrome, especially common in the dachshund, involves similar symptoms, but they're usually more severe.

Acupuncture, not surprisingly, is the treatment of choice to relieve immediate pain and restore some measure of flexibility, and is effective in reversing paralysis in those dogs who have had a severely ruptured disc. "Traumeel" or "Zeel" (Heel), injected at relevant acupuncture points, also helps address this condition. As therapeutic as it is, however, acupuncture may not be curative. I've found that these conditions respond better, with less likelihood of recurrence, when the following supplements are added: "Back" (BHI), Liquidamber 15 (Seven Forests), and Vetri-Disc (Vetri-Science Labs). Old male dogs with hind-leg weakness are especially helped by the homeopathic remedy conium maculatum (200 C is the potency I start with). Severe cases may need a three-day series of intravenous fluids, including high doses of vitamin C, to flush intracellular toxicity out of the body. There tends to be an associated elevated level of alkaline phosphatase in these patients, which the vitamin C's ascorbic acid buffers. At the site of pressure imbalance along the spine, I also inject a "cocktail" of B vitamins and adrenal cortex, along with injectable spinal cord ("Medulla Spinalis" by Heel) or intervertebral disc ("Discus Intervertebralis," also by Heel), if so indicated.

Spondylosis shows up on an X ray of the spine. A spinal infarction, or blood clot, does not, because it's within the spinal cord tissue itself. The symptoms, however, like those of a severely ruptured disc, are dramatically sudden paralysis and a rapid loss of deep pain perception. This is a debilitating condition that often ends with permanent paralysis, necessitating a wheelchair-like contraption for the pet, or euthanasia. However, in the one case of this rare condition which I've treated—an Old English sheepdog named Chloe—I had encouraging results from using intravenous fluids high in vitamin C, along with intravenous ozone and the injectable "cocktail"—plus phosphatidyl-serine, which appears to enhance the repair of the myelin covering of the nervous system. To supplement these therapies, I conducted sessions of electrical acupuncture: hooking the needles up to a battery generator to send electrical impulses through them to the relevant spinal acupuncture points. In twenty-four hours, the dog's deep pain perception, seemingly lost, began to return. In two weeks, the dog was actually up and walking. And continues to do so on her program of metabolic supplements and spinal-cord-specific products.

Trauma/Injuries

Any injury with potential severity, especially those caused by a motor vehicle, should be seen immediately by a veterinarian. The range of injuries that cause trauma is too broad to be considered here in detail, and the measures needed to address them are not, as a rule, ones that a layman should undertake. (Splinting a broken leg, for example, ought to be left to a veterinarian if at all possible.) The common thread in these conditions, however, is inflammation with associated pain. Almost invariably, once the medical emergency is eased, I use injectable "Traumeel" (Heel), as well as injectable adrenal cortex. Topical "Traumeel" ointment elicits good response. For pain and inflammation control orally, I use a combination of "Traumeel" and "Inflammation" (BHI-Heel). Professional Health Products has a good preparation called "Injury Drops," as well as one called "Post-Surgical Drops," when the inflammation is caused by surgery. Herbally, I've had success with myrrh tablets (Seven Forests), and "Anti-Flam"

(Crystal Star). "Anti-Flam" contains white willow bark, which has an effect similar to aspirin (indeed, aspirin is derived in part from white willow bark). As an old standby, echinacea, available from any health food store or pharmacy, is helpful.

Worms

Nearly all puppies and kittens are born with intestinal worms of one sort or another. Apparently the worms become chronic in the mother in an encysted form, like granules within a capsule. During the stress of pregnancy, the cysts break and the worms gain access to the fetus. Among kittens and puppies, the most presenting sign is a potbelly, which develops as the worms consume protein; because protein helps keep fluid in the blood vessels, a protein deficiency caused by worms leads to leakage into the patient's abdomen. Roundworms are visible as white, squiggly, spaghetti-like strings in the feces or vomit. Whip-worms and hookworms, on the other hand, are too small to be seen by the unpracticed eye. A fourth kind, tapeworms, are spread by fleas, though dogs in particular can get the other kinds of worms by licking another animal's feces, often from their paws. Tapeworms are usually seen as flat, rice-like granules appearing around the anus.

Of the four kinds, whipworms and hookworms are the most serious, the latter especially, as it's a bloodsucker that can bring on a severe bloody stool and anemia. Both kinds in extreme cases can be lethal. Roundworms, though less serious and rarely lethal, can cause chronic diarrhea and vomiting, and among mature pets lead to weight loss.

Some holistic veterinarians avoid chemical dewormers at all costs. I feel this is one condition that conventional medicine treats effectively, without undue toxicity, and so I'll use them, especially when alternatives I've tried produce little improvement. I don't use injectable dewormers for reasons that to me seem a matter of common sense: why go through the bloodstream to fight an intestinal worm when an ingested dewormer goes right to the source without using the blood as a delivery vehicle? I do, however, use any number of commercial ingestible dewormers (the brands are too numerous to name; obviously, start with the least toxic products available). For owners averse to inflicting even these modest chemicals on their pets, I recommend an herbal liquid dewormer called Wormafuge (Medicine Wheel). Among other ingredients, it contains black walnut and garlic, both central to any herbal dewormer because they kill parasites. (It also has cascara sagrada, a surefire stimulant of bowel function, to help expel the worms and some of the congestive toxins upon which the worms live that much more quickly.) The only reason I don't use Wormafuge more often myself is that it has a truly vile taste. Feed it to a pet and you get a reaction of real revulsion.

Whichever dewormer you choose, it becomes the first step in a two-step process. The first step is to kill the worms. The second is to clean out the intestines. A congested intestine is a breeding ground for parasites; a clean one provides protection from them. Other products I use are Homeo Helminth (Dolisos), which actually contains homeopathic onion, and the herbal Worm Parasite formula by an impressive new company called Quantum. Along with black walnut and garlic, the formula contains wormwood (an herb), pumpkin seeds, cloves, and male fern root—all top performers on the herbal deworming list. The herbalist Hannah Kroeger also has two good formulas, Rascal and Wormwood Combination (Kroeger).

If the worms become chronic, I favor using high levels of garlic, both in its liquid Kyolic form and as diced cloves put in a pet's every meal. A diet—natural, to be sure—ought to include a hefty share of fiber-rich grains, which help clean out the intestines. And if you've avoided the commercial dewormers in favor of an herbal approach, consider, in this case, trying the medicine. The fact is, I've seen no sign of ill effects from it, and it does get rid of worms. If the worms your pet has are hookworms or whipworms, you may have no choice.

CHAPTER EIGHT

Taking on Cancer

Every time I go to my clinic, I know I'm going to see cancer. There may be three cases, there may be five; on a bad day, there may be more. For better or worse, treating cancer is what I do more than anything else, and what I'm known for now. I guess it's what I'll do for the rest of my life, or until it's conquered. Believe me, there's no shortage of it out there.

This isn't what I intended when I chose to become a veterinarian years ago. I imagined extracting thorns from dogs' paws, setting broken legs, stitching wounds—in short, being the kindly vet who treated a pet with an obvious problem and made him feel better, probably in the mountains of Colorado (playing my guitar every night after work). As I began my practice, however, degenerative diseases were on the rise, both in dogs and in cats, with cancer emerging as the most prevalent of the lot. The cancers I saw were usually in old pets, as I'd been taught to expect. But that was beginning to change, too.

At first, I applied the therapies I'd learned in school, which meant surgery to remove cancerous tumors. Like other veterinarians, I found my success rate to be abysmally, depressingly low. Occasionally, I'd refer patients out for radiation and chemotherapy. The odds weren't much better. Nearly all pets with cancer died of it—unless they were put to sleep first. Out of desperation, I started experimenting with alternatives as part of my shift toward holistic therapy, working closely with my veterinarian brother, Robert, and his wife, Susan, who shared my frustrations about conventional medicine in general and cancer in particular. We began to get cases deemed hopeless by local animal hospitals—not so much by referral, since most veterinarians viewed our efforts with scorn, as by word of mouth, as owners sought us out on their own. We had some success from the first, but also more disappointments than triumphs. Then we discovered the missing piece—Dr. Lawrence Burton's Immuno-Augmentative Therapy (IAT)—and everything changed.

Today, our success rate with cancer patients stands at above 50 percent, a rate that would be higher still if we chose not to treat pets with truly bleak prospects, which we do as a matter of course. Because the program we've developed is available nowhere else in the U.S. as yet, we get cancer patients from around the country. Many pets are brought to us from out of state; many more we treat long-distance by serving as consultants to their attending veterinarians. Long-distance treatment is made easier than it might otherwise be because IAT therapy is based on analyzing blood samples sent to us, then formulating via computer a program of injections of isolated immune proteins, based on certain values in the blood, to be given at home. Dealing with cancer as much as we have over the years and delving into the histories of many patients, we've come to feel we understand many of the factors that help foster it, and to feel confident that its last secrets will soon be revealed.

I don't *like* seeing cancer every day. But I love helping cancer patients recover enough to lead happy, relatively normal lives. And I've come to appreciate how fitting it is that cancer should be the focus of my work. It is, in an odd, almost poetic way, the perfect disease for a holistic doctor to fight. In whatever part of the body it appears, it's the ultimate expression of ill health, a result of the body's failure as a whole—a *holistic* failure—to keep itself healthy. Which is also to say that with cancer, more dramatically than with any other disease I know, the road to recovery lies in restoring the integrity of health overall, and of the immune system specifically.

When I see a new cancer patient, the first thing I tell his owner is: Don't think of cancer as a foreign invader that's attacked your pet out of nowhere. Cancer doesn't really exist as an entity in itself, as a thing that attacks. It's not a cause so much as it is an effect. Think of it as the body out of tune with itself. Focus on health. See cancer for what it is.

Cancer is the ultimate excuse to get healthy.

In conventional medicine, of course, cancer *is* an invader that must be zapped as quickly and thoroughly as possible. I'm skeptical of radiation and chemotherapy for pets because the rationale behind them seems suspect. If cancer is the result of an immune deficiency or a suppressed immune system, then why use agents known to be immunosuppressive themselves to treat the condition? If part of your house was on fire, would you remedy the situation by putting a match to the other half? The drugs administered in chemotherapy attack *all* fast-growing cells, including white blood cells throughout the body, hair follicles, the lining of the intestine, and, in patients not altered, the gonadal cells. This is why the commonly listed side effects of chemo are hair loss, severe gastroenteritis with hemorrhaging, sterility, and suppressed white blood counts, low enough not to protect the body from routine bacteria. Radiation's risks are subtler. Treatment tends to be concentrated on a specific area, the rays can't be felt, and they cause no immediate systemic side effects. However, after a typical radiation protocol for a dog or cat of three treatments a week for six weeks, I've seen healthy tissue adjacent to the radiation sites become permanently damaged. I've seen cancers return and become more aggressive than they were before treatment. I've also seen tissue of the radiated sites literally fall apart. Are these risks worth taking?

But that's not all. Each radiation treatment is performed under general anesthesia. The radiation is bad enough, but then imagine aggravating it with general anesthesia eighteen times in less than a two-month period. Imagine having your own healthy young pet (or even yourself!) placed under anesthesia that many times in a short period, each time zapping him with high doses of radiation. How do you think he (or you) would feel? How much weaker do you think his (or your) immune system would be at the end of the day? In too many cases, *unacceptably* weaker, especially as the production of disease-causing free radicals is tremendously enhanced by the ionizing effect of the radiation.

Moreover, even if the tumor is eradicated through chemo or radiation, where does that leave the pet? In a lesser state of health than the one he was in before their debilitating effects. *A lesser state, that is, than the one he was in when he developed cancer in the first place.* To me, the only rationale for either of these treatments is to accomplish initial treatment of a cancer condition that is life-threatening, or when the statistics for success leading to healthier, prolonged lives support it for that cancer type. These cases certainly occur, and I do recommend radiation or chemo when I see them and know that there isn't enough time for alternative therapies to work. I have witnessed impressive benefits from conventional treatment for cancer. But my experience still cautions me against the use of the more invasive therapies. As soon as I can, I try to curtail them.

Mysterious as its origins are usually said to be, cancer simply begins in the body when one cell becomes corrupted: a cell that should replicate itself in the ongoing process of cell life called mitosis, but which instead spawns a mutant cell that runs amok with others. The mutant cells that radiation zaps are cancer's foundation. Its *cause* is whatever led that first cell to become mutant, as well as whatever kept the body from controlling cells *after* they mutated. Most likely, a combination of the two is involved. Unaddressed by conventional treatment, how likely is that cause to precipitate cancer again in a weaker host? *Very.*

What *is* the cause? The temptation is to picture some dark force from outside, pushing the cell to corruption. Certainly in people many cancers appear to begin that way: from chemically polluted drinking water or the radiation from overhead power lines to the effects of smoking and chronic stress. The forces are real, and if strong enough, a body subjected to them *will* get cancer. Pour enough PCBs into your daily drinking water and you'll get cancer. Live long enough near Chernobyl and you'll get cancer. Yet in situations less extreme, why do some people and pets become afflicted with cancer while others do not? A family history of cancer may suggest an inherited predisposition, but even in cancer-prone families, not everyone succumbs. In people, smoking may contribute, but again, not everyone who smokes gets lung cancer. (And pets, in any event, are pretty much exempt from the dangers of primary smoke.) To my brother and me, already drawn to the principles of holistic therapy, the cause of cancer in pets began to seem not so much an outside force as an absence of inner force—the inner force, that is, of the immune system.

Ironically, we arrived at that theory by means of a technique my brother had perfected to zap certain tumors considered inaccessible to surgery, more quickly and thoroughly even than radiation or chemotherapy. A longer discussion of cryosurgery appears in Chapter Five; essentially, it involves freezing a tumor with liquid nitrogen or special metal probes so that the diseased tissues get rejected and fall away, leaving healthy tissue behind. Unfortunately, while cryosurgery provided less invasive relief with few side effects or complications, the tumors tended to grow back. Perhaps, we thought, the immune system needed strengthening to do the work of keeping the body healthy after cryosurgery—the work we couldn't do.

At the time, the best way we knew to boost the immune system was through fasting or high doses of intravenous vitamin C. As soon as a fast begins, the body stops expending its energy on digestion and uses it instead to begin cleansing itself of toxicity that may be inhibiting the immune system. Vitamin C was the most immuno-supportive natural supplement we had at hand, and we were mindful of the success that holistic veterinarian Wendell O. Belfield was having in arresting or reversing other degenerative diseases with megadoses of intravenous C. One of our first test cases was a twenty-four-pound poodle. It taught us a lot.

The poodle had been brought to our clinic with a bone tumor in the mouth. Twice the tumor had been excised by conventional surgery; twice it had grown back more aggressively than before. More radical surgery would mean removing part of the jaw that adjoined the tumor, and for this pet, that wasn't a good option. Cryosurgery could freeze the tumor even though it was in the bone, so that it held special promise for oral cancers in pets. Unfortunately in the case of the poodle, my brother had no better luck than the operating surgeon. The bone remained intact after each of two procedures, supported by intravenous vitamin C, but the tumor grew back. At that point, we had nothing to lose. We decided to put the poodle on a liquid fast of juices, broths, and distilled water—the same fast that we had undergone to such good effect on our own health.

After ten days of fasting, the tumor showed a slower growth rate. After fourteen days, it began to soften. During this time, we monitored the poodle's vital signs and they stayed excellent. She had great energy and color, and her spirits, too, appeared very high. Finally, on the sixteenth day, the tumor began to shrink and break apart. We felt we were witnessing a natural miracle. On an almost hourly basis, we gathered to observe the tumor diminishing. By Day 18, we thought, the tumor would be gone.

On the seventeenth day, the poodle died.

In the somber aftermath, we realized our mistake. Holistic as our intent was, we'd retained our focus, as conventionally trained veterinarians, on wiping out the symptom—the tumor—as quickly as possible, in this case at the expense of the dog's overall health. The cancer, in breaking up, had flooded the body with more toxicity than it could handle, especially since the rest of the body had been so cleansed from the fast. The liver, the body's primary detoxifier, had been overwhelmed. The dog hadn't died of cancer. She hadn't starved to death, either; even on the next to last day she was full of energy, and she still had good muscle mass on her body. She had died of a sudden overload of toxicity which her liver simply couldn't handle.

Clearly we should have stopped the fast the day before. The process of detoxification would have stopped or slowed along with it, relaxing the pressure of tumor breakdown and allowing the liver to "catch up." Perhaps the tumor would have grown back a bit, but so what? The fast could resume later, when the liver would be ready again to process more of the tumor's toxicity. Later, we would see that a march of two steps forward, one step back, mimics the body's own healing process: first a strong attack on the cancer cells, then a modest retreat to let the body regain its balance, then another attack. We had fixated on beating the tumor in the shortest possible time. But why? If overall there was progress—two steps forward, one step back—what did it matter if we took three years, rather than three weeks, to neutralize the threat? The body as a whole, we realized, had to be our guide. We could treat cancer only as quickly as the body allowed.

At the same time, we felt sure now that we were on the right course—away from radiation and chemotherapy. I hit on an analogy that's stayed with me, about a high school janitor. As long as the janitor works his regular night shift, the school remains clean. What happens if he gets sick and fails to show up for work? Soon students and teachers arriving in the morning will find the school filled with papers and debris. But the garbage has not "attacked" the school any more than cancer "attacks" a body. How does conventional medicine respond? By burning all the papers! Not only does that put the whole school building at risk, it fails to solve the problem. Soon enough, more papers and debris will collect. Far more useful to get the janitor well, and put him back to work.

The janitor, in this analogy, as you may have guessed, is the immune system.

Other doctors, as it happened, were also starting to focus on the immune system's role in cancer treatment, and on the liver's importance in that effort. One was Max Gerson, whose book *Fifty Cures* recounted his success with fifty human patients using raw animal liver. Basically, Gerson put the liver in a blender and had his patients drink the result. Rich with unadulterated enzymes and other immune components, his concoctions seemed to support the liver, which could then do a better job of detoxifying the body, helping the immune system so that it, in turn, could better fight the cancer. We saw some success using Gerson's drinks, though when he died and his daughter took over his program, the drinks seemed to lose their potency for the patients. Finally the daughter realized why: instead of getting her livers from South American livestock, as her father had done, she'd used a U.S. distributor. Unfortunately, U.S. livestock absorbed far more toxicity—via commercial feeds, crop pesticides, and water and air pollution—than their South American counterparts, and their livers, as a result, were degraded and toxic. She switched back to Argentinian and Peruvian sources and her success rate rose again.

Eccentric as it sounds, we also found that coffee enemas stimulated the liver and helped it eliminate toxic wastes. An enema of body-temperature black organic coffee acts first as a solvent for wastes accumulated in the colon. The caffeine in it also excites the peristaltic action of the intestinal muscle, causing it to contract and expand more vigorously, removing more wastes. As the coffee filters up through the intestines, other wastes are sloughed off. And then, because the intestines work with the liver in a mini-circulatory system (called the portal circulation), the coffee actually goes directly to the liver, stimulating its function with caffeine and helping it break down the toxins the body has channeled into it. The cleaner the liver, the stronger the immune system. Coffee enemas are commonplace in the East; a prominent East Indian nutritionist, when asked at a lecture in Connecticut for his opinion on coffee consumption, grinned and said, "There's nothing wrong with coffee. It's just that you Westerners don't know what hole to put it in!"

In our search for a balance between fasting and immune support, we found coffee enemas to be a useful tool, and for a while administered them to several of our cancer patients. (We followed them with yogurt enemas, on the theory that the coffee might wipe out the colon's beneficial as well as its destructive bacteria, so that the yogurt, with its healthful bacteria, could restore the cleaned-out colon and intestine to perfect health.) When other alternatives appeared promising, we tried them, too, Laetrile (vitamin B_{17}) prominent among them. Each of these "miracle cures" had some validity; each had cured a few people of cancer, perhaps more than a few. Unfortunately, the vast majority of human patients—and pets—failed to respond to them. By using the "cures" in creative combinations, we pushed our success rate up to about 20 percent. These were pets whose local veterinarians had given up and recommended euthanasia, so 20 percent was a lot better than zero percent. But we wanted to do better than let four out of five of our cancer patients die.

The breakthrough came by chance. In 1982, my brother and his wife, Susan, went on vacation to the Bahamas. In a Bahamian newspaper, my brother saw an article about an American doctor named Lawrence Burton who'd set up a cancer clinic to treat human patients in a novel way. After years of research, Burton had isolated certain proteins in the immune system which played a key role, he felt, in controlling mutant cell growth. His approach, in essence, was to analyze the relationships between those proteins in a cancer patient and redress imbalances with a series of injections, so that the proteins could do the work of regulating the cancer themselves. He called his process Immuno-Augmentative Therapy because he managed to balance the proteins he found deficient or malfunctioning, *augmenting* or enhancing the immune system enough to battle the cancer into submission.

My brother was intrigued. On the face of it, this seemed exactly the means he needed to boost the immune systems of pets with cancer, so that his cryosurgery, along with our other complementary approaches, would have enduring results. He went over to the clinic, identified himself, and asked to see Dr. Burton. The receptionist grimaced. "Dr. Burton sees no one," she said. Later, my brother would learn that Burton had grown bitter and defensive after his ideas were rejected by the U.S. medical establishment, and perhaps a bit paranoid, too. Still, my brother left his card with the phone number of his hotel scrawled on it. Later that day, Burton called and invited him back. The two sat down to a talk that stretched over many hours. The result, for my brother, was the start of a satellite program of Burton's methods for pets at Smith Ridge.

The program started that year with a few pets for whom no other therapy, conventional or holistic, had worked. From Burton, my brother obtained a start-up supply of protein serums. In those precomputer, prefax days, the pets' blood samples were shipped to a mailbox in Miami, picked up for Dr. Burton by a courier who worked for a casino in the Bahamas, and analyzed at Burton's IAT clinic, with the results conveyed to Smith Ridge by phone, followed by express mail. For each case, a specific amount of each of the four proteins would be given, with each measurement changing on a daily basis as the balance of proteins in the blood changed. Over the course of one week, forty such measurements would be relayed—determining the content of forty injections.

To me, at first, the process seemed overwhelming, and possibly absurd. This was my brother's latest kick, not mine. I hardly had time to listen to him explain the basics of how the treatment worked, much less do the scientific reading that might have convinced me there was merit in it. In fact, I was juggling four jobs and still struggling to pay the bills. By now, most of what I preferred to practice was holistic medicine, and in the early 1980s, there was a price to pay for that: only truly desperate or eccentric pet owners sought me out. To make ends meet, I'd start the week at my brother's clinic—the genesis of what Smith Ridge is today, but in a space that was, I remember exactly, 298 square feet. Monday evening, after a full day working for my brother, I'd report for a night shift at an emergency clinic in White Plains, then work a third job at my friend Howard Rothstein's practice two hours away outside Woodstock, New York, only to put in another two-hour ride for another emergency-room shift in Queens, New York. Then one more shift at my brother's clinic. Which is to say that from Monday morning to Wednesday evening, I rarely slept. I could have found a full-time job as a conventional veterinarian, but I didn't want to do that. Holistic medicine felt right to me. I was sure it had enormous promise, and I was willing to make the necessary sacrifices until the right opportunity came up. I just wasn't sure that the Burton method was any better than simple fasting and intravenous vitamin C.

When my brother told me that five of the first eight pets on the program appeared to improve, I saw that he might be on to something. Then came the case that galvanized me, one that began not in his then tiny clinic but in the White Plains emergency room. A mid-sized, mixed-breed dog, twelve and a half years old, arrived one night in total heart failure. An electrocardiogram revealed only a few normal heartbeats; the dog's breathing was terribly labored. I recommended putting the dog to sleep, but her owner, a New Age-y woman, refused. She asked me, rather sternly, if I knew of any holistic veterinarians in the area. "Yeah, *me*," I said. "But an emergency room isn't the place for holistic medicine, and anyway I think your dog is too far gone." I said that if she wanted, she could take her dog to my brother's clinic for holistic therapy, but that my personal recommendation was euthanasia.

The owner was adamant. As a last resort, I sent her to the Animal

Medical Center, the area's largest conventional veterinary hospital, which also had twenty-four-hour emergency service. As an emergency measure, the sac around the dog's heart was drained of blood, but again the recommendation was euthanasia. Their diagnosis: pericardial hemangiosarcoma, or severe cancer of this area. Instead, the owner did take her dog to my brother's clinic, where she was put on Dr. Burton's Immuno-Augmentative Therapy, plus at least a dozen supplements. Months later, having forgotten about the case altogether, I began working at my brother's clinic. One of my first cases was that same mixed-breed dog, in for a routine follow-up visit to have a blood sample drawn for IAT monitoring. I was shocked. Here was a case I'd deemed truly hopeless, yet the dog appeared healthy, in clinical remission with a good-sounding heart.

That dog went on to live until the age of seventeen and a half—fully five years beyond the night of her trip to the emergency room.

With this case, seeing was believing. And yet no small doubt remained. This was *cancer*, after all. The big C. Even if Burton's program beat it in a few cases, the majority would probably die, and his protein injections would be put in the same category as all those other alternative therapies: promising, but hardly conclusive.

Then came the first case I put on the Burton program myself. Pinky was a white standard poodle, eleven years old. I'd just taken over ownership of the clinic from my brother—this was April 1984. The Burton program was mine to continue or perhaps not, depending on what results I saw with Pinky and the next dozen or so cases.

Certainly Pinky presented a formidable test-case challenge. In a course of conventional treatment which had cost his owner more than $7,000, he had had a malignant tumor of the abdomen called an anaplastic sarcoma excised surgically, then gone on chemotherapy. A ruptured spleen months later had seemed a sorry coincidence until doctors, in removing the spleen, discovered lymph cancer. When they removed a bit of bone marrow for analysis—a bone "aspiration"— they learned that the dog also had grade III lymphosarcoma. This dog was *sick*. And to the veterinarians at the University of Pennsylvania, where he was being treated, his case came to be seen as hopeless.

When the case was presented to me, Pinky's red blood cell count, which in a normal dog is about 40 percent of total blood volume, had dropped to 17 percent. As a result of all the chemotherapy he had received, the skin was literally sloughing off his muzzle. Often when the dog defecated, he fainted. I finished my examination, looked hard at the medical history, and also recommended euthanasia. The owner, a Peekskill, New York, woman named Ann Bland, refused. "I just love this dog too much," she said. "If you love this dog," I said, "put him to sleep." But Ann said no.

Reluctantly, I gave a sample of Pinky's blood to my brother, who was headed down to Burton's clinic in the Bahamas with samples from other ongoing cases to pick up a new supply of therapeutic serums. Over the next three days, I tried homeopathic remedies and supplements on Pinky; his condition remained the same. Then my brother called from Burton's clinic to give me the blood results from all the patients. About Pinky, he said, "Burton thinks this dog is going to do well."

"If that's what he thinks, then get the next plane off the island," I said. I was flabbergasted. How could I possibly represent his prognosis as good to Ann when the dog's condition was so obviously terminal? Instead, I shared my grave doubts with Ann, but did tell her that Burton felt Pinky's immune system was blocked, and that if "released," he might respond. I thought we should go ahead with the injections Burton prescribed—but only because we had nothing to lose.

Within twenty-four hours of his first series of injections, Pinky got up unaided, began walking around his home, and ate a full meal. He also stopped fainting.

I couldn't believe it.

In retrospect, Pinky's recovery was unusual even by Burton's standards: only about 2 percent of the cases treated by IAT do so well so dramatically fast. But Pinky's woes weren't over. Seemingly on the mend for two months, he suddenly slipped into a coma, the result of a sudden drop in red blood cells. Again I recommended euthanasia. Again Ann Bland refused. This time Pinky was given a transfusion at the emergency clinic in White Plains where I'd once worked. Pinky perked up for another month or so, then dropped into another coma. For the third time, I recommended euthanasia; for the third time, Ann refused. When Pinky defied the odds and perked up again, only to plummet after nearly six months, I gave the next and last transfusion he needed. At last, the recovery took: Pinky died at almost fifteen, not of cancer but of old age.

Six months after Pinky's initial series of injections, I harbored no more doubts about continuing Burton's program at Smith Ridge. Our success rate with cancer, especially with cases deemed hopeless, had nearly tripled since we started on it. To my knowledge, no other veterinarian in the country could report results anywhere near as good. As yet, however, I'd still not met the mysterious doctor himself. Clearly it was time to pay a visit.

The clinic lay in downtown Freeport, not far from the Bahamian Princess hotel. Uncontrolled tourism and the casinos had taken their toll: Freeport even then was a rambling hodgepodge without much civic beauty, and as I'd been warned, it wasn't too safe. Yet Burton's clinic proved to be a clean, modern, low-rise building imbued with a sense of sanctuary. Inside, the clinic was immaculate, with all the professional decor of a top-tier U.S. facility. From my brother, I knew that Burton worked not in some beautiful corner office but in a windowless cubbyhole redolent of pipe smoke. When I knocked on his open door, he was just lighting one of perhaps two dozen pipes he kept in a rack on his desk, the lit pipe protruding from a thick gray beard beneath very intense, rather suspicious eyes. Short and barrel-chested, he had the wary demeanor of a barroom regular who wouldn't hesitate to leap into a fight. Pinned to the wall behind him were two posters. One was a drawing of Albert Einstein's head and wavy curls, with what had already become my favorite declaration: "Great spirits have always encountered violent opposition from mediocre minds." The other showed a hawk descending with talons extended on a mouse. One talon was labeled the American Cancer Society. The other was labeled the National Cancer Institute. As for the mouse, it bravely stood its ground, making a rather obscene gesture at the hawk. It wore a sweatshirt that read "Dr. Burton." I looked from Burton to the posters and back again into those eyes. *This guy is right on,* I thought.

As we began to talk, Burton swung around to demonstrate the hulking computer at his side. For months, I'd received printouts from this machine. When the blood samples for each cancer case were analyzed, a computer model churned out exact measurements for each of the four critical cancer factors in the blood which the pet in question should be given by injection, day by day, week by week, to redress the imbalances that were allowing the cancer to grow. The therapy seemed eminently logical, and to hear Burton go on about it—once started, with a sympathetic audience, he would talk for hours—I felt its effectiveness was beyond question.

As a medical researcher at St. Vincent's Hospital in New York City in the late 1950s and early 1960s, Burton had made steady, quiet progress in a new approach to understanding cancer using fruit flies, then laboratory mice. The premise he sought to prove was that animals (including man) possess a network of proteins in their immune systems whose job it is to quell cancer. Most animals do develop mutant cells, Burton felt, but in most, the special proteins avert the threat before it leads to the runaway effect we know as cancer. Burton isolated one of these proteins, which he called a tumor antibody, and injected it into mice with significant mammary tumors. He saw tangible improvement.

From there, Burton theorized that a second substance must be involved, one that emanated from the cancerous cells to alert the antibodies to the need to go into action. This second substance he named the "tumor complement factor."

That led him to a *third* player in the process. When the antibodies did their job and destroyed the mutant cells, they might do it too well: too many mutant cells, that is, might be broken up and passed down for elimination, overwhelming the liver as they accumulated and, in extreme cases, killing the animal—as we'd seen with the poodle we'd put on an eighteen-day fast. To protect the liver, Burton theorized, this third factor—he called it the "blocking protein factor"—shielded the mutant cells like a candy coating, so that not too many mutant cells broke up at once.

The fourth and last factor in this elegant balance was the one that regulated the blocking protein—that made sure the candy coating was coming off at the right rate. When the liver had caught up and was ready to process more toxicity, this fourth factor—the "deblocking protein"—eroded the blocking protein factor from the mutant cells so that the antibodies could go in for the kill.

Though only a Ph.D., not a medical doctor, Burton managed to isolate and extract his four factors and then patent the process. All he needed now was to test his theories on human cancer patients. Unfortunately, he was a small fish in a small pond. Had he worked as the head of a research lab at Harvard, he felt, he would have commanded enough respect to have his theories accepted. Instead, his papers were rejected by medical journals, his grant requests either refused or granted in such winnowed amounts as to constitute insults. The FDA refused his request to conduct human clinical trials on an experimental basis. As for the American Medical Association, it insisted that in order to win its blessing, Burton would have to conduct strict double-blind tests: putting one-third of a test group of cancer patients on his own program, the next third on conventional therapy, and the final third on placebos. To Burton, that was nothing less than being asked to instigate needless deaths. When he refused, the entire U.S. medical establishment turned its back on him, and Burton, in a cold fury, moved down to the Bahamas—this was 1977—where he received support to open a cancer research lab and outpatient treatment center in a building on the grounds of Rand Memorial Hospital. The government welcomed him eagerly: Burton would bring in tax dollars, and tourists, albeit tourists with cancer. "Here I am," he declared happily, "protected from the American Cancer Society by the entire Bahamian navy consisting of five gunboats."

That year and the next, 20 percent of Burton's patients recovered enough to go home and lead normal lives—not necessarily tumor-free, but with their cancers no longer aggressive and, in most cases, in remission. Most of the early successes were with cancers of the head and neck, bladder, colon, and prostate. Those cancers with which Burton was least successful—bone cancer, for example—were also those most resistant to conventional therapy, and in any case, the patients he saw had been told by American doctors that their prospects were nil. To all, upon arriving, Burton acknowledged that the treatment might fail. But it also might work. And unlike chemotherapy or radiation, he emphasized, IAT inflicted no pain or side effects—no more than the pinprick of a hypodermic needle.

For that first stay, I'd made a hotel reservation. Almost as soon as we met, however, Burton insisted I be his guest in the sprawling, waterfront home he shared with his wife Betty, whom he'd first met when she came to him for treatment. (Betty had had six CAT-scan-confirmed, inoperable tumors called chondrosarcomas at the base of her skull, and had been told by U.S. doctors that she would die imminently. That was a decade before.) The house was in a high-fenced compound, guarded by five Rottweilers. Inside were marble floors and antiques, a sunken living room with a six-foot-high TV hooked up to a satellite system, and the most beautiful seashell collection I'd ever seen—picked by Burton, Betty, and their occasional guests—in every room of the house. Adjacent to the master bedroom was a hot tub, in which Burton would often soak at 2:00 or 3:00 a.m. while playing chess with an IBM computer. (Most games, he won.) He was a sybarite, I suppose, though he didn't profit in any other visible way from his work, and certainly charged his human patients modest rates: $5,000 for the first month of analysis and treatments, $2,000 for each month thereafter. He used the house as a place to think—and *think*: by the next day, I knew I was in the presence of a genius whose mind raced so far ahead of mine that I felt like an awkward child. But also, the house served as his refuge, a kingdom in exile, not only from criminal elements on the islands but from the U.S. medical establishment, which had done all it could, he felt, to keep him from bringing IAT to needy people in his own country.

Soon enough, I learned firsthand how stinging that rejection could be. My brother and I had begun reporting on our IAT work to holistic veterinary societies, and word got out. When an invitation came to address an audience of conventional veterinarians, we showed up with slides, IAT treatments, computer printouts—and Pinky, whom we brought along as Exhibit A. As I took the audience through Pinky's case step by step, I could hear an angry muttering grow. Some in the audience walked out; others began asking scornful questions. To my surprise, attention focused not on Pinky's obvious terminal cancer but on a purplish tumor of the neck which I'd ignored initially because it wasn't life-threatening. After nearly three years of treatment, the tumor had shrunk and begun to drain, so I'd chosen to remove it. As a matter of course, I'd sent it in to a lab, where it was revealed to be fibrous tissue. *Scar* tissue. Which suggested to my brother and me that as a dividend of our treatment, a malignant neck tumor had turned benign.

Why, the veterinarians demanded, hadn't I biopsied the neck tumor when I first saw Pinky, so as to confirm that it was malignant then? How unprofessional could I be? I said that at the time, we'd just focused our efforts on three different confirmed cancers that were actually killing the dog, and had chosen not to impose additional physical stress and pain by removing the small neck tumor. But our reasoning fell on deaf ears. And so was established, for my brother and me, a new reputation: as "those Goldsteins," the good veterinarians gone insane.

For nearly a decade, that sting of rejection hurt more than I cared to admit. Finally one of the East Coast's most distinguished veterinary surgeons, Martin DeAngelis, formerly of the Animal Medical Center in New York and now in private practice in Ardsley, New York, made me see it for what it was. Though traditional in his outlook, DeAngelis had become enthusiastic about the holistic work my brother and I were doing, and referred an increasing number of patients to us. "You just have to realize that what you were doing was scaring them," DeAngelis said. "After all, these were veterinarians who would have recommended euthanasia for Pinky—and there was Ann Bland, the dog's owner, sitting right there in the audience with him." To take in what we were saying would have been more than unnerving; it would have invalidated much of what they did in the treatment of cancer. "You can't shove it in their faces," DeAngelis counseled. "Just do your work and let them come to you."

At that moment, the anger and frustration of years lifted. I realized, too, that some of the fault was mine. Like Burton, I'd let the pain of rejection make me arrogant, and had actually provoked much of the adverse reaction I'd felt was so unfair. In so doing, I'd made life more difficult than it had to be, not only for me but for my brother. Most important, I'd kept Burton's vital work from being accepted as quickly and widely as it deserved to be.

So that's what I do now: just focus on the work. And when colleagues ask about it, I share it without taking offense at their logical doubts and concerns. I see them as allies, not enemies. I see that they have experience and knowledge that may help me administer IAT better. On an almost daily basis, I see what a difference that attitude makes.

These days, operating the IAT program between Smith Ridge and the Bahamas is as routine as dealing with a local laboratory. We no longer send samples to the Bahamas, as we now have our own, in-house testing facility. High-speed computers communicate the results in seconds. Nothing in the years since we began the program has shaken my faith in Burton's theories, or in the value of his isolated proteins for the treatment of cancer. At the same time, we keep trying new remedies and procedures with it, in new combinations, envisioning a time when *all* the pets we see with cancer will survive it.

For the IAT program, a dog or cat with serious cancer typically receives three to four injections each morning (spaced an hour apart) and three to four injections in the evening, five days a week. That adds up to more than one hundred injections a month—an annoyance, but hardly on the same scale as the discomfort of chemo or radiation (and, as Burton emphasized, with no side effects or complications). The same four immunoprotein factors are administered to all patients, and yet each patient's regimen is unique, determined by the imbalances seen in his blood sample and by his type of cancer. The amounts of each protein factor vary from patient to patient. So does the order of the injections. And daily, the dosages change, based on ongoing analyses of each patient's blood.

If a pet reaches the clinic in an extreme condition, I'll usually start him on high doses of intravenous vitamin C as soon as I see him. I don't regard it as the cure-all that Wendell O. Belfield declared it to be a decade or so ago, but I'll use it for two or three days to pull a patient back from the brink—sort of like jump-starting a car with a weak battery. (I'll also inject B vitamins and adrenal cortex, plus injectable homeopathics from Heel if appropriate.) Once the patient is stable, good immunological and metabolic support can maintain him. And, of course, all patients go on full supplemental programs based on their BNAs in conjunction with good-quality diets (see Chapter Three).

We no longer use some of the therapies we did in the late 1970s—the Gerson liver "shakes," coffee enemas, or Laetrile—only because so many natural supplements have since come on the market to address those needs. Along with the vitamins and enzymes discussed in Chapter Five, we have homeopathic remedies to support each of the internal organs, from the liver, needed to fight all cancers, to the thymus, the gland that helps program the immune system in youth and then mysteriously (and, I think, unnecessarily) atrophies. A boost of homeopathic animal "thymus" is immunosupportive, and in my experience a helpful measure against all cancers. A more recent addition to the arsenal, bizarre as it sounds, is injections of homeopathically succussed cancer types from the German company Heel. For a dog with mammary cancer, for example, we'll give injections of homeopathic mammary adenocarcinoma. As discussed in Chapter Five, the homeopathic principle of "like cures like" appears to work in this newest spin on Hahnemann's original revelation.

In conjunction with IAT, I'll start a cancer patient typically on six or seven supplements as specified by the BNA. Along with these, I'll add in one or two of several supplements that have direct immune supportive effects. Among my favorites are: Immuno Complex (Professional Health Products), Betathyme (Doctors Mutual), herbal Astragalus 10 Plus or Gymnostemma (Seven Forests), the antioxidant Cell Advance (Vetri-Science), and homeopathic Thymus Drops (Professional Health Products). Also included in this arsenal will be one or more of the supplements newly promoted as anticancer agents: cat's claw, Carnivora (an injectable extract of the venus flytrap plant), and shark cartilage.

Regarding the last of these, I've used shark cartilage extensively in my practice. As documented in the book *Sharks Don't Get Cancer*, by Dr. I. William Lane, and then aired on *60 Minutes* twice within one month, shark cartilage has an antiangiogenesis effect, which means it actually diminishes the blood supply to both cancerous tumors and arthritic joints. I have personally witnessed beneficial effects with the use of shark cartilage on both cancer and arthritis patients. My one big concern is the destruction of sharks to obtain their cartilage. Their diminishing numbers, especially in the Pacific Ocean, threaten to disrupt the food chain and unbalance the ecology, since sharks are among the Pacific's primary predators. Potentially, the harvesting of sharks may have global environmental implications. While I'm grateful for the good it does to my patients, I continue to search for other natural products to replace it. One new promising product is called inositol hexaphosphate (IP-6). Available through some health food stores, it is derived from plants, and has proven anticancer effects.

To a conventional doctor, this grab-bag approach will seem unscientific at best. But since virtually everything we use has no side effects, why not throw in the works? In my experience, especially in dealing with debilitated cancer patients, giving more supplements rather than fewer does produce better results—which makes sense, given that all, in one way or another, help boost the immune system. Someday, double-blind studies will doubtless be done to determine exactly which of these supplements helps fight cancer to exactly what degree. But they won't be done by me. Like Burton, I deeply object to the practice of giving placebos to one group of cancer patients, be they people or pets, when their chances of survival are so much greater with the therapies the treated group gets. If there's an ethical dilemma here, I think it lies in the court of conventional medicine—not in the heartfelt effort to fight cancer with as many promising, nontoxic measures as possible.

That conflict informs everything from the means used to fight cancer to the end each side pursues. In conventional cancer therapy, the goal is complete and permanent removal of the malignant tumor. Zap! And the faster the better. What I seek with my cancer patients is *good quality of life*. When, through IAT and other holistic measures, we can help the body eliminate the tumor altogether, we're thrilled. But I've also had pets run around for years on treatment with some portion of their tumors intact. As long as we've contained the tumor, reduced or eliminated any pain, and enabled the pet to lead a happy, energetic life, who cares if he has a tumor or not? Certainly the tumor will need to be monitored on a regular basis, but if it remains dormant, it need not arouse our concern or provoke an all-out assault with surgery, chemotherapy, or radiation. With pets more often than not, that's the way to win the battle and lose the war: to eradicate the tumor and so ravage the pet's immune system to such a degree that he's left diminished, more susceptible to cancer and other diseases than before.

As anyone knows who's dealt with cancer either as a doctor or as a patient, there isn't just one "big C." Among the more than three dozen standard varieties we treat, the range of aggressiveness and treatability is as wide for pets as it is for people. In my experience, one of the most responsive to therapy is brain cancer, surprising as that may seem. Among cats, in particular, we've had a string of successes, of whom Jupiter, a nearly twelve-year-old black domestic shorthair, is perhaps the most dramatic example.

When Jupiter was first brought to the clinic, he was totally blind. His pupils, overly dilated, showed no response to light. Why? Because, as a CAT scan revealed, a huge tumor had wiped out at least a third of his brain and put debilitating pressure on his optic nerve area. The Animal Medical Center had scheduled surgical removal of the tumor, but the attending surgeon had changed his mind, declaring that even if the operation was successful, removing a tumor of that size would leave Jupiter in a vegetable-like state. Instead, he recommended euthanasia. When I took blood samples, Jupiter's eyes rolled back in his head and he fell backward. I thought he'd died right there. Asked by his owners what his chances of survival were, I guessed 2 percent—and a zero percent chance of regaining his vision, since that section of the brain was already gone.

But Jupiter proved to be one of those 2 percent miraculous recoveries. Within the first week he showed rapid response to IAT and all the supplements we could get into him. After thirteen months of therapy, we had him reevaluated by the Animal Medical Center. The AMC could detect only a "slight deficiency" in his nervous system, which might suggest the presence of the "former tumor." As doctors at the AMC stated to me, Jupiter's restored vision and obvious energy were proof enough that the tumor was gone. Yet, they requested that another CAT scan be performed so they could know for sure. To their considerable irritation, I counseled Jupiter's owner to refuse—and she did. Why put a thirteen-year-old cat under general anesthesia and take all the X rays constituting a CAT scan of his skull if they weren't needed to save his life? As much as I would have liked to have had those results, I couldn't sacrifice the well-being of my patient in the name of science. Consequently, the AMC's final report on Jupiter concluded that he *seemed* to be in remission, but added that that probably had nothing to do with the treatment we'd given him. On the other hand, the report added drily, as long as the treatment wasn't toxic, it might as well be continued. Indeed!

One other point here: I tend not to draw a strict line between benign and malignant. Medically speaking, Jupiter's good news was that he had a benign tumor in his brain. But his bad news was that his recommendation was euthanasia. I feel that a tumor is cancer and ought to be addressed, regardless of its classification. For that reason, I also disagree with conventional doctors who often suggest that a patient with a small benign tumor should be left alone. Any tumor is a sign that something has gone wrong with the immune system: it's a wake-up call that ought not be ignored. At the same time, any tumor *may* respond to treatment. And that includes the tumors classified as malignant.

Though different in kind, cancers that affect regions near the brain—such as the mouth and face—tend to respond well, too, in part because they're localized. One of my most memorable cases involved a golden retriever named Brunzi, whose owner, Carol Marangoni, has since become not only a good friend but a representative of Alternative Solutions to Animal Health, Inc., the foundation I've helped start to further research into holistic therapies. Carol tells the story better than I can:

In October of 1992 I was devastated when I received a biopsy report on a lump that had been removed from Brunzi's face. The lab report said "Diagnosis: squamous cell carcinoma. Prognosis: guarded." I read that report over and over with mounting anxiety. The thought that I might lose "my little boy" at five years of age was unbearable to me.

When I first spoke with Marty Goldstein about Brunzi's diagnosis, he was remarkably calm. Too calm, I thought. He advised me to keep Brunzi on a supplement program and periodically monitor his progress through blood testing. He did not recommend any formal cancer treatment and he implored me not to panic—telling me that my fearful emotional state would be conveyed to Brunzi with detrimental effect. My initial reaction when I hung up the phone was "Is this guy nuts?" How could he be so calm? How could he not recommend an aggressive treatment program? Above all, how could he expect me not to panic?

So I immediately took Brunzi to a different vet. Not just any vet, but the chief oncologist at a prestigious veterinary teaching hospital. After examining Brunzi and reviewing the lab report, he recommended a course of therapy that involved surgically removing all seven lumps that were on his body, implanting small metal disks at each incision, and administering pinpoint radiation at all cancerous sites. (The reason for the metal disks was to precisely identify each site to radiate.) The oncologist told me Brunzi would need to be anesthetized and radiated approximately three times a week for six to seven weeks, and that I could expect ulcers to develop internally and externally at all radiated sites. At the same time, he outright dismissed my inquiries about Marty Goldstein's alternative treatment for cancer.

Please understand that I was not predisposed to look kindly upon "alternative" health care. I come from a very conventional background—my father was a conventional physician, I myself was trained as a research scientist, and I was surrounded by conventional-approach colleagues in the pharmaceutical industry in which I worked for years. So it was with great fear and trepidation that I considered Marty's alternative form of treatment for Brunzi's cancer.

When I told Marty that the oncologist wanted to remove all the lumps on Brunzi's body, he asked some very straightforward questions. "Suppose you remove all these bumps—you still haven't addressed the underlying cause. Why did Brunzi develop these cancerous bumps in the first place? And what's going to stop him from growing seven, fourteen, or fifty more cancerous bumps just like the ones you want to remove?" Marty went on to explain that all living beings have cells with the potential of becoming cancerous, but that these cells don't take control and become cancer if the body's immune system is functioning properly. What caused Brunzi's immune system to function poorly? Probably a variety of factors: genetics (Brunzi had allergies and even mange as a puppy, both of which are considered immuno-suppressive diseases); poor nutrition (dog foods made from pesticide- and chemical-laden crops, with preservatives, additives, and meat from diseased animals that are considered unfit for human consumption); and possibly too many vaccines.

Marty's approach, which I decided to follow after all, was a multifaceted one, designed to enhance Brunzi's debilitated immune function. He put Brunzi on a variety of glandular, enzymatic, vitamin, and mineral supplements, based on his metabolic nutritional analysis. He monitored Brunzi's progress through blood testing and put him on a course of Immuno-Augmentative Therapy (IAT). In accordance with his advice, I also changed Brunzi's diet. Whenever possible, I began cooking fresh foods for him, using organically grown grains (mainly brown rice), veggies, and free-range meat. I used a super-premium dry dog food, and continued with his food supplement program as Marty recommended.

Brunzi never received radiation, chemotherapy, or additional surgery. He was retested approximately every six months, and his supplement regimen was modified accordingly. He was also routinely tested for immune function (IAT retesting), but did not need to repeat that course of treatment. Over the next four years, Brunzi often developed new lumps or bumps, but they all wound up being either benign or cystic, or just went away as I worked on his health and immune system. When Brunzi finally died in 1997, at ten years old, he'd lived twice as long as expected by his conventional veterinarian—as long, indeed, as golden retrievers without any debilitating disease tend to live. Of equal importance, he'd lived a happy and pain-free life, free from the adverse effects of additional cancer treatment.

High on the list of other cancers that respond particularly well to IAT is bladder cancer. One of our star patients was Sophie, a black rag doll of a pooch, whose bladder cancer was declared so aggressive by a board-certified veterinary surgeon from New York City that surgery was ruled out as an option. Sophie would be lucky to live at most nine months afterward, and should be put to sleep instead. I had a sonogram performed to see just what I had to deal with: a tongue-shaped tumor, undulating in the bladder like a flag, 2.3 by 2.7 centimeters. In this case, I thought surgery might help. If the tumor could be reduced somewhat, IAT might have a better chance.

So the referring veterinarian did what he could, managing to remove 75 percent of the tumor. A biopsy confirmed that the cancer was transitional cell carcinoma, and a follow-up sonogram showed, as expected, that what remained of the tumor was already beginning to grow again. So in late April 1986, with the tumor at 1.1 by 1.1 centimeters, we started in with IAT and a slew of supplements. A month later to the day, we had another sonogram done. It showed no evidence of cancer. The summer passed, the therapy continued. Still no tumor. In a sonogram that fall, the tumor was back, at about half its size presurgery, but the sonographer added that while the lump appeared large enough to be the malignant tumor, it looked fibrous—like scar tissue. From a sonogram done a month later, the sonographer concluded that the tumor was "definitely fibrous, indicating chronicity." In other words, the tumor was dead.

One day about four months after that last sonogram, Sophie excreted blood and a chunk of tissue. We assumed the worst, and immediately had another sonogram done. The chronic mass was still there, but we could see on the sonogram that a chunk of it was missing. We submitted the excreted chunk for biopsy; it came back as fibrous scar tissue. Sophie, her immune system augmented by IAT, had not only beaten her cancer but eliminated it. Instead of being euthanized or dying a few months after surgery, she died years later—of old age.

Burton never did determine why in a healthy person or pet those four critical immunoproteins that govern mutant cell growth first fall out of balance with one another. Or, to put it simply, why cancer begins. He suspected that nearly all cancers are genetically based, and that a key factor was the discovery and use of agents like penicillin, which kept alive weak patients—pets or people—who otherwise would have succumbed, and who instead passed on their growing genetic predilection for disease. Of all the cancers he studied, the only one not inherited to some degree, Burton felt, was the asbestos-caused cancer called mesothelioma. As poorly as it responds to conventional therapy, by the way, Burton achieved surprisingly positive results with mesothelioma patients on IAT. We too treated two dogs with mesothelioma; both responded well on IAT.

Because generations turn so much more quickly with pets than with human beings, the cancers I'm seeing now appear more and more often, I'm sorry to report, in puppies and kittens—a sure sign, to me, of their genetic origin. Not long ago, a fifteen-month-old Scottie named Scarlet was brought to me after her third surgery to remove malignant tumors. So malignant was her cancer that it was diagnosed as undifferentiated sarcoma, which is to say that it was growing so wildly it hadn't even differentiated into a specific cell type. Both Cornell's veterinary school and the Animal Medical Center received biopsies. Both agreed that the dog would not live to see her second birthday. Nevertheless, we started her on IAT and supplements. On the fifth day of therapy, a tumor resembling the one she'd just had removed grew right at the incision of the last surgery. On the seventh day, it was gone—and no more malignancies appeared. Despite the fact that Scarlet moved to Atlanta, Georgia, and we lost hands-on contact with her, her owner stayed in touch and let us know, in the end, that Scarlet lived nine years past her two-year life expectancy. Which to me suggests the silver lining in cancer cases that hit pets so young: genetically based as they are, inevitable as the first tumors may be, a young dog or cat may also be strong enough to fight his way back to health, and even to heal his genetic tendency to manifest a malignancy, so that his offspring may not inherit it. Believe it or not, I have actually witnessed the reversal of conditions considered genetically based so that their symptoms don't manifest.

Of all the cancers I treat, among the least responsive to holistic therapy, even among young pets, are lymph cancers. They usually hit so quickly, often appearing over much of the body's lymph tissues, that chemotherapy is often necessary. In fact, this cancer is so responsive to chemotherapy, with relatively few lingering side effects, that it can be eradicated clinically overnight. I see it as buying time, getting a patient into clinical remission, in order then to support him with IAT and supplements. One tendency I've noticed again and again is the "potentiating," or enhancing, effect of alternative therapy on conventional therapy. Chemo used to treat lymph cancer works far better, with fewer side effects, when alternative therapies are used, too, which enables a doctor to administer lower doses of it at less frequent intervals.

Happily, this double-barreled approach has proved unnecessary with atypical lymph cancer. One of the first cases to indicate that was Jake, a Labrador–Great Dane mix who was, despite her name, female. At the Animal Medical Center, an X ray had shown a tumor eroding the bones of her hip, lower back, and tail, fusing them together. She couldn't squat, she had difficulty defecating and urinating, and when I did a rectal exam, the tumor felt as big as a lemon, pushing down into the rectum from above. Because of the location, surgery wasn't an option. In removing the tumor, a surgeon would have severed the connection between the pelvis and the back—the pelvic carriage that actually supports the legs. Dr. Cindy Wasserman at the AMC, in charge of the case, advised me that she had ruled out a biopsy. The tumor was so inaccessible and, she said, therefore untreatable.

To Jake's owners, a nice young couple, I put the prognosis in no less blunt terms after sending a blood sample down to the Bahamas. Jake's prospects were slim, all right. But I felt she stood a ghost of a chance, if only because the tumor might not be bone cancer, which would make it about 100 percent untreatable, but rather another cancer type invading the bone. And if it was bone cancer, I told them, maybe Jake would be my first success.

Within the first three weeks of therapy, several lumps appeared on Jake's skin around her rectum, almost like an allergic reaction. Sensitive to the criticism I'd received in the Pinky case for not taking a biopsy of an incidental tumor, I submitted one of the lumps to a laboratory. It was diagnosed as round cell sarcoma, most likely lymphosarcoma. I reported this to Burton when sending a follow-up blood sample. He advised that we just keep on with the therapy protocol, as Jake's follow-up immune report looked good. Over the next several months, the tumor shrank steadily, centimeter by centimeter. Finally after two and a half years, I did take a follow-up X ray and sent it to the radiology consultant service affiliated with the Cornell veterinary school. The head of the service, Dr. Victor Rendano, reported, in writing, the following: "The follow-up X rays show that the lytic [or eroded] area is no longer identified in the sacrum [back] and the bone. The appearance of the bone in the back would be compatible with bony remodeling consistent with a healing process, and change would be consistent with the satisfactory response of the cancer to therapy." In his own dry, medical terms, the radiologist was telling us that Jake's cancer of the bones was not only gone but had healed to a point where normal tissue had regrown in the formerly cancerous region. She lived two and a half cancer-free years and died at almost thirteen years old, a ripe old age for a Great Dane.

With primary bone cancer, medically known as osteosarcoma, the only stories I could tell until about two years ago were unremittingly negative. The success I've had since then is due, I'm convinced, to the introduction of ozone therapy in treatment. As discussed in Chapter Five, ozone therapy involves the intravenous channeling of ozone through the bloodstream, predicated on the idea that ozone breaks into pure oxygen, which promotes healing. I believe that disease is associated with, and further fosters, an oxygen-depleted environment. Whether the lack of oxygen allows it to grow or the disease destroys the oxygen, the relationship between the two is what has spawned ozone therapy. Because bone cancer was so impenetrable, I began using ozone therapy as an adjunct to IAT—essentially because I had nothing to lose, and no other treatment, conventional or alternative, was affecting it. In three or four cases, it appeared to be a swing factor in producing results superior to those I expected when dealing with a bone tumor and to those predicted by veterinarians or institutions that saw the cases before I did. So I started doing more of it.

Ozone therapy requires an ozone generator, which few veterinarians have as yet. It also requires practicing in one of the few states that allow the use of ozone for therapy. New York State does allow it, and if the results I achieved with a ten-year-old Rottweiler named Sassi can become more widely known, perhaps other states will start to recognize ozone for the extraordinary therapy it is.

Sassi had a tumor in the gum of her upper jaw. At Virginia Polytechnic veterinary school, near where her owners lived, she was examined, her tumor biopsied as a squamous cell carcinoma, and radical surgery recommended. If the owners approved, the operation would remove a whole section of Sassi's upper jaw, and she wouldn't be able to eat well for weeks. Her owners knew about the cryosurgery done at Smith Ridge, and brought Sassi up to see me. I examined her, did cryosurgery, and actually sent her home that night with her tumor destroyed but her jaw intact. That night, she ate a regular meal.

For well over a year, there was no recurrence of the tumor. Sassi was on supplements and appeared healthy and well. Then came the call that Sassi had developed a bone tumor in the upper part of the bone that connects the shoulder to the elbow, the humerus. This was confirmed at VPI by X ray and biopsy. The recommendation there: amputation or euthanasia. Once again, Sassi's owners brought her up to Smith Ridge. First I put her on high levels of intravenous vitamin C as a "jump start" and started her on IAT. Along with the usual supplements, I used the homeopathic remedy silicea at high potencies, since I'd heard reports of its success in helping reverse bone cancer. I also added injectable homeopathic bone, "Os Suis" from the German company Heel. Now, I sensed, was also the time for intravenous ozone. In all previous cases of bone cancer for which I'd used ozone, I'd injected ozone gas directly into the tumors. But due to this tumor's location, deep in the musculature of the upper arm, I couldn't reach it directly. Instead, Sassi was given ozone intravenously, and by painless enema into her rectum.

For months afterward, Sassi did well. Her tumor remained totally unchanged, as shown by follow-up X rays at VPI—astounding with such an aggressive cancer—and remained small enough not to be painful, enabling her to lead a normal life. A year after her visit, her health appeared to falter. Up she came again for another "pick-me-up" round of intravenous vitamin C and ozone. The bone cancer appeared not to have grown at all. During that period, though, it was clear she had developed some sharp, undefined pain in her neck. The obvious conclusion was that the bone cancer had spread to her upper spine, but a full X-ray series, again at VPI, revealed no evidence of any growth, progression, or spread of the tumor. At VPI, the best guess was that Sassi might have arthritis—by now, she was eleven years old—and so she was put on Rimadyl, a drug I warn against in the "Arthritis" section of Chapter Seven. Though classified as one of the NSAID's—nonsteroidal anti-inflammatory drugs—which are considered to have milder side effects than steroids, Rimadyl has produced side effects that are very disturbing indeed, and appeared to lead to at least three deaths among dogs in my practice. Within several weeks, Sassi was euthanized.

I don't know whether Rimadyl contributed to Sassi's death. Perhaps some other cause is to blame. She was, after all, eleven years old, and her unspecified pain was so acute at times in that last stage that the relief she did get from Rimadyl may have warranted its use. But the last report I received about her, just prior to her death, indicated no spread of the original cancer.

For my brother and me, the IAT program has proved more rewarding—and exciting—than either of us could ever have imagined. For the man who created it, driven as much by anger and paranoia as by intellectual genius, the results were more contradictory, controversial, and ultimately sad.

By 1985, Burton had been operating his clinic nearly a decade, his reputation growing with each seemingly miraculous remission. Harry Reasoner from *60 Minutes* had swooped down to do an exposé, only to be so favorably impressed by what he saw that the segment became a strongly positive one, giving Burton some national recognition and bringing him more patients. Yet his rising profile also caused problems. That year, a Seattle, Washington, laboratory tested a Burton patient's serum supply and found antibodies to the AIDS virus. Though the antibodies may have only indicated a blood donor's *immunity* to AIDS, the dread word did real damage. Soon after, pressure was exerted on local health organizations, and Burton's clinic was shut down.

Among patients who'd been treated successfully by Burton, the outcry was swift and loud. Nearly all of these patients were still on IAT, either on full therapy at the clinic in Freeport or on a maintenance program of home injections. With the clinic closed, they felt their lifelines had literally been cut. In more than a few cases, a cancer in remission reappeared. One eleven-year-old boy, saved from certain death by IAT a year before, died without his injections; I heard reports of other deaths, too. The clinic reopened on a limited basis to deal with severe cases, on the condition that Burton strictly screen his donors' blood. Still, protests mounted. An extraordinary open-court hearing sponsored by Congressman Guy Molinari was held in a Brooklyn federal court. Burton's patients testified, telling what IAT had done for them and demanding their freedom of choice to continue with the treatments. My brother and I came to that hearing, bringing success stories like Jupiter and Pinky with us to help dramatize our presentations. The hearing led to a decision by the Office of Technological Assessment (OTA) to investigate alternative cancer therapies, particularly IAT. Burton's therapy were neither validated nor condemned, but he was able to operate the clinic without constraints.

The patients came back, and Burton presided, but the shutdown had taken an emotional toll. Even an apparent peace offering by the National Cancer Institute failed to mollify him. Presented with a proposal to let the agency try IAT at its own clinics—as an independent treatment, and part of a double-blind study—Burton angrily refused. If the NCI wanted to see how IAT worked, he thundered, why couldn't its doctors come down to the Bahamas?

As rewarding as it was to know and learn from Burton's genius, I have to admit that he was frustrating at times. Burton's relentless war with the U.S. medical system had definitely made him somewhat paranoid, and exasperatingly rigid in dealing with the animal IAT program that my brother and I had started. Because his father and brother had both died as vegetarians in their early forties, Burton was convinced that nutrition has nothing to do with health, and was thus opposed to all the other work my brother and I were doing with our patients. He went so far as to shut down Smith Ridge's IAT program on several occasions, forcing us to plead with his very responsible Bahamian business partner for reinstatement. The same scorn for nutrition, unfortunately, led to the deterioration of Burton's own health. Still in his sixties, he died in 1994 of diabetes, kidney failure, and heart disease after quadruple bypass surgery.

As much as I wish he were still alive to consult on cases and answer questions, and as much as he's missed, the clinic he created appears to run smoothly and successfully without his irascible presence. Open to new ideas, its directors now appreciate in particular what we're doing at Smith Ridge to complement IAT with our other therapies, and are observing our success with keen interest. It's my hope that as our success grows, it may bring to Burton, though indirectly and belatedly, the Nobel Prize he so deserves.

I tell Burton's story in my seminars and to the owners of pets I treat with IAT. I also tell them something I've learned about the nature of cancer—something that always helps.

No matter how quickly the disease may appear to be growing clinically, it's a disease which has taken time to develop—over either years in an older pet's lifetime, or generations in the case of a young pet born with a genetic predisposition. *It takes time to treat.* We live in a society that expects instant results, but there is no quick fix for cancer. Even if a pet has a single tumor which treatment appears to remove, reestablishing the pet's immune system and easing him through waves of detoxification is a process, not a procedure. There are ups, and there are downs, which is why I often use the analogy of a roller coaster to describe the process of recovery. The down periods are discouraging, but less so if an owner remembers that on a roller coaster, we go back up again.

The other analogy I use for cancer recovery is a marathon. You may be the fastest marathon runner in the world, but in this race a serious rival has started six miles ahead of you. Chances are, by the end of the race you'll still be first over the finish line, but at mile eight out of twenty-six, you may be trailing. It's the same with cancer treatment. At the outset of treatment, your rival is ahead of you, and you've got a full race to run. But put one foot in front of the other steadily, patiently, without getting discouraged, and some day you'll win the race.

For more information, see Appendix A (page 350).

PART THREE

Understanding
Your Pet

CHAPTER NINE

The Spiritual Realm

Most of my patients have a physical problem. A problem you can see, feel, and treat with a physical result. Either it diminishes or it doesn't; either the patient physically improves or he declines. Yet now that you've followed me this far, and perhaps read enough case histories to believe that alternative therapies may often produce physical healing better than conventional ones, I have a confession to make.

I'm not sure illness always begins as a physical condition.

At the start of Chapter Five, I explained that I always consider a pet's emotional as well as his physical being, that the two are both important in diagnosing and treating disease. Because that chapter was devoted to actual therapies I use to treat my patients, I let the implications of that statement go unsaid. But I feel this book would be incomplete—and less than honest—if I failed to acknowledge them.

Consider, as a starting point, this credo: "Illness exists first in the nonphysical realm of spiritual need, emotional confusion, or mental aberration. It is never primarily physical. The body is the reactor. It vibrates to stress and is an outward manifestation of inner turmoil." The person who wrote those words is not a veterinarian, not even a medical writer. She's a channeler named Pat Rodegast, whose *Emmanuel's Book* is so wise and wondrous that I keep it on a shelf right above my desk and often use it with my clients to lend inspiration.

In many readers, no doubt, the word "channeler" sends off warning bells. (I hear them ringing even now.) I won't try here to make the case one way or the other for channelers' claims: believe, or disbelieve, as you like. My own feeling is that whether or not Emmanuel exists as an actual being or as part of Rodegast's own higher self, the book conveys such illuminating insights that they're worth embracing. Among them is one that I've observed again and again in my practice. Illness in pets really does appear to begin with the emotions—and, yes, the spirit—at least as much as it does with genes, germs, and the immune system.

I have no double-blind studies to support this intuition. I cannot prove that disease begins in the nonphysical realm, or draw you a Venn diagram illustrating how and where the physical and nonphysical origins of disease overlap. I do know that healthy animals radiate a vital energy—a life force; a spirit, if you like—so evident that the Chinese have a word for it: chi. And I know that in sick pets, the chi is dulled. Does the chi diminish or get blocked first, allowing disease to take hold? Or is it the other way around, as conventional medicine would have us believe? I happen to think that often the chi dims first. My sense, moreover, is that a pet is intuitively aware of the ebbing of that force, and understands that the illness which follows is a natural consequence. That, to me, is definitely spiritual.

I can suggest that a pet's illness starts with his spirit, you can agree or disagree, and there we are, with nothing more to say. The longer talk we can have is about what might best be called spiritual interdependence. I think that a pet and his owner both have spirits, that those spirits interact, and that the interaction affects the mental and physical well-being of both. For that, I can give you all the anecdotal evidence you'd ever want to hear. The stories are interesting in themselves; they also make a practical point. Open yourself to the possibility of a spiritual realm in your relationship with your pet, be aware of what its effects might be, and your pet's physical health may be improved. As, indeed, may be your own.

Let's start with the obvious. Is there anyone who hasn't observed the startling physical resemblance between some pets and their owners and wondered what's behind it? One of the first examples I remember was a lady who bred boxers and looked exactly like a boxer herself. Same jowly look to her face, same masculine manner; she even had a rough voice like a boxer's bark. I've seen men who look like their cocker spaniels, women who look like their Afghans (even a man and wife who *both* looked like their Afghan); I knew someone once who not only looked like his standard poodle but had the same black curly hair, cut the same way as his dog's.

As most of us would confirm from personal experience, the resemblance between pets and their owners is usually not just physical.

Whether the individuals are high-strung or laid-back, playful or glum, the affinities of temperament and character are often remarkably clear. You can say that owners are drawn, subconsciously or not, to pets who mirror themselves. Or you can wonder, as I do, if pets choose us more than we choose them—and in so doing, take that first little tentative step toward the spiritual.

If you've never gone to an animal shelter to choose your next pet, you may not appreciate what I mean. If you have, do you remember how you felt as you walked past cage after cage of needy dogs or cats? Probably every one of those caged animals tugged at your heart. Yet when you reached a certain cage that held a certain pet, something deeper was stirred. Was it just a greater degree of desire, like settling on a shirt at the Gap, or one of Baskin-Robbins's thirty-one flavors of ice cream? Or did the pet that would become your own recognize *you* as a kindred soul, and look at you in a way that made you realize you needed each other?

From my first days in practice, I noticed that this affinity often reached a deeper level between pets and owners who had become part of each other's lives. It affected their *health*. An overweight woman who had a crippled right leg and used a cane came into my clinic, accompanied by an overweight dog who had a severe limp in her right hind leg. The heavyset, potbellied man who looked like an ex-wrestler came in with his equally heavyset, muscular, and aggressive bulldog. The visibly nervous woman in her forties clutched a visibly anxious tiny poodle.

It began to dawn on me that a pet's internal conditon might duplicate his owner's, and vice versa. A beagle was brought to me with an arrhythmic heartbeat that defied easy diagnosis. Concerned, I sent the dog over to a major animal hospital to be examined by a cardiologist, who concluded that the beagle was suffering from some newly reported heart condition I'd never heard of, and prescribed three different medications. When the dog was sent back to me, I had the owner come in and ticked off the cardiologist's recommendations. "That's odd," the owner said. "My wife and I are on the same medication. Not only that—my daughter is, too." The beagle, it turned out, had lived problem-free with the owner's brother a year before. Only when the beagle had been placed in his new home had the symptoms of his heart condition begun to appear.

At first, I assumed this was coincidence. But as I spent more time in practice, coincidences no less striking appeared. I'd just begun practicing acupuncture, and was still one of the few veterinarians to do so, when a dog was referred to me with neck pain that medication seemed unable to ease. She responded very well to an initial acupuncture session, and I heard nothing more for months. Then the pain returned, so the owner brought her dog back in. On a hunch, I asked the owner if she'd been having any neck problems herself. "As a matter of fact, I have," she said. "Why do you ask?" I figured that practicing acupuncture made me seem eccentric enough, so I responded with some noncommittal comment about relationships between owners and pets, and started my physical examination of the dog's back, manipulating each of his vertebrae from the top down. When I reached her lower back, the dog jumped back in pain.

"Oh, I know what you're going to say," the owner told me. "You're going to ask if I have lower-back problems, too. Well—I don't."

I continued my exam.

"Wait a minute," the owner said. "My husband has chronic lower-back problems, and his back went out yesterday. Which is when the dog's back went out. . . ."

The owner was, in fact, a nurse, and more open to the implications of what I'd taken to calling "resonance" than another owner might have been. Curious, we rigged our own little experiment. Instead of working on the dog's neck, which was the source of the chronic pain that no therapy but acupuncture had helped, I massaged acupuncture points on the owner's neck. She felt instant relief. The next day, she called to say the *dog's* neck was fine. Two days later, when her husband's chronic lower-back pain eased in response to his medication, so did the dog's.

I came across an odd little book at that time which made my suspicions seem more credible. *Your Pet Isn't Sick—He Just Wants You to Think So* was written by Herb Tanzer, an extraordinary veterinarian who, as it happened, had been my brother's first employer. Tanzer made the case that there is a tremendous subconscious interplay between owners and their pets which often manifests itself in disease. I also became aware of Kirlian, or infrared, photography. Take an infrared picture of a person and you'll see an energy field surrounding the body. This isn't mysticism, it's science. The energy field, also called the aura, is communicated on a wavelength we can't see with the naked eye. Yet it's clear in infrared photographs, and when two human beings are photographed by this special camera in close proximity to each other, we can see that their energy fields overlap. As do those of a person and his pet. The fact that our five senses are too limited for us to perceive auras makes them no less real than the high-pitched sounds that animals, but not humans, can hear. Similarly, electromagnetic waves are passing through us right now from our computer monitors, our television sets, and our overhead utility wires; we just can't perceive them. In fact, our bodies are being bombarded by signals right now that you can't hear or see, signals you remain oblivious to until you turn on the radio that can convert and broadcast them.

We know that couples who live together for many years often develop sympathetic symptoms, as do female college students who after several months of rooming together find that their menstrual cycles are aligned. How less likely is it that pets, whose whole worlds are defined by their owners, should acquire sympathetic symptoms as their energy fields overlap with those of their owners? After all, they can hear sounds we can't hear, smell scents we can't smell, and sense fear or danger to a degree we can't begin to understand. Why not absorb an emanation of illness and then express its symptoms, perhaps out of empathy, perhaps as a way to help the owner by holding a mirror up to his own condition, perhaps just as an instinctual adjustment to the new relationship between the owner's physical being and the surrounding environment?

I came upon another astounding example of this phenomenon when treating the dogs of a woman named Gabe, who owned a farm with many different animals. One day I began a routine neutering procedure on an eighteen-month-old black Labrador that Gabe had adopted. As I castrated the dog, some uncharacteristically dark blood appeared around the testicles. Because that part of the scrotum is actually connected to the abdominal cavity, I wondered if something might be wrong in that area. A needle inserted into the belly yielded pure blood, indicating internal bleeding. When Gabe gave me permission to perform an exploratory surgery, I discovered a ruptured spleen. Gabe thought one of her horses might have kicked the dog earlier that morning. That sounded plausible to me, too.

A while later, strangely enough, another of Gabe's dogs, a German shepherd, collapsed, and was so deathly pale by the time he reached the clinic that I suspected internal bleeding. He too, as it turned out, had a ruptured spleen, this time secondary to a tumor. A few months after that, Gabe's short-haired pointer also ruptured his spleen. Oddly enough, just at that time Gabe asked me to recommend a holistic doctor she could see for her own health. When he examined her, he found that she, too, had an enlarged spleen.

What could possibly cause four spleen problems within one family? Gabe was sure the drinking water was to blame. I told her to get it tested, but I had my doubts, since the houses in her immediate area were on the same line from the same aquifer. Sure enough, none of the neighbors had enlarged or ruptured spleens. To this day, no medical explanation fits the facts. But I sure would have liked to have taken an infrared photo of Gabe and her dogs in their home to see how their energy fields interrelated.

The pet who made me realize just how far-reaching these relationships can be was a cat named Sneezely May. Sneezely was brought to me some months after she'd been hit by a car. Her hip had healed in an awkward manner, with a bone pushed into the pelvic canal, so that she couldn't defecate easily and had to be put on a daily regimen of stool softeners. Sneezely was an outdoor cat, or at least fancied that she still was, and sometimes managed to escape for a couple of days into the neighboring woods. When she returned, we'd have to tranquilize her and manually remove the stool that had accumulated, then give her an enema. It wasn't a terribly pleasant procedure, but we all got used to it, and otherwise Sneezely appeared fine.

One day Mrs. Sneezely, as we called her owner, came into the clinic because Sneezely's two-year prescription for stool softeners had run out. I examined Sneezely, then wrote a new prescription and handed it over to Mrs. Sneezely. "Hey, isn't this funny," she said. She took out another prescription from her pocket. It was for the exact same medication—to be given to Mrs. Sneezely's mother.

"Wow!" I said. "How come we never thought of that?"

"Because my mother lives in England," said Mrs. Sneezely. "She just happens to be visiting now."

"Where was she when this happened to the cat?"

Mrs. Sneezely paused. "That was the last time she visited us. Several years ago. I know that for sure because it was my mother who found Sneezely by the side of the road after she'd been hit by the car." Believe it or not, Mrs. Sneezely's mom turned out to have also had a car accident injury that fractured her hip.

That's what I call acute physical resonance. Less dramatic, but no less real, is chronic resonance. Its manifestations are physical, but more subtly so, over a longer period of time. More often than not, in these cases the causes are emotional.

A classic example was my own dog Daniel, a red-haired golden retriever who liked to shamble into neighboring villages and properties, making friends wherever he went. One day he met a woman named Cathy Soukup, who was sitting on the hill behind her house, watching some local children play. The two got along so well that Daniel began sleeping over at Cathy's house on a regular basis, which pleased Cathy enormously, and pleased me, too. (That first day, Cathy called the phone number on Daniel's dog tags, which was the Smith Ridge clinic, and we had the first of many chats without actually meeting.) Soon enough, the clinic staff began referring to Cathy as Daniel's mom. For Cathy, Daniel became more than a dog companion. He seemed to understand exactly what she was feeling—more than she did herself.

"I was in a very destructive relationship," Cathy wrote later in a tribute to Daniel. "And of course I didn't want to see it, feel it, or know it. When it came time for the relationship to come to an end it took three years to do it. Daniel stayed close beside me through it all, watching me cry, scream, get drunk, get sick, and fight, to keep this relationship. During this time Daniel got so sick he couldn't get up. He acted as though he had aged one hundred years. It was as if all the life had been sucked out of him. I called Marty the first time it happened. He did the normal things: blood analysis, supplements, fasting—and Daniel improved. Then I'd get sucked back into that relationship and Daniel once again would sink into this lethargic state. Finally Marty said, 'I'm taking Daniel back until he gets well.' It took several months before Daniel was well enough to return to me. When he did, I realized he was mirroring my pain and agony, and manifesting it in a physical form to show me that continuing the relationship was life-threatening. Daniel's sacrifice actually helped me to walk away from that relationship—an incredibly generous gift of unconditional love."

I'm sure that pets I had earlier in my life demonstrated similar shows of chronic resonance. But the first one who made me aware of such "mirroring" was my Siamese cat Scrimshaw in the mid-1980s.

That was my frantic period, of too much work and too little pay and stress that wouldn't quit. At four years old, Scrimshaw developed the heart condition known as cardiomyopathy, the chief symptom of which was congestive coughing. I was often congested myself at the time. When Scrimshaw's coughing worsened, I would stay home more often to tend to her; when I did that, my own congestion would improve, too. I was too busy to think much about it. In fact, I was at the end of a two-year stretch in which I'd taken only four days off (including weekends). Finally, even I realized I needed a vacation.

By the time I was scheduled to leave, Scrimshaw's condition had worsened. So had mine, though I tried not to notice it. Indeed, both of us were in such bad shape that I worried that Scrimshaw might not be alive in two weeks when I returned. Yet I was so run-down myself that I felt I had to get away for my own survival. Guiltily, I found a friend to cat-sit for me and headed off to Jamaica.

The first question I asked my friend when I returned was: Is Scrimshaw alive? My friend looked at me strangely. "Of course," she said. "She did really well." Scrimshaw appeared from around the corner, purring contentedly, her congestive coughing gone. My cat-sitter hadn't heard her cough once.

Coincidence? Perhaps. But to me, the lesson was clear. Scrimshaw had mirrored me. I'd thought I was caring for her because she was in bad shape; in fact, I was caring for myself. And as my own condition improved, so did Scrimshaw's. My absence had helped, too. By removing my run-down energy from the house, I was allowing Scrimshaw to heal in a healthier environment. One can read more into this than may be the case: I have no idea if Scrimshaw got sick in order to force me to take care of myself. But I did see then, and have seen in other cases since, that when you care for an ill pet, you're sometimes led to take better care of yourself, too.

Maybe because I see so many patients with cancer, the incidence of corresponding cancer in their owners' families or environment seems that much higher. Perhaps if most of the pets I treated had cardiomyopathy, I'd hear of more owners with heart disease or corresponding symptoms. But everything I know about cancer makes me think that it too easily serves as the perfect example of the phenomenon of resonance.

Let me be very clear about this: neither people nor pets "catch" cancer from each other. As discussed in Chapter Eight, most cancers have genetic origins, to which environmental factors and general health contribute. If pets do have the ability to mirror their owners' medical conditions, however, then a dog or cat with a genetic predisposition to cancer might have a greater chance of developing it by living in close contact with an owner who has cancer than with an owner who's in excellent health. Call it fantasy if you like, but I've treated many, many pets whose owners turn out to have some form of cancer in their family. To be sure, I've treated many more whose owners don't have cancer, so the fact that your dog develops a mammary tumor shouldn't be taken as a sign to rush out for a breast exam. These are just indications worth considering, given that resonance between pet and owner with cancer seems to occur. Anyway, why *not* get a breast exam?*

Skeptics may feel free to disregard the above. But even they must acknowledge that in the treatment of cancer, a patient's attitude is fundamental to his prognosis. What I've found is that with cancer in a pet, the *owner's* attitude is fundamental. To me, the ramifications of that are definitely spiritual.

By the time I see a pet with cancer, the owner has likely heard the diagnosis from his own veterinarian and had days, perhaps weeks, to ponder the news. Chances are he's become frantic, depressed, or just plain pessimistic. If the pet has gone through a regimen of chemotherapy or radiation which hasn't eradicated the cancer, the owner is likely to be all the gloomier. How can a pet whose life is devoted to pleasing his master be unaware of this attitude? Of course he feels it, and interprets it in the only way he can: as rejection. And when nothing he can do seems able to make his master happy again, how does he react? By growing depressed! Maybe not outwardly, but inwardly. Which, especially after the assault to his immune system from chemo or radiation, diminishes his will—and his ability—to survive.

That's why, during a cancer patient's first visit, even before I take a blood sample to have it sent out for analysis, I deal with the owner, too. I show him albums of before-and-after pictures of terminally ill dogs and cats we've saved with Immuno-Augmentative Therapy and other holistic measures. I tell him the stories I've told in this book. I make him understand that the word "cancer" is not a death sentence, that patients do get well. That there is, in a word, hope. And always, I read aloud this quote from *Emmanuel's Book*: "If we could launder the word 'cancer,' hang it out in the sun to dry and bring it in bleached

---

*Call it another coincidence, but those of my clients who do see their pets' cancers reverse tend, in my observation, not to get cancer themselves. Is it possible that the spirit of optimism they gain from witnessing their pets' improvement is powerful enough to help them stave off this dread disease, too? Or as Emmanuel puts it so wisely, "Illness is a teaching, a message from the soul. When the lessons are learned, the illness becomes a thing of no moment."

white and beautiful, I promise you that there would be less cancer and less death from it. Souls would choose other ways. The issue of cancer is the issue of fear—cancer brings a message of fear—that is so prevalent in all your world. And so the illness must be dealt with squarely as fear. Once cancer is cured there will be something else. People have to deal with fear because it is one of the greatest denials of the reality of God." I can't tell you how often clients have called the next day to obtain initial blood results only to tell me, before treatment has even begun, that their pet seems a little better. The owner's new optimism has lifted the pet's spirits, with real, physical results.

A first-time client named Debbie Ewing provided a perfect example of this one Saturday morning, when she arrived at the clinic with a cat diagnosed as having terminal leukemia. As I examined the cat, Debbie launched into an anguished speech about all the New Age measures she'd taken to try to save him. It was everything I'd ever learned in the holistic field. Homeopathy, diets, crystals. Even pyramids: one of her measures involved pointing the cat under a prismatic pyramid at a certain hour, facing a certain direction. Suddenly she broke down in tears. "I don't understand!" she said. "This is the third cat I've owned, and it's the third cat that's dying of cancer."

"Whoa," I said. "I want you to understand something. Every time you have a cat, it dies of cancer. Think about it."

"What are you saying?" she said. "That I'm to blame?"

"Forget about whatever caused the deaths," I said. "Forget about blame. Just consider that there's a pattern, and that now we have an opportunity to break it."

By then, I'd come to see that there are three steps involved in addressing any problem: to identify it, to accept it, and then to handle it. The steps work in conjunction with each other, and in that particular sequence. Ignore any one of them, or follow them out of order, and the problem persists. Try to handle a problem before identifying it— you won't be able to. So often, owners come to Smith Ridge obsessed with getting their animals better right away. "What can we do to get him well today?" They want a quick fix without even knowing what's wrong. A quick fix may alleviate symptoms, but it won't address the underlying problem. What's really wrong with their pet? With Debbie, the problem wasn't that this cat was dying of leukemia. It was that one after another of her cats was getting cancer.

The second step is probably the most difficult to follow. You have to accept the condition as it is—its severity, and the reality it has in your pet's life and your own—in order not to be at the mercy of it. This was the step that Debbie had stumbled on. Rather than accept the fact that her cats had cancer, after considering why they might have gotten sick in the first place, she obsessed about how to make the problem go away. As soon as most owners hear that their pets have cancer, they assume the worst and become driven by the disease. In this way, they surrender control, and the disease almost inevitably wins. When they can see their pet's condition exactly as it is—when, that is, they can accept it— they can take charge. Which means going to the next step.

Once the first two steps have been surmounted, the third is easier to climb. The need here is simply to gather knowledge, learn all that one can about how to address the condition, and then apply that knowledge in working toward a cure.

Within a day of his visit to Smith Ridge, Debbie's cat died. The leukemia had been too advanced to be treated by any measures. I told Debbie that until she could identify the pattern in her own life that seemed to create such similar tragedies and fully accept it, she shouldn't get another cat.

Debbie began calling me regularly, as if I were her therapist, asking questions I couldn't answer. "Could it be the diet?" "Something about my rugs?" "Am I really a bad person deep down?" Then one day I got a different kind of call.

"I think I got it," Debbie said. For the first time in months, she seemed calm.

"I was walking down the street and I passed this pet store, and there were these kittens in a cage," she said. "They looked at me, and I saw my entire life flash in front of me. I saw the anxieties and fears and all the baggage I'd been carrying with me, but then I had an epiphany. Life, even with all the baggage, seemed okay. Suddenly, it all just lifted off my shoulders. I looked at those cats, and named them, and saw them as healthy—as staying healthy, in my care."

Sixteen years later, we are working long-distance on one of the cats she chose from that pet store. He's been healthy all that time. Now he has cancer, most likely from a rabies vaccine. I've treated it successfully for three years—a fibrosarcoma that kills most cats in a few months—and I'm convinced that part of what's pulling him through is his owner's positive attitude. You can't put into a medical textbook what Debbie felt, either before or after her revelation at the pet store. I see it as a shift in her energy, which in turn must affect the energy of her cat. Whatever it is, it seems to have helped keep Debbie from doing something that may have nudged cancerous cells into replicating in her cats. And if her change in attitude, after three dead cats, is merely coincidental with her next cats' long and healthy life spans, why *not* believe?

If owners can help ill pets by adopting a positive attitude, their pets can help them, too. Carol Marangoni, mother of Brunzi—discussed in Chapter Eight—now visits old-age homes with her other two goldens, Chaos and Barnes Berry. The dogs come dressed in outrageous costumes: as Dallas Cowboys with bandannas and football uniforms, or in dress appropriate for Halloween, Thanksgiving, or Christmas. Carol is convinced that the laughter and affection her dogs provoke has a salutary effect, not just on the elderly residents' spirits but on their physical health. And the nursing-home administrators agree. Hospitals are increasingly making use of pets to cheer up their patients. And in one recent study publicized on *60 Minutes*, animals from dogs to ducks were put in prisons where hard-core felons were allowed to care for them. The number of violent incidents among prisoners declined dramatically.

Almost every day in my practice, I see owners who've come to depend on their pets not merely for company but for an essential, life-affirming connection. Older owners who live alone and, for whatever reason, seem to have no friends or relatives. Younger owners who have emotional difficulty communicating with other people and practice, in effect, with a family dog or cat. Owners who have an illness and draw sustaining comfort from an affectionate pet. These last, in my experience, provide the most dramatic examples. I could give you dozens; I'll settle for one.

My acquaintance with a client named Jessica began with a frantic Saturday phone call from Trenton, New Jersey. Jessica's little dog Sally, a tan-and-white terrier, had been diagnosed with an aggressive cancer called neurofibroma on one of her legs. Veterinarians at the University of Pennsylvania had removed it, but after just weeks it had grown back. Now the veterinarians wanted to amputate Sally's diseased leg and put her on chemotherapy. I told Jessica that with a tumor this aggressive, she should bring Sally to my office Monday morning.

"I can't do that," Jessica told me.

"Why?"

"Because I'm admitting myself to a mental hospital tomorrow."

Great, I thought. And we're worried about the dog?

"Even if I did," she said, "I have a phobia about driving over bridges, and there are at least two bridges between me and where you are."

Great!

For twenty minutes, I stayed on the phone with her, trying to reason out a solution while my schedule backed up. Finally I said, "Look, you just have to be here Monday if you want to save your dog. And that's that."

Monday morning at about 11:00 a.m., I was in my examining room and called for the next patient. A very spooked-looking woman entered with her little dog. Beside the woman was a young, jovial-looking guy who seemed completely incongruous. It took me a minute to connect this woman with the one who'd called two days before.

"Congratulations on not admitting yourself to the hospital," I said. "How'd you get over those bridges?"

"Ralph, my neighbor, drove me," Jessica said, indicating her sidekick.

I examined Sally and then showed Jessica my photo album of before-and-after cancer cases. She barely looked up at them, and not once did she look up at me. "It's not going to work on my dog," she said more than once. "I don't even want to look at those pictures because I'll just get depressed knowing my dog couldn't be saved."

If Jessica was unreachable, though, Ralph was beaming as he looked at the pictures. He really got it. As for Sally, I realized that this little twenty-two-pound bundle, despite her cancer, was delighted, too—by the pictures, or just by the sheer fun of taking a trip, who knew. For some reason, seeing how happy that dog was made me a bit slaphappy, too. Still unable to get through to Jessica, I tried a new tactic. "Do you realize that if it wasn't for your dog's cancer, you'd be in a nuthouse now?"

Jessica suddenly looked up. "What?"

"So maybe there's a reason Sally has cancer." I was really winging it here, just looking for any reaction.

"Wait a minute," Jessica said. "I never thought about that."

"So do you think that maybe this dog grew this tumor to save your life?" I said. "Because without this tumor, you'd be on drugs now. Hell, you'd probably be having electroshock therapy."

"Wow," said Jessica. "I never thought of that. Show me those pictures again!"

As soon as Sally's blood samples were analyzed, we started IAT long-distance, sending Jessica the appropriate dosages and having her inject Sally herself. Jessica reported that the tumor was diminishing. Then she told me it was gone. Uncertain about her judgment, I arranged to speak with her local veterinarian. He confirmed the absence of the tumor. I never saw Sally again, because Ralph moved to Cincinnati and Jessica still had her phobia about bridges, so she couldn't get up to the clinic. After several years, Sally came off IAT and I lost contact with her—until a new client told me that she had been referred by Jessica, who sent her regards. From home, not a mental hospital. I assumed Sally was dead by now, and refrained from asking about her, but the client volunteered that Sally was doing fine.

Six years later, a dog whose leg would have been amputated and whose life expectancy even after surgery was said to be a year at best, was healthy and cancer-free—at about twelve years old. And Jessica, whose own lease on life had been nearly as tenuous, sent her regards.

Had Sally kept Jessica from entering a mental hospital? Had she saved her life? At the least, some very real emotional bond had enabled pet and owner to help each other profoundly.

For many pet owners, the issue of spirituality and pets is a literal one. Not only do pets have spirits; animal communicators can connect with them. I guess I feel the same way about animal communicators as I do about channelers of human spirits: I'm not totally persuaded, but not closed-minded. I admit that the idea of an animal communicator talking on the phone long-distance to a dog at the other end and purporting to divine his thoughts may seem dubious. But I have to report that I've been staggered by what some communicators "learned."

One incident involved a shih tzu named Barney, who belonged to two of my now-dearest friends, Suzen Ellis and her husband, Bob. Barney had a melanoma in his mouth, which I'd removed with cryosurgery. Unfortunately, it had grown back, and after a lot more therapy we began to fear that Barney might die. Suzen, who had always been open to New Age ideas, took it upon herself to contact an animal communicator, and to tape the conversation. I listened to the reading later and found much of it vague. Toward the end, though, came a message that was specific—and baffling. "He's really upset," he said, "because you took his view away."

Suzen was mystified until the next morning, when she turned in her bed to look out a window that extended from the floor nearly to the ceiling. There, at floor level, was the large air conditioner that had just been installed for summer. Barney's bed was right by that window, overlooking Suzen's beautiful wooded landscape. There was no way the communicator could have known that.

A second occasion was more personal. In the early 1990s, I was married to a woman named Quenya, who loves dogs as much as I do. One day, while we were still engaged, I went out to Port Jefferson, Long Island, to conduct one of the all-day seminars that I'd begun to give on my holistic therapies, and Quenya came along. The seminar's sponsor was a woman who bred papillons, the Thumbelinas of dogs. With her was an eight-week-old puppy, all of one pound. Quenya fell in love with him immediately. "We *have* to have him," she declared.

Unfortunately, the papillon cost $800, and for me at that time, finances were tight: I was counting on the $900 I would get from the seminar to pay for a number of upcoming wedding expenses. More-over, Quenya already had a dog named Kico who was in the final stages of old age, and getting a new dog now seemed disloyal. Endur-ing Quenya's hurt and resentment, I said no. Some days later, the breeder called Quenya, who then gave me the good news: the papillon was to be given to us as an engagement present, so impressed was the breeder by my seminar. (The breeder had merely given Quenya a mod-est discount. But I didn't learn that until later.) And so Alexander, as Quenya named him, joined our growing menagerie.

Not long afterward, Kico's condition declined and Quenya con-tacted an animal communicator to see if she could understand better what he was going through. A lot of the comments were along the lines of "Well, he's tired, but he wants to fight. . . ." Then Quenya asked about Alexander. "He was one of your dogs in a past life," the commu-nicator declared. Quenya then identified this dog as a dog named Julie she had when she lived in Colombia. "By the way," the communicator said of Alexander. "He wants you to know he was really upset when you left him behind the first time."

This communicator lived way up north, near Syracuse. She knew no one we knew, so how did she know *that*?

A word of warning, though, on using animal communicators. A client whose pets I'd treated before came into the clinic with a dog who seemed to have some serious respiratory problem. I was leaning, reluc-tantly, toward taking an X ray when the client announced that before I did so, she would contact a world-famous communicator who had experience with animals. The communicator did her thing long-distance, channeling a sense of the dog's condition by phone, and then reported her findings to me. A lot of what she said sounded plausible, and when she suggested that the dog's lungs were cancer-free, I put off the X ray. When the dog failed after weeks to improve on nutritional supplements, I finally heeded my instincts: X rays showed that the dog was riddled with lung cancer.

That was the first and last time I've let an animal communicator affect my medical judgment to any degree. I will second a client's decision to seek one out, simply because the communicator's report may make the owner feel better and even shed some light on the overall situation. And I do keep an open mind. But I proceed with caution when channeling and veterinary medicine are combined.

That said, I've come to believe more and more strongly that pets and their owners do communicate in a nonphysical way, one that's not just emotional but spiritual. The concept as I sense it defies easy definition—that's part of what makes it spiritual!—but I can say one thing about it. As far as I'm concerned, a basic principle of holistic veterinary practice is that there are no coincidences.

I was reminded of that just last week when my friend Andrea Eastman, a Smith Ridge client of long standing, called to report that Oliver, her fourteen-and-a-half-year-old black-and-white mixed-breed dog, was having worsening eye problems. Another holistic veterinarian had prescribed some natural products that elicited no response. He then referred Andrea and Oliver to a board-certified ophthalmologist, who examined the dog and decided that surgery was necessary to save the troubled eye. Just to get another opinion, Andrea asked me to talk to the ophthalmologist, so I did. He seemed to have weighed the options with due care, so I agreed with his decision that Oliver needed surgery. Before I rang off, I also agreed to help him by stopping by Andrea's house to take a presurgical blood sample, and to make sure Oliver could withstand surgery.

In my office at the end of the day, I gathered the tools I would need to take the blood sample and happened to notice a bottle of Cosequin, the natural supplement discussed in Chapter Seven for the treatment of arthritis and other joint problems, sitting unexpectedly in the middle of my examining-room counter. "What's that doing there?" I mused. Suddenly I remembered having seen an article, many months before, on the *topical* use of an injectable substance similar to Cosequin—

known as Adequan—in the treatment of corneal ulcers. Why not give it a try?

I made up a solution of Adequan with sterile water and added it to my doctor's kit. When I got to Andrea's house, I administered a couple of drops to Oliver and took the blood sample. An hour later, she called me amazed. "What did you do?" she said. Oliver's eye was already better.

We canceled the surgery and kept on with the Adequan. Within three weeks, Oliver's eye was completely healed.

So was it a coincidence that that bottle of Cosequin happened to be on my desk, and that I happened to notice it, and that I happened to remember an article about the topical use of Adequan for corneal ulcers?

I don't think so.

Now consider an even more mind-bending thought: What if Oliver somehow communicated to me a plea not to undergo invasive surgery? What if that helped nudge me to think of the Cosequin? If that seems bizarre, consider Carlyn's story.

Carlyn Clayton, whom I mentioned in Chapter Two as having had a cat die of FIP, later suffered the loss of her dog Blackjack from mast cell cancer. Before Blackjack died, she asked him to come back to her in another dog's body, and to let her know when he did. Months later, Carlyn found herself walking past West 71st Street in Manhattan, near where she lives, en route to her dentist. A strong image came into her mind as she did—the image of a black bear cub. She went on to the dentist. Two hours later, as she was returning home, she envisioned the bear cub again, just as she was crossing 71st Street. She turned up the street, not quite knowing why she did, and found herself drawn toward her local pet store. In fact, she had bought all her supplies at the store just two days earlier.

"What are you doing back here?" the proprietor said with a smile.

In a cage behind him was a black puppy with fluffy hair.

"What's the story on that dog?" Carlyn asked. The puppy looked *exactly* like Blackjack.

"Oh, I sold him a while ago, but he got sick, so his owner returned him to me," the proprietor said. "He does seem very sick; he hasn't moved since he came back. I'm afraid we may have to put him to sleep."

Carlyn peered in at the inert dog. "Blackjack," she whispered.

The dog sat up.

"Hey," said the proprietor. "What did you do?"

"You'd never understand," Carlyn said, "but I'm taking him home."

As soon as the new puppy entered her apartment, he seemed to know its every corner as well as Blackjack had. He sought out Blackjack's special places; he curled up with Carlyn in just the same way. As far as Carlyn is concerned, he *is* Blackjack.

Far-fetched as it sounds, I do suspect that dogs and cats—and perhaps all animals—have powers of consciousness that we don't understand. And that along with those powers, they may be able to communicate on levels we can't perceive. After all, if dogs can hear high-pitched sounds that entirely elude us, who's to say they can't transmit sounds or signals outside our conscious range of perception, either? Consider this notion from the naturalist Henry Beston, which appeared in his book *The Outer Most House* in 1928:

> We need another and a wiser and perhaps a more mystical concept of animals. . . . In a world older and more complete than ours they move finished and complete, gifted with extensions of the senses we have lost or never attained, living by voices we shall never hear.

There's one other phenomenon that I think of as spiritual, because it occurs among some pets with no explanation except, possibly, that their spirits have prevailed.

With every serious case, I do what I can to instill hope in a patient's owner. Holistic medicine is nothing if not a therapy of hope: until an animal actually dies, there's hope of recovery from even the direst condition, because when you allow for miracles by persisting with the right natural supplements, sometimes they occur. Keep up hope, I tell those owners, for hope breeds perseverance, and perseverance, I'm convinced, is often the element that makes the difference in desperate cases. Yet privately, even I perceive some cases as hopeless, and send a sick pet home expecting to see no improvement, or to hear, soon enough, that he's died. And then, once in a while, the unimaginable occurs.

So it was with Annie, a bichon frise already paralyzed by the time I saw her. When you have a dog with a severe spinal problem, you have to decide whether to try acupuncture first or to send her right in for surgery. As a determining test, you stick a needle in the tip of the dog's tail. If you get a detectable movement from the tail, that's enough to make acupuncture the right first treatment. If you don't, into surgery she goes. With Annie, there was no tail movement. "Get her over to Dr. DeAngelis," I told the owner.

Martin DeAngelis, the well-known board-certified surgeon who's referred at least as many cases to me as I have to him over the years, started by doing a myelogram: injecting a radiographic dye into the spinal canal to see which of Annie's spinal discs was causing the paralysis. He injected the dye from both directions, yet the dye streams failed to meet; in between there was a space large enough to indicate that she had two ruptured discs, a very uncommon condition.

Still, Dr. DeAngelis went in surgically, actually removing the part of the backbone over each ruptured disc, then sewing the muscles back over them. After such operations, you hope for obvious signs of improvement within three weeks. With Annie, some feeling did return—but no movement, despite follow-up acupuncture treatments at Smith Ridge. Unfortunately, we told her owner, Annie would be paralyzed for life.

Over a year later, I got a call from the owner. "Annie's started walking," she said. "Right," I said. "No—she is!" the owner protested. "I don't believe it," I said. I felt sure she was mistaking a reflex reaction for conscious movement. "Bring her in."

In came Annie, walking slowly, but on all fours. I called Dr. DeAngelis and reminded him of the case. He laughed. "Do you know why she did that?" he asked.

"Why?" I said. I expected some complex medical analysis.

"To show you it could be done!"

"Far-out!" I said. Here was a distinguished veterinary surgeon celebrating the unexplainable. Acknowledging the spiritual. Suddenly, as a holistic veterinarian, I didn't feel so alone anymore.

As remarkable, in its own way, was the story of Shiki, a sixteen-year-old white poodle diagnosed as having terminal cancer of several internal organs and declared a hopeless case by the Animal Medical Center. Shiki belonged to a writer named Pat Lazarus, who was no stranger to holistic practices, having interviewed a number of holistic veterinarians, including my brother and me, for a book called *Keep Your Pet Healthy the Natural Way*. The following account is in her words, and begins with the first call she and her husband Joe made to Smith Ridge about Shiki.

Dr. Goldstein had, oddly (or so we thought at the time), urged us *not* to take Shiki immediately to him, but to "keep her at home with you for two days. The first thing we need to do is let her recover from the stress of separation and all the fright she's felt being in a hospital. Give her a few days to feel all comfy and safe with you again."

When we saw her crumpled there on the hospital floor, we felt that Dr. Goldstein was wrong. Shiki wouldn't last another two days without any medical care at all. Then again, the only medical care the center offered was to put her to sleep. We carried her down to the street and propped her up on the ground while we waited for the car service to take us home. (She couldn't bend her legs to lift forward as animals do, you see. If you didn't hold her up, she toppled onto her side, which distressed her so much.) Joe and I took turns kneeling beside her and holding her upright. Then I decided to test Dr. Goldstein's idea that "once Shiki feels she's going to be safely back home with you, you'll see improvement." Gingerly, I took one of my hands off her body. If she was going to topple, as I was sure she would, my other hand could still keep her basically upright.

Eventually Joe said, "Let me know when you get tired holding her up. The last thing we need right now is for her to fall over and hurt herself."

"Joe," I said, "she's been standing on her own for ten minutes."

Shiki did indeed improve further in the two days of Dr. Goldstein's prescribed "cozy time" with us at home. In those two days, he received all the Animal Medical Center's tests and records. . . . Using his training as an animal chiropractor, Dr. Goldstein found a point on Shiki's spine "that's really out of whack," he said. . . . [He] slightly twisted Shiki's neck in a way that looked as if he'd just gently nudged her to look to her left. Then he lifted her off the examining table and put her down on the floor. "Who's her favorite parent?" Joe was, as much as I hated admitting it. "Okay, Joe. Hold your hand up high in the air, and let's see if she'll try to get to it."

Shiki stood up on her hind legs grasping toward Joe's fingers. When she realized the fingers were too high, she made a straight-up leap in the air. Shiki wasn't going toward food, because Joe had none. She wasn't even repeating a trick she had been taught. She just saw her person obviously wanting her to do something, for some strange reason, and—since she was now physically able to do it—she did it.

Shiki's recovery wasn't quick or without cost. It was several weeks before she was back to her old spunky, bullheaded self. And the therapy was more complex than holistic therapy often is: it involved a rigidly controlled diet, several vitamin and mineral supplements, enzyme tablets, and two homeopathic remedies. But the cost of all this was about the same as it would have cost us to bury her.

Even Shiki's case pales next to that of Snoopy, whose story is so remarkable that he's become the poster boy for my affiliated foundation, Alternative Solutions to Animal Health, Inc., and a testament, more broadly, to the therapy of hope that holistic medicine is.

In 1994, Snoopy was an eleven-year-old terrier mix who one day fell down the stairs of his house. At first, he seemed fine, and his owners, a lovely couple, thought he was merely being clumsy. Soon, however, he began walking with difficulty. As his condition worsened, his owners took him to their local veterinarian, who referred them to a board-certified neurologist. The diagnosis: a tumor of the spinal cord in the neck region which was, the neurologist said, cancerous and inoperable. There was nothing to be done.

In despair, the owners came to Smith Ridge. Initial blood tests indicated cancerous activity in Snoopy's immune system, which aligned with the neurologist's diagnosis. So we started him on IAT, as well as supplements based on a nutritional analysis. Then—perhaps this was in bad taste—I asked the owners to videotape him over time as we treated him. Most likely the owners would end up with a videotape that simply showed the sad, irreversible decline of their beloved dog—hardly a tape they'd want to keep. But we had seen so many cases of "inoperable" tumors which we hadn't documented, and experienced such success with them on IAT, that it seemed a shame not to have a visual record of the treatment. If Snoopy did improve, what a testament that videotape would be.

Month after month, we treated a dog who remained paralyzed in all four legs. To transport him, Snoopy's owners took one of those firewood carriers made of canvas and cut four holes in it, one for each of his legs. When he wasn't being carried that way, Snoopy would be wheeled in a baby crib. Or just hung in the firewood carrier from a low branch of a tree in the yard. In this period, his weight dropped from twenty-five to fourteen pounds. In his neighborhood, he acquired a nickname: "Road Kill." And yet, as unlikely as it seemed, Snoopy remained one of the happiest little dogs I'd ever worked on. His mood was just always up—due in large part, I realized, to his owners' determination to be optimistic. And at least he could wag the tip of his tail, so I knew that his nerve system wasn't completely shot; somehow, a neural message was traveling from his brain to his tail.

After about six months of IAT treatment, blood tests showed that Snoopy's immune system had improved. Indeed, it seemed so healthy that we stopped the IAT program. He did remain paralyzed. At that point, I put him on intravenous vitamin C for three days. At the same time, I administered intravenous ozone. I'd just begun to work with ozone, and I'd read reports that it could be effective with canine paralysis.

Within a couple of weeks, Snoopy experienced a little movement in all four legs. Encouraged, his owners tried to make him walk by propping him up, then letting him stand free—letting the video camera run as they did. Every time, he just plopped down like a rag doll. Then came the unbelievable moment. An in-law pulled into the driveway; Snoopy, propped up, turned to see who had arrived; and then, on four shaky legs, he walked over to the visitor's car to see for himself.

Almost seventeen years old, Snoopy now walks normally. All evidence of the cancerous tumor is gone. He is, incredibly, a healthy dog. And happily for Smith Ridge, his remarkable odyssey, from paralysis to full recovery, including his first miraculous walk, was captured on videotape. That makes him a poster boy of a very different sort from those that sadly represent the fight against muscular dystrophy and other dread diseases. The poster need not illustrate a campaign in search of a cure.

It illustrates that the cure *is* here.

CHAPTER TEN

The Death of a Pet

With every pet, there comes a time when no therapy, holistic or conventional, can stave off the inevitable. No one who hasn't lived with a pet can appreciate how painful the leave-taking is, or how profound the mourning. Nor does the experience grow any easier from one pet to the next. I've lived with cats and dogs for nearly forty-five years, usually several at a time, and had to deal with the deaths of more than a dozen—sweet creatures all, who took joy in every day of their lives and brightened my own life with their loyalty and love. Each loss hurts as much as the last. In most cases, an owner suffers the added pain of having to serve—so it can seem at the time—as his own pet's executioner. Choosing euthanasia can provoke guilt, remorse, and often doubts. *Is this really the right time to have my pet put to sleep? If heroic measures give him a little more time, should I choose them instead? Do I want to pay the thousands of dollars those measures cost? Can I be so heartless as to let financial considerations determine whether my pet lives or dies?*

I can't help you avoid the difficult issues surrounding a pet's dying and death. What I *can* do is to share some thoughts about pets at the end of their lives, and the owners who love them, that may help you make decisions more easily, and to experience the leave-taking, when it does come, with less sorrow and anxiety. If I can manage to convey what I feel, from what I've seen at the clinic and experienced at home, you may even find yourself applying a word to the death of your pet you never expected to use. *Celebration.*

I'll say more about that word later on in this chapter. But let's start by considering the pet who still has a chance to live longer, either by enduring a gradually worsening condition or by undergoing a complex medical procedure. His owner has no time to think about celebration. He needs to know what to *do*.

If his pet is being treated by a conventional veterinarian who recommends a complex procedure, an owner should at least solicit another opinion from a holistic veterinarian. As these pages have shown, holistic therapies with very sick patients are often less invasive than those of conventional medicine; they may be less expensive, too. If the conventional veterinarian advises euthanasia, all the more reason for another point of view. A conventional veterinarian's judgment may be very wise indeed. But as several case histories in this book underscore, the call for euthanasia occasionally proves premature. At the least, holistic medicine is worth a try when a pet's prospects have been declared hopeless. At that stage, as I tell worried clients, there's really nothing to lose.

If a complex medical procedure does seem capable of prolonging a pet's life, I urge owners not to let their guilt—and their love—prevent them from making a rational decision that takes every factor into account. If I see a sixteen-year-old dog with terminal cancer who might gain two or three more months of compromised life by a complex operation, I'll tell the owners, bluntly, that they should at least consider not going through with it. The dog may be debilitated by the surgery, and will probably suffer residual pain, which, added to the discomfort he already feels, will leave him miserable during those extra three months, if he lives that long. Is this the kind of life that God or nature intended him to have? I don't think so. Let's try something noninvasive.

As for cost, it *is* a factor that no owner should feel guilty about considering. I personally feel that it should never be *the* factor for either owner or veterinarian. If it is for the owner, he'll live to regret his choice. (For couples, a euthanasia decision based on money often becomes a bitter issue.) I suppose there are veterinarians who will let an owner's lack of money determine the decision, but I'm certainly not one of them. I've never put a pet to sleep because his owner lacked the money to pay for his medical needs. (In fact, the foundation I've started is dedicated in part to helping finance the care of pets, especially those with cancer, whose owners can't afford proper therapy.) But sometimes money becomes an entrapping factor. Owners who spend $2,000 on conventional therapy and still have a very sick pet may feel that much more obligated to spend additional thousands of dollars, both to justify their investment and to make it all come out right in the end. Sometimes it just can't come out right; sometimes they may be unwilling to acknowledge that they can't afford to keep spending money this way, and that the consequences for their own lives will be catastrophic, both financially and emotionally. I do what I can in each individual case, listening until I begin to understand the circumstances. In all, I know that money *is* a factor, one that must be recognized and balanced against the others.

If money provokes one kind of guilt in owners, a reaction I call "If/Should" leads to another, often as painful and potentially long-lasting. Every owner desperately wants to do all he can for his pet. His love for his pet is pure; so is his intention. Yet as carefully as all his decisions are made about treatment, his pet will eventually be confronted by an illness or condition he cannot overcome. That's life—and death! Unfortunately, an owner tends to blame himself at this point. *If* only he had chosen that other course of treatment. . . . He *should* have recognized those telltale symptoms so much sooner than he did. Then, he anguishes, often for years, his pet would still be alive. But for *every* course taken, we can imagine another: an *"if"* and *"should"* not pursued. That's needless self-punishment; it is, in fact, neurotic behavior. All we can do is make decisions that seem best at the time. And in cases where death really is imminent, there is no "better" decision than the one you chose to make. Don't dwell in the house of ifs and shoulds. The fact is: you can't second-guess death.

A complex procedure, at least, offers a clear choice. What about the ill pet who can't be helped by surgery, whose condition is deteriorating steadily but slowly? How can we know in these situations when to let the pet go on until he dies at home, and when to concede that euthanasia is best?

When a pet is in little or no pain and his illness isn't severely impeding a life-sustaining function—like breathing—I'll work toward natural passage, which is to say letting the pet die peacefully when he's ready, preferably at home. Sometimes, if he's been in the hospital and I've sent him home to die, I'll get a baffled call from the owner two days later. "He's getting better!" he'll report. "He's almost normal again!" The miraculous recovery, when it does occur, may in part be a result of giving the remedies time to take effect. But also, as we saw in Chapter Nine with the little white poodle named Shiki, a sick pet put into a veterinary hospital comes to feel depressed and abandoned, which has to affect his condition. Restored to his family, he may just find the energy and hope to fight his way back to health.*

Euthanasia is never preferable to a natural passage. If a pet is suffering, however, it seems as merciful a choice to a holistic veterinarian as it does to a conventional one. One injection of a very strong anesthetic, usually sodium pentobarbital, will end a pet's life painlessly in one or two seconds. (Usually, by the time the first cc is injected, the pet is already gone.) For a pet who's really suffering, with no hope of feeling better, euthanasia comes as a blessing. The question is: How do we know when a pet has reached that stage?

I wish I could put a nice neat chart on the opposite page showing exactly when a very ill dog or cat should be euthanized. Across the top would be numbers to indicate the animal's age. Down the side would be every disease we've discussed, in various shadings to show degrees of severity. In the appropriate box for your pet would be one of two words: Yes or No. All the uncertainty removed. No more second thoughts. Unfortunately, every case is different. The hardest decision you will ever have to make concerning your pet will always be an individual one, not quite like any other, and you will feel, as a result, conflicted about what's best. At the same time, I'm convinced you can make a decision untroubled by doubt.

How? I have a rule that's stood me in good stead throughout my practice. When a client calls me and asks if he should have his pet euthanized, I'll say let's discuss it. Usually, as the conversation unfolds, I'll know it's not yet time to put the pet to sleep. Why? Because a client who's asking questions is still in doubt. So I'll suggest to the client that we talk again in a few days after advising him on some treatment to help his pet's symptoms. If when he calls back he says, "It's time," then I'll know it's time, too, and I'll agree. I'm just the veterinarian, the out-

---

*The question of whether or not to keep a pet who seems terminally ill in the hospital is actually as complex as it is crucial. I usually recommend that a pet should be admitted to a hospital for a short stay. Aside from the constant care and monitoring a pet will receive, the chance to rest quietly, away from his owner, serves as a form of isolation, which is what he would choose to do naturally. At home, the pet has been expending vital emotional energy reacting to his owner's anxious presence. In the hospital, he can concentrate entirely on his own condition—and just possibly begin to improve. But that logic only applies for so long. All too often, I hear of terminally ill pets hospitalized for two or three weeks—essentially, until they die. That's completely unjustifiable. Because at a certain point, a pet is cut off from his family for so long that he loses his will to survive. At what point? One week is a good benchmark, but a veterinarian needs to be sensitive to each case and judge accordingly.

sider to an intense, emotional relationship that's lasted the pet's whole life and probably a decade or more of the client's own. The communication about ending that relationship is between *them*. They have to decide between themselves. And when the owner makes that decision—really makes it—there's rarely any doubt. The exception is when those questions are accompanied by a dire report—of bloody stools, of severe vomiting, labored breathing, and other symptoms that suggest rapid and irreversible decline in the patient's condition. In those cases, I'll nudge the conversation toward euthanasia, hoping the client is the first to actually come to that conclusion.

Granted, this is a rule with exceptions. Occasionally, I'll encounter an owner who's so emotionally attached to his pet that he's lost the capacity to conduct that communication, and may, as a result, keep a deeply suffering pet alive for his own emotional needs. Then I'll say, gently but firmly, "You must let go." Far more often, an owner comes to sense that his pet is tired of suffering, that his vital energy has drained away, that he is, with some instinctive awareness, ready to cross over.

Still, euthanasia is a difficult decision, and inevitably we hesitate about making it. Do we really have the right to decide if an animal should live or die? At first, the decision may seem beyond our scope. How presumptuous of us even to consider it! But what, really, are we bringing to an end? Only an animal's physical suffering. Your only intention is to do good for your pet. The prospect may cause sorrow; it may bring lingering grief. But it should not provoke guilt, anxiety, or even confusion. And when it's done, the reward, invariably, is relief.

In other words, if you feel anguished about euthanizing your pet, understand that the anguish is mostly yours—and not so much your pet's. You have a rational awareness of death; your pet doesn't, which is also to say that he has less fear of it. He lives more in the present than you do, and if he's presently suffering, he realizes instinctually what he needs to do. And I doubt that he blames you for the decision you're making. He loves you completely and irrevocably; he can't imagine not loving you. If you locked him in a closet by mistake and discovered your mistake three days later, he'd bound out of the closet, wagging his tail, *still* loving you. (Lock a family member in the closet by mistake for even an hour, and, believe me, you won't get that love when the door is unlocked. . . .) Can you really think that he would resent you now? If you do, just remember: That's what *you* think, not what *he* thinks. He's not the one who tries to deny the reality of death by cloaking it with mourning, funerals, and black limousines. You are.

Often, even owners who understand this feel a fierce sense of obligation to accompany their pets to the clinic or hospital where euthanasia is to occur, and to be with them during the procedure. This, in my experience, is not necessary. Just as an owner need not imagine that his pet is nurturing feelings of betrayal, nor should he think that his pet will feel hurt that he's not there for the pet's final moments. Remember: Animals in the wild go off on their own to die. They want no other being with them when they do; for them, this is a private and solitary act. If we have to deprive them of that dignity, as creatures in our urban society, we can at least respect their inclinations enough to say our good-byes at home.

If possible, I suggest that an owner then have a friend drive his pet to the clinic for euthanasia. This is for the owner's benefit, too: as painless as euthanasia is, an owner doesn't need to have that memory. It can actually blot out all the fond memories of his pet as a vigorous being and leave him haunted by sad associations. Over the years, I've had clients who've had more than one pet euthanized, and handled the leave-taking both ways. So many times, they've called to say that not going to the clinic with their pet, or just dropping him off with good-byes already said, worked better for them in the end. Still, paradoxically, a natural passage at home can be more comforting to a pet and his family. If the owners view it with the right attitude, it can even become the start of that curious word I mentioned earlier: *celebration*.

Years ago, a dear client, a young man who had a form of Hodgkin's disease, showed me a lot about celebration. He went out to Arizona with his fiancée to try a new kind of therapy, and had to leave his beloved old golden retriever behind. His parents cared for the dog back east, and at Smith Ridge, we checked her regularly. The client responded so well to the Hodgkin's therapy and to the Southwest that he decided to settle there; by then, we knew his dog had cancer, and we were battling it. "Just keep her alive until I can get her out here," the young man said. The dog made it through an intense surgery involving the removal of her spleen and part of her liver, and poked along in passable health until she turned fifteen, when she headed gently into an irreversible decline. "I can take her now," he reported. His parents put her on a plane to Arizona. Within a day or two of being reunited with her owner, the retriever died. The owner wasn't surprised, having heard our reports, and he chose not to dwell on the sadness of his dog's death. Instead, he arranged for a desert funeral service with a local tribe of Native Americans. At dawn the next day, they lifted up the retriever's body onto a celebration pyre that burned for hours while they all chanted and sang. It was, as the owner told me later, a celebration of the dog's spirit, not a mourning of the dog's physical life. And the owner, whose own sense of mortality had been sharpened, clearly, by his battle with Hodgkin's, said it was one of the most incredible days of his life.

If you live in a less rural setting, funeral pyres and Indian ceremonies may not go over well with your neighbors. But a simple burial service in a back garden can become a celebration, too. My coauthor, Michael Shnayerson, and his wife, Cheryl Merser, buried their terrier Annie a few days after New Year's in a spot within sight of their kitchen windows. "Light was one concern," Cheryl reports of the spot they chose. "When it was cool, Annie would seek out the sun, then seek out the shade in the heat. Shelter was another; she was tiny, and we didn't want a plot too exposed." The place they chose was sheltered by a lilac, in a corner of a garden bed set off by railroad ties. As Michael dug the hole and Cheryl held Annie wrapped in a favorite blanket, both were in tears. Yet by the time the burial was completed, they also felt grateful, even happy, that they could put Annie to rest in a place so close to them. Early that spring, Cheryl planted Annie's corner with flowers as vibrant as Annie had been: primroses, forget-me-nots, pansies, and a fragrant daphne. As they came into bloom, the flowers became an ongoing form of celebration: not of Annie's death but of her life and spirit.

Spirit is a word we touched on in Chapter Nine, but only in the broad, loosely defined context of spirituality. The bond between some owners and their pets might seem spiritual to one reader; to another it might seem emotional, or just instinctive. To my mind, though, the ways in which animal spirits appear at death and beyond are so tangible and vivid that I have no doubt, personally, of their existence. Doubt if you like, but I'm telling you: they're *there*.

Almost every natural passage of a pet I've witnessed has affirmed that belief for me. Often, as a pet dies naturally, his back arches and his legs go out straight, almost as if he were adopting a yoga position. At this point, the physical body is actually discharging its electrical neurons. As it does so, the energy, or chi, that was the pet's vital spirit is released. I can't tell you that I see it issuing upward. But I sure can feel it. And so can owners who've also witnessed it as their pets died. It's like a bolt of electrical current that displaces the ions around it as it shoots upward, as tangible in its way as the white light that so many people on the brink of death have described upon their return. Just before and during this phenomenon, a pet may appear to be suffering. Sometimes he may even have a tremor, or emit a howl of seeming anguish. In fact, these reactions are just physical, secondary to the electrical discharge (a process called "depolarization"). The sound is nothing more than the reaction of air passing through his larynx as his body contracts. By the time his back arches, spiritually and consciously the pet has crossed over, so that what appears to be a flexing due to pain is merely the final passage of his spirit from his body to the spiritual world.

One of the most vivid examples of this, for me, was the death of my ex-wife's dog Kico, at fifteen years old. Kico, a little white poodle, had had a great life despite the development of tumors in his old age. He'd remained a pain-free, happy dog with a healthy appetite. Suddenly he stopped eating. Somehow, Quenya and I just knew that Kico would die that night. So she slept with him in our bed, and, to give them space, I slept on the living room couch. At about 2:15 a.m., I suddenly woke up and went running into the bedroom. At the same moment, Quenya woke up, too. Within ten minutes, Kico died: his body arching up, in a reverse curve, his tail and head up, his legs splaying out. Then, just as abruptly, he relaxed.

As soon as that happened, it began to rain. It rained nonstop until about 11:00 a.m., when we had a garden burial service of our own, right outside the house. Just as the service began, the rain stopped. We put Kico gently into a freshly dug grave; when it was filled in, we planted a perennial on top. With the last shovelful of dirt, the rain resumed. It would keep on, steadily, through the day. "It's okay," Quenya told Kico, without any sadness now. "You'll be okay. And it's okay for you to come back to us." And truly, we both knew he *would* be okay.

So often, in the hours after a pet dies, his spirit seems to hover nearby. Other pets in a family seem preternaturally attuned to this: creatures who science tells us are incapable of comprehending death go out to a new grave, lie beside it, and solemnly cross their paws over the freshly turned dirt, communing, I'm convinced, with the spirit of their newly departed friend. I can't tell you how many times an owner who's lost a pet has told me, too, that he's felt the pet brushing against his leg, usually the first night after the pet's death. (So common is this feeling that I now counsel clients, in advance, not to think they're hallucinating if it happens.) Nor is it unusual for a pet's spirit to make itself heard through telltale sounds. Two sisters I know suffered the loss of Max, one of their shelties. They were watching television one night soon afterward, and heard a knock at the dog door—the same exact knock their shelty had been accustomed to making. When they checked, they found nothing. They even called their neighbor, who had a perfect view of the yard. The neighbor saw nothing. Astounded, they called me the next morning. "You won't believe this . . ." they started. "Well, maybe you *will*."

My own most startling experience occurred, in fact, during the writing of this book. Only three weeks before Christmas 1997, I'd adopted Terry, a little Pomeranian, by responding to a Humane Society plea aired on a local television show. As my friend Meg and I started out for home with him, we noticed a road sign for Tarrytown; that was how Terry got his name. In just three weeks, I bonded more closely with that little dog than any, I think, I'd ever known in my life. There was just something about him. Then, on Christmas Day, he was killed instantly by a car.

I guide so many people through the deaths of their pets that I'm rarely rattled by the experience. This time, though, I was devastated. I buried him in the other side garden, across from Kico, and then I called my friend Dave, who's always good for advice when I'm down. Dave heard me describe how Terry had been hit by a car right outside my house.

"Here's what I perceive," Dave said. "Terry was just flying around having a great time, and suddenly—boom—his body died. And without his body as a reference point, he's confused! He doesn't understand what's going on. You have to go back to the spot where he was killed and get in touch with him. Not verbally but—on the level of thought. Let him know what happened. And then guide him to safety. You'll know the process worked when you feel a weight lift off you."

At first, when I tried, nothing seemed to happen. I felt sort of foolish, to tell the truth, standing there by the roadside late on a cold Sunday afternoon, trying to commune with a dog spirit. I started walking back to the house, and then I thought—no. Do it right. So I tried again. And this time, the strangest feeling came over me. Not just a feeling of peace or relief but giddiness. I walked back to where he was buried and just laughed as I stood by the grave, because I felt Terry's presence right beside me. It was just as if I were taking him for a walk and actually saying "Come on, boy."

That night, I fell asleep on the couch with the Christmas tree lights on. I got up at about 4:30 a.m., and at first I felt sad, remembering Terry's death. Then I looked on my mantel, at the four Christmas socks I had put there, one for each of my pets. Suddenly the one we'd put up for Terry started playing "Jingle Bells." Now mind you, it was one of those socks that's got a little electronic chip in it which does play "Jingle Bells"—but only when you squeeze it in the right place. I was lying on the couch when it started playing. At first, I thought nothing of it. I stayed there, and then, ten minutes later, it started playing again! I got up, finally, and went over to make it play the song by squeezing the sock. Nothing happened—until I bent Santa's arm ninety degrees, as the toy was designed. How could this sock have started playing on its own?

I'm a sane person with a reasonably high IQ. I wasn't hallucinating, or sleepwalking, or drunk. Terry's spirit was in the house, that's all there is to it.

After a while, when you've heard enough stories of animal spirits and witnessed enough evidence of them yourself, you realize that death really *is* a celebration—and so ought to be viewed that way.

"Death is like taking off a tight shoe," writes Pat Rodegast of Emmanuel in her book. "Even when you're dead you're still alive. You do not cease to exist in death, that's only illusion. You go through the doorway of death alive, and there is no altering of the consciousness. It's not a strange land that you go to, but a land of living reality where the growth process is a continuation." I like that passage enough to have inscribed it, many times, in condolence cards to clients whose pets have died.

A lot of owners ask me if their animals have individual spirits, and if so, whether those spirits can evolve and reappear in other life forms. I certainly think so, and here again, Emmanuel puts it best: Of course they have evolving spirits, he says. "Consciousness must create what it is from the posture of its own existence. When a consciousness expands, it will grow to where it can reach beyond its present under- standing into greater wisdom. There is no end to evolution. You, yourselves, will evolve into beings far more brilliant, far more beautiful, and far wiser."

I've heard tell over the years from several sources that animals come from what's called a group spirit or soul, and that upon death they lose their individuality. Having lived and worked with so many dogs and cats, getting to know them as well as I have, and hearing so many accounts of their return, I believe that animals definitely have individual spirits. Are their spirits like ours? I think they're less complex. Humans have greater intelligence; the power of the animal spirit is its simplicity. We make ourselves miserable with our fear of death, and have an almost constitutional inability to live in the moment. Our pets have no vices. They love without qualification, exhibit loyalty and courage, have no fear of death, and live every moment fully for itself. Who's purer?

In that spirit—forgive the pun—consider this lovely passage posted on the Internet and credited to "Anonymous." One of my clients sent it to me as a tribute to a beloved dog, Bailey:

If you can start the day without caffeine,
If you can get going without pep pills,
If you can always be cheerful, ignoring aches and pains,
If you can resist complaining and boring people with your troubles,
If you can eat the same food every day and be grateful for it,
If you can understand when your loved ones are too busy to give you any time,
If you can overlook it when your loved ones take it out on you when, no fault of yours, something goes wrong,
If you can take criticism and blame without resentment,
If you can ignore a friend's limited education and never correct him,
If you can resist treating a rich friend better than a poor friend,
If you can face the world without lies and deceit,
If you can conquer tension without medical help,
If you can relax without liquor and sleep without the aid of drugs,
If you can say honestly that deep in your heart you have no prejudice against creed, color, religion, or politics,
Then, my friend, you are almost as good as your pet.

To which I'll add just this: if pets ruled the world, I have to believe that it would be in better shape than it is today. We've applied scientific intelligence to the earth—and all but destroyed it! How smart are we, anyway, to destroy our own home?

Emmanuel, for one, has no doubts about the higher purity of animal spirits. I went to hear Pat Rodegast lecture once on man's struggle up the mountain of spirituality, and how he's just beginning his climb "out of the valley." When she invited us to ask questions of Emmanuel—which she relayed to him psychically, or so she said—I asked if animals have spirits, and if so, how those spirits are different from human spirits. "Animals definitely have spirits," Emmanuel relayed back through Rodegast. "In fact, the animal spirit is already on top of the mountain we are ascending."

So we celebrate. And yet, to be sure, we continue to mourn. If losing a pet is hard at first, sometimes the harder time is later: a month later, three months, a year or more. If our pets were loved and loving members of our families—and what pet was ever not?—we cannot help but keenly feel their absence long after the shock of their death. Unfortunately, no one outside our families can appreciate that grief—at all! Your closest friends may be genuinely sympathetic when they first hear the news. A week later, if you tell them you're still feeling sad, they'll listen with barely masked impatience. Still grieving, a week later, over a *dog*? Come on, they're thinking: life goes on! A fellow pet owner may extend more sympathy, but the truth is that too many of us must bear the long-term sorrow of a pet's passing alone. Once we realize that, we often feel that much more reluctant to *stop* mourning. If beings live as long as they're remembered, we reason, then our pets' last vestige of existence is the memories we cherish of them. We ought not forget them, it's true, but if animals do have spirits, as I know they do, those spirits are zipping around happily free of their worn-out bodies, and we need not cling to our memories of them in a bleak or sorrowful way. That's one comfort to get us beyond mourning. The other is to find a new pet.

Most of us, when we first consider the prospect of a new pet to replace our "old" one, feel sharply conflicted. The very idea seems disrespectful to the pet we loved. That pet was an individual being, unique on this earth. You don't bring in a new one to take his place as you'd buy a new sofa to replace the one you carted off to the dump.

And what about us? We can't just transfer our love from one animal to the next. Anyway, no pet could be as loving, intelligent, and communicative as the pet we recently lost.

I sympathize with those feelings, but in my experience, both personally and professionally, they're misguided. Getting a new pet, rather than not, has proved to be, without exception, the right decision to make. And the sooner the better.

Consider, first, that in so doing, you're probably saving that next pet's life, or at the least assuring him a happy home. Not enough people in this world are willing to take on the responsibilities of properly caring for a pet. You are—and so you should. Moreover, having read this book, you're in a position to keep a pet healthier than he'd likely be in many other pet owners' homes. If you can make such a positive difference in another being's life, don't you want to do that?

You may feel unwilling, or unable as yet, to open your heart to a new pet, but as strongly as you may feel that, you are—fortunately— wrong. Start looking, and I *promise* you that sooner than you can imagine, you *will* find a pet you can love (or, more correctly, he will find you). When you do, you may also experience the phenomenon that proves to me, if any doubts remained, that pets do have spirits. I refer to the experience so many owners have related to me, and that I've had myself, of finding their departed pet's spirit alive and well, residing cheerfully—and knowingly—in their new pet.

When our little white poodle Kico died, my ex-wife Quenya and I felt too glum to replace him immediately. Several months later, a woman came to Smith Ridge with a standard poodle named Bernie suffering from lymphatic cancer of the intestines. As treatment got under way, I saw the woman and her dog regularly. When she mentioned that she also raised small white poodles, and took out a snapshot of a young litter, I was amazed. "They really look like Kico," I told her. Quenya actually chose one of the pups, a small female, to have the breeder bring back to show her. Instead, weeks later, the woman brought up a different pup, a male who, upon entering my hospital, made a beeline to Quenya, who happened to be sitting in the back office. Before she even realized that this was the breeder's dog, she exclaimed, "This is my dog! I want him!" As soon as we brought him to the house for the first time, he went zipping down the front yard, put on his brakes, and stared at Kico's grave site. Then he went into the house and felt right at home. "That dog doesn't just look like Kico," my ex-wife said. "That *is* Kico." More important, Clayton, as we named our new dog, simply removed the sharp feelings of grief which we'd lived with since the loss of Kico. How can you mourn the loss of a pet who's back in your life?

More recently, after Terry was killed, I decided to look for a Pomeranian to replace him. Because the clinic was consuming most of my time, I asked two of my employees, Meg and Julie, to follow up on an available litter in Pennsylvania. The two drove down one day and met the puppies' breeder in the town nearest his house. He directed them to follow him. As his car swung out ahead of theirs, they gasped: the breeder's car had a bumper sticker that read "Another Goldstein." The slogan, as it turned out, referred to a car dealership. Or did it? At any rate, the puppy they brought home not only looked and acted like Terry but had the same taste in music. This is Kooper, my newest family member. And it's true: with his arrival, our sense of loss over Terry has lifted.

By coincidence—or not—as I was finishing this chapter, I ran into a client named Angela Porpora at a business meeting. Angela had owned Wrinkles, the Rottweiler whose cancer I described in the introduction. So fast-growing was Wrinkles' rectal tumor, despite two cryosurgeries, that I'd had to put her to sleep. "You won't believe it," Angela said as she greeted me, beaming. "Wrinkles is back."

"What do you mean?" I asked, a bit warily.

"My new black-and-white cat," Angela said. "His name is Michael. Michael *is* Wrinkles."

At first, when Angela brought Michael home, she'd thought of him as a cat to replace one she'd lost to feline AIDS a few years ago. Anyway, he was a *cat*. There seemed no reason to assume a connection, spiritual or otherwise, between a black-and-white cat and a dead Rottweiler dog. Soon enough, however, Michael began to make the connections himself. He started playing with a stuffed animal toy in just the way Wrinkles had. He slept in Wrinkles' spot, batted Angela's legs with his paws just as Wrinkles had done, communicated with her as Wrinkles had, and even ate the same dog food Wrinkles had eaten, having shown no interest in the cat food first given him.

"That's when I started thinking about the essential connection," Angela explained. "Michael was born April 1, 1997. Wrinkles died six days later. Yet you know as well as I do that her spirit had started to leave her several days before she was put to sleep. The transfer of souls took place within that time, I'm convinced.

"All this time, I haven't let go of Wrinkles," Angela said. "In fact, I haven't washed my sliding glass doors in the bedroom because Wrinkles' nose prints are still on them, and I didn't want to lose that last connection with her. But you know what? I'm going to wash those windows now."

All pets die. All pet spirits, I truly believe, fly free when they do, into a sphere we can't begin to understand or perceive; in time they reappear in other newborn pets. And if we, as the stewards of those newborn pets, can feed them well and care for them holistically, we can ease their journeys through this next life, as they, with their utter delight in the world, ease ours.

Death, for most of us, is the hardest reality we have to face. Because animals' life spans are so much shorter than ours, their crossing over offers us the most extraordinary lesson, one we learn with every pet as we ourselves age. It may be that the most profound benefit of having a pet is that we come to understand better the experience of death, and, perhaps, lose some of our fear of it in the process. When our pets die and other pets come into our lives, the lesson becomes that much more inspirational, one that truly calls for celebration: death, our pets teach us, is necessary for new life to appear. Both for our pets and, eventually, for us, too.

EPILOGUE

One day, when I was about halfway through the writing of this book, my old cat, the Geeter, hobbled feebly into the woods behind my house as he always does. This time, he disappeared. My guess is that he was acting on a primitive instinct, going off to die in isolation as animals in the wild still do when they sense it's their time to go. At twenty-four, the Geeter could have died from any one of several specific ailments associated with old age. I have no idea which one he succumbed to, because I chose not to subject him to invasive procedures that might have provided the answer. I can say that the Geeter was not *suffering* from cancer or any other degenerative disease. He was feeble, he spent most of his time sleeping, he stopped grooming himself and would get matted with fleas, but he was eating well and would purr when you petted him. He was, as far as I could tell, about as happy and healthy as a very old cat can be, and it pleased me to think that by caring for him holistically, I might have added several years to his life span. It's not every cat that lives to the age of twenty-four.

And yet, I couldn't claim that I'd raised the Geeter from kittenhood using the holistic methods I practice today. He'd been with me for two decades, but he'd come to me as an adult. Though I don't know what vaccines or antibiotics he was given before he came into my life, I have to assume the list was considerable. At the least, the toxins he absorbed had to be expelled over a very long period by a strengthened immune system and the right diet. Moreover, he didn't get that diet as soon as I took him in, because my own perspective was different. I had begun exploring alternative therapies, and was already certified in acupuncture, but I hadn't begun to work seriously on my own health, and my practice was more conventional than alternative. In those two decades, everything changed, both for me and for the animals whom I treat.

As I sit here finishing this book at last, my youngest cat, Squeeki, wanders over to rub against my leg. Two and a half years ago, a friend went to drop her car off at the local gas station, and saw a week-old kitten in the hands of one of the young men pumping gas. The young man told her he couldn't keep the kitten himself, and didn't really know what to do with her. My friend said she knew a veterinarian who might help, and brought her over to Smith Ridge. The day I saw her, Squeeki looked more like a rat than a kitten. She was rodent-gray, with speckles of white and orange, her fur was dull, and her ribs were showing. And instead of purring, she squeaked, which is what inspired her name. But she was willing to be bottle-fed, and she ate well.

Over the next several days, she had various discharges. She coughed and sneezed, and produced a lot of phlegm. Her nose dripped, and her eyes were runny. I gave her an occasional homeopathic remedy but I did not take her in, as most owners would have, to a clinic to receive antibiotics. And when she was six weeks old, I didn't vaccinate her.

Besides protecting her from rabies, I have given Squeeki no other vaccines in those intervening months, either. At six months I gave her an anesthetic so I could spay her without causing any pain, but her body has absorbed no other drugs. She eats only the fresh food, cooked or raw, that I prepare for her, and drinks only distilled water. Her health is perfect—she hasn't been sick once—and she looks extraordinary. Her eyes glow, she doesn't have a speck of tartar on her teeth, and her coat is thick and shiny to the touch. Free to come and go as she pleases, foraging through the woods and padding back inside the house on her own schedule, she is living, to the fullest extent a domesticated cat can, the life that her forbears led thousands of years ago.

Often, when I look at Squeeki, I think: Here is the result of all I have learned in those decades since I began exploring alternative therapies. Here is a cat so clearly and radiantly healthy without drugs and low-grade commercial pet food, so happy and content in the purity of nature, that I *know* the lessons I've learned are true, and that the time it took to put them into practice was time well spent. And then I think of all the other dogs and cats not fortunate enough to enjoy such good health, whose immune systems struggle daily against the barrage of vaccines and drugs administered so often to them, and I think: *so much more to do*. So much getting out the word that another way is here. So many more animals to reach. The challenge seems overwhelming sometimes, but we have to keep at it. Dog by dog, cat by cat.

One animal at a time.

SOURCE GUIDE

This source guide is in three parts. Listed first is a compendium of holistic resources. What follows is a listing of veterinarians with whom I've interacted or have become familiar. The third section lists the manufacturers whose products I use in my practice.

As any reader of the preceding pages knows, many of the products I administer are packaged for humans and readily available at health food stores. Several of those products, however, are available only to licensed practitioners through distributors. I've mentioned these products throughout the book to be forthcoming about what I use, and I offer the following list of manufacturers in the same spirit. *Please do not call or write those manufacturers who, as noted, sell only to practitioners or wholesale.* Instead, show the source guide to your veterinarian, and let him or her use it as needed.

Since my full-time job is veterinarian, not product sampler, there may be other manufacturers whose holistic products are first-rate but are not listed here, simply because I haven't heard of them or haven't had a chance to try them yet. Please don't assume that a manufacturer omitted is necessarily inferior to those on the list. Ask around, get second opinions—and if you're impressed with the results, let me know!

Section I
COMPENDIUM OF HOLISTIC ANIMAL CARE RESOURCES

Organizations

Alternative Solutions to Animal Health, Inc.
400 Smith Ridge Road
South Salem, NY 10590
(914) 533-6269
(845) 734-4490

Alternative Solutions to Animal Health, Inc., is the nonprofit foundation that I founded. Some of the goals of this corporate endeavor are to investigate and compile all of the data accrued over twenty-five years of alternative veterinary practice into retrospective studies to be published in referred veterinary journals; to conduct prospective scientific veterinary research for the purpose of preventing, controlling, remediating, and, indeed, even "curing" cancer and other chronic degenerative diseases using holistic treatment modalities; and to disseminate this information for the purpose of educating and informing both veterinarians and laypersons alike about the efficacy of cancer treatment strategies that minimize the use of drugs and other widely used toxic treatment methods. Furthermore, the foundation would like to conduct a certain percentage of pro bono cases, such that viable non-toxic therapies can be made available to cancer patients whose owners could otherwise not afford them. All donations are gratefully acknowledged.

American Holistic Veterinary Medical Association (AHVMA)
2214 Old Emmorton Road
Bel Air, MD 21015
(410) 569-0795
Fax: (410) 515-7774

American Veterinary Chiropractic Association
623 Main
Hillsdale, IL 61257
(309) 658-2920
Fax: (309) 658-2622

American Veterinary Dental Society
708 South Owyhee
Boise, ID 83705
(208) 344-0194
Fax: (708) 344-7333

Canine Companions for Independence
P.O. Box 446
Santa Rosa, CA 95402-0446
(800) 767-BARK
Assistance dogs for the disabled.

Hemopet
17672-A Cowan, Suite 300
Irvine, CA 92614
(949) 252-8455
Fax: (949) 252-0224
Nonprofit animal blood bank and facility for vaccine titer testing.

Humane Society of the United States
2100 L Street, NW
Washington, D.C. 20037-1598
(202) 452-1100

International Veterinary Acupuncture Society (IVAS)
P.O. Box 2074
Nederland, CO 80466-2074
(303) 682-1167
Fax: (303) 682-1168

Morris Animal Foundation
45 Inverness Drive East
Englewood, CO 80112-5480
(800) 243-2345

Pet Savers Foundation, Inc.
14 Vanderventer Avenue
Port Washington, NY 10050
(516) 767-1627

Therapy Dogs International
6 Hilltop Road
Mendham, NJ 07945
(201) 543-0888

World Society for the Protection of Animals (WSPA)
29 Perkins Street, P.O. Box 190
Boston, MA 02130
(617) 522-7000

Recommended Publications

The Bark
(510) 704-0827
Published quarterly out of Berkeley, California, a really high-class magazine focused on the animal kingdom.

Best Friends Magazine
Best Friends Animal Santuary,
Kanab, UT 84741
(801) 644-2001

Canine Health Naturally
(604) 921-7784 (Canada)

Country Living's Healthy Living
Magazine
(800) 925-0485
Primarily for humans, but has a column addressing holistic health issues.

Enchanted Connections Review
18 Josephine Lane
Fort Salonga, NY 11768
(516) 269-7641
"Healing the Earth through Education."

Journal of the American Holistic
Veterinary Medical Association
2214 Old Emmorton Road
Bel Air, MD 21015
(410) 569-0795

Love of Animals
(800) 711-2292
Natural care and healing newsletter
by Dr. Robert and Susan Goldstein.

Natural Rearing
(541) 899-2080 (OR)
An excellent source for the latest
information on holistic pet care.

The Whole Dog Journal
(800) 829-9165
A type of *Consumer Reports* on holistic pet products and services.

BOOKS

All You Ever Wanted to know
About Herbs for Pets
Gregory Tilford and Mary
Wulff-Tilford
Bowtie Press

A comprehensive resource guide that
presents the theoretical underpinnings
of herbal medicine as well as the practical use of herbs for a wide variety of
pet ailments. An indispensable resource
in a "coffee-table book" package!

A Primer to Herbs for Animals
Gregory Tilford and Mary Wulff-Tilford

Are You Poisoning Your Pets?
Nina Anderson and Howard Peiper
Avery Publishing Group

This guide identifies household and
other daily toxins our pets are exposed to that contribute to poor
health and shortened life spans.

The Bach Remedies Repertory
F. J. Wheeler, M.D.
C. W. Daniel Company

Beyond Obedience: Training with
Awareness for You and Your Dog
April Frost
Harmony Books

A unique dog training approach that
focuses on the spiritual and psychological aspects of the human-animal
bond.

Cats: Homeopathic Remedies
George Macleod, M.R.C.V.S., D.V.S.M.

Dogs: Homeopathic Remedies
George Macleod, M.R.C.V.S., D.V.S.M.

A Veterinary Materia Medica and Clinical Repertory with a Materia Medica of The Nosodes
G. Macleod, M.R.C.V.S., D.V.S.M.

Cats Naturally
Juliette de Bairacli Levy
Faber & Faber

The Complete Herbal Handbook for the Dog and Cat
Juliette de Bairacli Levy
Faber & Faber

A forerunner in the natural rearing movement, de Bairacli Levy stresses the importance of a raw diet, natural rearing (no vaccines and other common toxins), and herbal remedies to treat a vast array of animal ailments.

Dogs Never Lie About Love: Reflections on the Emotional World of Dogs
Jeffrey Moussaieff Masson
Random House
A heartwarming look at the emotional lives of our canine companions.

Dr. Pitcairn's Complete Guide to Natural Health for Dogs & Cats
Richard H. Pitcairn, D.V.M., Ph.D., and Susan Hubble Pitcairn
Rodale Press

The classic book of natural therapies and homemade pet foods. No holistic library is complete without this book.

The Encyclopedia of Natural Pet Care
C. J. Puotinen
Keats Publishing

Extensive encyclopedia covering holistic health topics from A to Z.

First Pulse: A Personal Journey in Cancer Research
Dr. Merrill Garnett
First Pulse Projects, Inc.

By the developer of POLY-MVA, this is a fascinating discourse on the life force and cancer and how to battle this dreaded disease.

Food Pets Die For
Ann Martin
Newsage Press

Extensive investigation of the commercial pet food industry reveals horrifying details of the ingredients—not for the faint hearted! A must-read for people who are still feeding their pets commercial pet food.

Four Paws Five Directions: A Guide to Chinese Medicine for Cats and Dogs
Cheryl Schwartz, D.V.M.
Celestial Arts

Application of traditional Chinese herbal medicine to our animal companions. Also covers acupuncture, accupressure, and diet.

Give Your Dog a Bone
Ian Billinghurst, B.V.S. c[Hons],
B.S. cAgr., Dip. Ed.

Promotes the BARF (bones and raw food) diet for optimal health.

Grow Your Pup with Bones
Ian Billinghurst, B.V.S. c[Hons],
B.S. cAgr., Dip. Ed.

Advocates using the BARF diet to produce healthy puppies free of skeletal diseases such as dysplasia.

Heal Thyself
Edward Bach, M.D.
Sun Publishing

Herbal Remedies for Dogs and Cats
Mary Wulff-Tilford and Greg Tilford
(406) 821-4090

Holistic Guide for a Healthy Dog
Wendy Volhard and
Kerry Brown, D.V.M.
Howell Book House

An updated holistic health guide that covers raw diets, the vaccine controversy, homeopathic remedies, and more.

The Holistic Veterinary Handbook:
Safe, Effective Treatment Plans for
the Companion Animal Practitioner
William G. Winter, D.V.M.
Galde Press

Although targeted primarily for veterinarians, it is also useful for the nonprofessional. Contains client handouts on how to treat a variety of ailments using natural and holistic methods.

Homeopathic Care for Cats and Dogs:
Small Doses for Small Animals
Don Hamilton, D.V.M.
North Atlantic Books

It's for The Animals! Natural Care &
Resources
Helen L. McKinnon

Original, easy "big batch" method to make food that is fresh, wholesome and varied. It contains an extensive resource directory of interest to care-givers who want to provide holistic care for their pets. A portion of proceeds is donated to shelters and rescue.

Keep Your Dog Healthy
the Natural Way
Keep Your Cat Healthy the Natural Way
Pat Lazarus
Random House

Discusses holistic methods to keep your pets healthy and long-lived. A revision of one of the classical standards in holistic veterinary medicine.

Love, Miracles, and Animal Healing: A
Veterinarian's Journey from Physical
Medicine to Spiritual Understanding
Allen M. Schoen, D.V.M., M.S., and
Pam Proctor
Simon & Schuster

Heartwarming animal companion tales and holistic advice for the pet owner.

Natural Cat Care and
Natural Dog Care
Celeste Yarnall
Journey Editions

Natural rearing for dogs and cats, with emphasis on raw diets. I highly recommend these books.

The Natural Dog: A Complete Guide for
Caring Owners
Mary L. Brennan, D.V.M., with Norma
Eckroate
Plume

Comprehensive manual of natural pet care, from choosing the dog that's right for you to common health problems.

Natural Healing for Dogs and Cats A-Z.
Cheryl Schwartz, D.V.M.
Hay House

Alphabetical listings of animal ailments with holistic methods of treatment for each.

The Ultimate Diet: Natural Nutrition for Dogs and Cats
Kymythy Schultze, A.H.I.
Hay House

Promotes what the author calls a "species appropriate diet" for ultimate health. Includes a holistic animal Yellow Pages.

The Natural Remedy Book for Dogs and Cats
Diane Stein
The Crossing Press

Extensive number of animal ailments listed alphabetically, with a discussion of natural and homeopathic remedies for each.

The New Natural Cat
Anita Frazier and Norma Eckroate
E.P. Dutton

Natural rearing for cats.

Pack of Two: The Intricate Bond Between People and Dogs
Caroline Knapp
Delta

Wonderful story of the relationship between a human and her dog that illustrates how our canine companions can provide love and connectedness at the lowest points in our lives. A book for people who revel in delight when in the company of their dogs.

Pet Allergies: Remedies for an Epidemic
Alfred Plechner, D.V.M., and Martin Zucker

Pottenger's Cats
Francis M. Pottenger, Jr., M.D.
Price-Pottenger Nutrition Foundation, Inc.

A comparative study of feeding raw vs. cooked foods to generations of cats, documenting the detrimental consequences of a cooked/processed diet.

Rational Fasting
The Mucusless Diet Healing System
Arnold Ehret
Ehret Literature

Discusses how aging and disease are a function of diet, and the benefits of fasting.

Reigning Cats and Dogs: Good Nutrition Healthy Happy Animals
Pat McKay

A good introduction to raw-food diets for animals.

The Twelve Healers
Edward Bach, M.D.
C. W. Daniel Company

Super Nutrition for Dogs N' Cats: Preventive Medicine for Your Pet
Nina Anderson and Dr. Howard Peiper
Safe Goods

Vibrational Medicine: New Choices for Healing Ourselves
Richard Gerber, M.D.

Comprehensive coverage of energy fields, from acupuncture to radionics.

Source Guide

*Your Pet Isn't Sick—He Just
Wants You to Think So
Herb Tanzer, D.V.M.
Wharton Publishing*

Explains how the concept of pet illness must be expanded to include the entire family dynamics, and illustrates how the human caregivers unwittingly contribute to their pets' ailments.

BEREAVEMENT

*Animal Death, A Spiritual Journey
(Audio Tape)
Penelope Smith*

*The Courage to Grieve
Judy Tatelbaum*

*Pet Loss: A Thoughtful Guide for
Adults & Children
Herbert A. Nieburg and Arlene Fisher*

*Questions and Answers on Death
and Dying
Elisabeth Kubler-Ross, M.D.
Simon & Schuster*

*The Wheel of Life: A Memoir of
Living and Dying
Elisabeth Kubler-Ross, M.D.
Scribner*

Herbs and Flower Essences

*Anaflora Flower Essences
by Sharan Callahan
(530) 926-6424*

*Animals Apawthecary
(406) 821-4090*

*Crystal Garden Herbs
(802) 885-5500*

*Day Creek Herb Farm & Learning
Center
(530) 878-2441*

*Green Hope Farm Guide
(603) 469-3662*

*Healing Herbs for Pets
(888) 775-7387*

*Healing Spirits
(607) 566-2701*

*Herb Pharm
(800) 599-2392*

*Woodland Essence
(315) 845-1515*

Vaccinations

*Immunizations: The People Speak!
Neil Z. Miller
New Atlantean Press
Santa Fe, NM 87504
(505) 983-1856*

*Tetrahedron, Inc.
P.O. Box 2033
Sandpoint, ID 83864
(800) 336-9266*

*Vaccinations Do Not Protect
E. McBean, Ph.D., N.D.
Life Science*

*Vaccination the Silent Killer
Ida Honorof and E. McBean
Honor Publications
Sherman Oaks, California*

Source Guide

Who Killed the Darling Buds of May?
(What Vets Don't Know About Vaccines)
Catherine O'Driscoll

Natural Toys

Planet Dog Outfitters
(207) 761-1515
ECO-Buddy chew toy made from ecofleece, with ecofill stuffing.

Thunder Paws, Inc.
(717) 272-9977
Ecofleece organic catnip toys shaped like mice and rats, made from 87% recycled materials.

Supplements

ESSENTIAL FATTY ACIDS (EFA's)

Barlean's Organic Oils
(800) 445-3529
Products include Animal Oils, Flaxseed Oil, and Omega Twin.

Merritt Naturals Animal Essentials
(888) 463-7748
Contains marine lipids, organic flax oil, and spirulina. Available in a twist open gel cap form that keeps the oil fresh. Necessary supplement to maintain healthy skin, strong heart, and nervous system.

Vita Treat
(800) 929-0418
Certified organic flaxseed oil.

TREATS

Doggie Divines, Brunzi's Best, Inc.
toll-free: (877) Brunzi's, (877) 278-6947

Organically correct health food snacks. To drool for!

Coastside Bio Resources
(800) 732-8072
Sea Jerky treat containing sea chondroitin and glucosamine, for older dogs with joint discomfort.

KITTY LITTER

Some cat litters can be extremely hazardous, e.g., certain clumping litters. Many safe litters are available but are too numerous to list here. Please consult with your holistic veterinarian for recommendations for what is available in your area.

Affiliates for Natural Pet Care

Ambrican Enterprises Ltd.
(541) 899-2080
Wonderful resource for the latest information on supplements and homeopathic remedies. Certified in NAET and bioset techniques (allergy-elimination methods).

Harvey Cohen, D.C.
Noah's Kingdom
(800) 662-4711
Specializes in herbs and homeopathy. Has excellent supplements for dogs, cats, birds, and horses. Offers a unique pre-mix dog food, consisting of organic grains, vegetables, and herbs. You just add meat and essential fatty acids to create an excellent fresh meal.

Dynamite Specialty Products
(509) 697-4647

328

A company out of Washington State that has been producing quality supplemental products for the animal kingdom for many years. Products include nontoxic, earth-friendly fertilizer.

Earth Animal
(800) 622-0260

A wonderful mail-order catalogue and retail store in Westport, Connecticut, featuring the finest holistic pet care products. They offer the Bio-Nutritional Analysis program, designed to identify specific nutritional deficiencies and imbalances that may be present in your animal. This program can help supplement and support those deficiencies and/or imbalances by working with the animals' natural healing system to guide them back to health and to maintain wellness.

Susan Marino, R.N.
Angel's Gate Hospice for Animals
(516) 269-7641

First nonprofit hospice for animals in the country. Cares for terminally ill animals and animals in need of constant supervision. Donations welcome.

Barbara Meyers
Holistic Animal Consulting Center
(718) 720-5548

Human-animal bond consultant, flower essences expert, and certified grief therapist.

PetSage: A New Wisdom in Pet Care
(800) 738-4584

Very knowledgeable in holistic care for animals. An excellent comprehensive mail-order catalogue featuring a wide variety of natural-care products, including western and Chinese herbs, homeopathic remedies, nutritional supplements, and nonpesticide flea products. Specializes in care of senior animals.

Lynn Vaughan
(914) 764-8389

Licensed massage therapist who frequently works with holistic veterinarians to provide massage, energy work, and physical therapy for animals.

Whiskers
(800) Whiskers (944-7537)

Another must-have catalog filled with holistic products for pets. Whiskers offers their own homemade raw food diet for pet guardians who want to serve the optimal diet but do not have the time to prepare their pets' meals. Whiskers also has a great little store located in New York City for direct customer service.

ANIMAL COMMUNICATORS

This is a list of the animal communicators that I and/or my clients have found to be helpful, inspirational, and comforting.

Sharon Callahan(CA)
(530) 926-6424

Gail De Sciose (NY)
(212) 831-4666

Sonya Fitzpatrick (TX)
(281) 364-0608

Dawn Hayman
(315) 737-9339

Megan MacPhearson (MA)
(978) 456-8473

Sue Marino (NY)
(516) 269-7641

Marlene Sandler (PA)
(215) 491-0707

Marta Williams (CA)
(707) 829-8186

Section II
Holistic Veterinarians

The following is a listing of the holistic veterinarians with whom I've interacted or have become familiar. It is not intended to show favoritism.

There are many more highly trained and experienced consultants, but a complete listing would stagger this section.

A more comprehensive list is available from the American Holistic Veterinary Medical Association.

Thanks so much for your support.
Marty

American Holistic Veterinary Medical Association Directory

2214 Old Emmorton Road
Bel Air, MD 21015
(410) 569-0795
Fax: (410) 515-7774
E-mail: AHVMA@compuserve.com

You can also find this directory on the following Web site: www.altvetmed.com/ahvmadir.html

How to use this directory:

This referral directory of Holistic Veterinarians has been organized by state. Please look for your state, and then for telephone area codes that are in your area. You may also wish to check states adjoining yours. At the end of each veterinarian's listing are initials that tell you what modalities the doctor in question uses.

Modalities

AC—Acupuncture
AC(IVAS)—Acupuncture (International Veterinary Acupuncture Society certified)
Acuscope
AK—Applied Kinesiology
BF—Bach Flower Remedies
BI—Biotron II
CH—Chinese Herbs
CR—Chiropractic
CR(AVCA)—Chiropractic (American Veterinary Chiropractic Association certified)
CN—Clinical Nutrition
CT—Color Therapy
CM—Conventional Medicine
EAV—Electroacupuncture according to Voll
GT—Glandular Therapy
H—Homeopathy
HC—Homeopathy Classical
HC(AVH)—Homeopathy (Academy of Veterinary Homeopathy Certified)
HO—Homeopathy Other

IAT—Immuno-Augmentation
  Therapy (Cancer)
IN—Interro
NAET—Nambrudripad's Allergy
  Elimination Technique
NU—Nutrition
MA—Massage Therapy
MT—Magnetic Therapy
PMT—Pulsating Magnetic Therapy
Reiki
VOM—Veterinary Orthopedic
  Manipulation
WH—Western Herbs

ALASKA

Jeanne Olson, D.V.M.
1684 Palomino Drive
North Pole, AK 99705
(907) 488-2906
Small Animal, Equine, Farm Animal,
Avian, Exotic
AC(IVAS), BF, CH, WH, CR(AVCA),
CN, CM, GT, H, NU, MT

ARIZONA

Deborah C. Mallu, D.V.M.
215 Disney Lane
Sedona, AZ 86336
(520) 282-5651
Fax: (520) 282-3586
Small Animal
AC(IVAS), BF, CH, WH, CN, CM,
GT, HO, NU, Energy Healing, Animal
Communication, Medical Intuitive

CALIFORNIA

Robert A. Anderson, D.V.M.
1695 Clara Avenue
Fortuna, CA 95540
(707) 725-2472
Fax: (707) 725-2472
BF, CM, H, HC

Marc Bittan, D.V.M.
11673 National Blvd.
Los Angeles, CA 90064
(310) 231-4415
Fax:(310) 231-4418
Small Animal
AC, BF, CH, WH, CR, CN, CM, GT,
HC, HO, NU

Steve R. Blake, D.V.M.
12436 Grainwood Way
San Diego, CA 92131
(619) 566-3588
Fax: (619) 566-3588
Small Animal, Equine
AC(IVAS), BF, CN, CR, GT, HC
(AVH), NU, Aromatherapy

Gloria Dodd, D.V.M.
P.O. Box 1010
Boonville, CA 95415
(707) 895-3020
www.everglo-naturalvet.com
Small Animal, Equine
AC, AK, BF, WH, CR, CN, CT,
CM, EAV, GT, HC, HO, NU, MT,
MA, PMT, Crystal healing, Deray-
ing noxious energy fields, Radionics,
Dermatron

W. Jean Dodds, D.V.M.
938 Stanford Street
Santa Monica, CA 90403
(310) 828-4804
Fax: (310) 828-8251
Small Animal
BF, CH, WH, CN, CM, NU, Animal
Blood Bank

John B. Limehouse, D.V.M.
10742 Riverside Dr.
Toluca Lake, CA 91602
(818) 761-0787
Fax: (818) 761-0719
Small Animal
AC(IVAS), AK, BF, CH, WH,
CR(AVCA), CN, CM, EAV, GT, H,
HC, HO, IN, NU, MA

Priscilla Taylor-Limehouse, D.V.M.
10742 Riverside Drive
Toluca Lake, CA 91602
(818) 761-0787
Fax: (818) 761-0719
Small Animal
AC(IVAS), AK, BF, CH, WH, CR
(AVCA), CM, EAV, GT, HC, HO,
NU, MA

Richard Palmquist, D.V.M.
721 Centinela Ave.
Inglewood, CA 90302
(310) 673-1910
Fax: (310) 673-8089
Small Animal
AC, CN, CM, GT, H, NU

Nancy Scanlan, D.V.M.
13824 Moorpark Street
Sherman Oaks, CA 91423
Small Animal
(818) 784-9977
Fax: (818) 784-0293
Small Animal
AC(IVAS), CH, WH, CR, CN, HO,
NU, MA, Trigger point therapy

Cheryl Schwartz, D.V.M.
San Francisco Vet Specialists
3619 California St.
San Francisco, CA 94118
(415) 387-6844
Small Animal
AC(IVAS), BF, CH, WH, CT, HC,
HO, NU, MA

Neal K. Weiner, D.V.M.
P. O. Box 222
Mt. Shasta, CA 96087
(530) 242-0911
Fax: (530) 242-0195
Small Animal
AD, BF, WH, CR, CN, CM, GT, HO,
NU, Enzymatic Therapy

COLORADO

David H. Jaggar, M.R.C.V.S, D.C.
5139 Sugar Loaf Road
Boulder, CO 80302-9217
(303) 449-7936
Fax: (303) 449-8312
Small Animal, Equine, Farm Animal,
Avian
AC(IVAS), CH, WH, CR, NU,
Manual Therapy, Intra-Muscular
Stimulation

David McCluggage, D.V.M.
9390 Rogers Road
Longmont, CO 80503
(303) 702-1986
Fax:(303) 702-9602
Small Animal, Avian, Exotic
AC(IVAS), AK, BF, CH, WH, CR,
CN, CM, GT, HC, NU

Robert J. Silver, D.V.M.
685 S. Broadway Suite A
Boulder, CO 80303
(303) 494-7877
Fax: (303) 494-4496
Small Animal
AC(IVAS), BF, CH, CR, CN, GT, HO,
NU, MT, WH, Therapeutic Touch,
Crystal Healing, Human Animal Bond

CONNECTICUT

C. Christian Benyei, D.V.M.
199 Post Road West
Westport, CT 06880
(203) 226-1231
Fax: (203) 222-8601
Small Animal
AC, BF, HC, NU, CM

Marcie Fallek, D.V.M.
248 Alden St.
Fairfield, CT 06430
(203) 254-8642
Fax: (203) 255-0703
Small Animal
AC(IVAS), BF, WH, GT, HC, NU

Robert Goldstein, V.M.D.
Northern Skies Consultants
Bio-Nutritional Diagnostics
606 Post Road East
Westport, CT 06880
(203) 222-0260
Fax: (203) 227-8094
Bio-Nutritional Analysis (BNA), IAT,
BF, CH, CN, CM, GT, H, HO, NU,
WH

Allen M. Schoen, D.V.M.
15 Sunset Terrace
Sherman, CT 06784
(860) 354-2287
Fax: (860) 350-3482
Small Animal, Equine
AC(IVAS), CH, WH, CR(AVCA),
CM, CN, GT, H, NU, MT

Stephen Tobin, D.V.M.
26 Pleasant St.
Meriden, CT 06450
(203) 238-9863
Fax: (203) 237-2334
Small Animal, Equine, Farm Animal,
Avian, Exotic
WH, CN, CM, HC(AVH), NU

Neil C. Wolff, D.V.M.
530 E. Putnam Ave.
Greenwich, CT 06830
(203) 869-7755
AC(IVAS) BF, CH, CM, H, HC, HO,
NU, Laser AC

DELAWARE

Greig Howie, D.V.M.
21 Muirfield Ct.
Dover, DE 19901
(302) 734-8425
Small Animal
AC(IVAS), BF, WH, HC(AVH)

FLORIDA

John H. Fudens, D.V.M.
Affinity Holistic Clinic
(813) 446-3603
Fax: (813) 446-3546

Anne Lampru, D.V.M.
14923 N. Florida Ave.
Tampa, FL 33613
(813) 265-2411
Fax: (813) 962-4477
Small Animal
AC(IVAS), BF, CH, WH, CM, GT,
HC, NU

Russell Swift, D.V.M.
7154 N. University Dr. #86
Tamarac, FL 33321
(954) 720-0794
Fax: (954) 720-0978
Small Animal, Equine, Avian, Exotic
BF, GT, HC, NU

Arthur Young, D.V.M.
3003 S. Federal Highway
Stuart, FL 34994
(561) 287-2242
Fax: (561) 287-0089
Small Animal, Equine, Avian, Exotic
BF, WH, CN, CM, GT, HC(AVH), NU

GEORGIA

Mary Brennan, D.V.M.
965 Bobcat Court
Marietta, GA 30067
(770) 612-0318
Fax: (770) 916-9809
Equine
AC(IVAS), AK, BF, CH, WH, CR,
CN, CT, EAV, GT, HC, HO, NU,
MT, PMT, NAET

Michelle Tilghman, D.V.M.
1975 Glenn Club Drive
Stone Mountain, GA 30087
(770) 498-5956
Fax: (770) 498-3458
Small Animal
AC(IVAS), BF, CH, CR, CM, HO,
NU, MA, NAET

Susan Wynn, D.V.M.
1080 N. Cobb Parkway
Marietta, GA 30062
(770) 424-6303
Fax: (770) 426-4257
AC(IVAS), BF, CH, CN, CM, CR,
HC, HO, NU, WH, BI

HAWAII

Ihor Basko, D.V.M.
P. O. Box 159
Kapaa, HI 96746
(808) 828-1330
Fax: (808) 822-2452
Small Animal, Equine, Farm Animal,
Avian
AC(IVAS), BF, CH, CR, CN, CT,
CM, GT, HC, HO, NU, PMT, WH,
Laser Therapy Massage

IDAHO

Debra J. Mack, D.V.M.
3660 Flint Dr.
Eagle, ID 83616-4534
(208) 939-4800
Fax: (208) 939-7304
Small Animal
AC(IVAS), AK, BF, CH, CR(AVCA),
CN, GT, NU, NAET, Vibrational
Therapy

Heather K. Mack, D.V.M.
P.O. Box 597
Mountain Home, ID 83647-0597
(208) 366-7992
Small Animal, Equine
AC, BF, CH, CR, CM, HC, WH

ILLINOIS

Deborah M. Mitchell, D.V.M.
2237 W. Schaumburg Road
Schaumburg, IL 60172
(847) 893-8944
Fax: (847) 891-9040
Small Animal
AC(IVAS), AK, BF, CH, WH, CR
(AVCA), CM, GT, H, HO, NU MA

Judith Rae Swanson, D.V.M.
1465 W. Catalpa Ave.
Chicago, IL 60640
(773) 561-4526
Small Animal
AC(IVAS), BF, CN, GT, HO, NU, MA

Sharon L. Willoughby, D.V.M.
623 Main Street
Hillsdale, IL 61257
(309) 658-2920
Fax: (309) 658-2622
Small Animal, Equine, Farm Animal,
Avian, Exotic
CR

INDIANA

Terry Durkes, D.V.M.
909 N. Western Ave.
Marion, IN 46952
(755) 664-0734
Fax:(765) 851-9158
Small Animal, Avian, Exotic
AC(IVAS), CR, CM, MT

Mark P. Haverkos, D.V.M.
22163 Main St. Box 119
Oldenburg, IN 47036
(812) 934-2410
Fax: (812) 934-2410
Small Animal, Equine, Farm Animal,
Avian, Exotic
AC, AK, BF, WH, CR, CN, CM, HC,
NU, Laser Therapy

IOWA

William Pollak, D.V.M.
1115 East Madison Ave.
Fairfield, IA 52556
(515) 472-6983
BF, CH, WH, CN, CM, HC, NU,
Ayurvedic Medicine

KANSAS

Randy Kidd, D.V.M.
16879 46th Street
McLouth, KS 66054
(785) 863-3425
Fax: (785) 863-3425
Small Animal, Equine, Farm Animal,
Avian, Exotic
AC, BF, CR, CN, CM, HC, NU, WH,
Network Chiropractic

KENTUCKY

Joy Dunn, D.V.M.
236A Rd. 3
Mt. Vernon, KY 40456
(606) 256-5360
Small Animal
BF, CN, HC, NU

MARYLAND

Christina B. Chambreau, D.V.M.
908 Cold Bottom Road
Sparks, MD 21152
(410) 771-4968
Fax: (410) 771-4094
Small Animal
BF, CN, HC(AVH), Courses and
Workshops

Monique Maniet, D.V.M.
4820 Moorland Lane
Bethesda, MD 20814
(301) 656-2882
Fax: (301) 656-5033
Small Animal
AC(IVAS), BF, CH, CR, CN, CM,
GT, H, HC, NU, WH

Carvel G. Tiekert D.V.M.
2214 Old Emmorton Road
Bel Air, MD 21015
(410) 569-7777
Small Animal, Equine (Acpuncture,
Chiropractic)
AC(IVAS), BF, CR(AVCA), CN, CM,
GL, H, HC, BI, PMT, NU, AK

MASSACHUSETTS

Brian Corwin, D.V.M.
96 Inverness Lane
Longmeadow, MA 01106
(413) 565-5104
1-888-567-3840
Small Animal
AC, BF, CH, CN, CM, GT, HC, NU,
WH, Homotoxicology, Dr. Reckewee

Jeffrey Levy, D.V.M.
RR 01 Box 178-G
Williamsburg, MA 01096
(413) 268-3000
Fax: (413) 268-0333
Small Animal
H, HC, CN

Margo Roman, D.V.M.
72 W. Main St.
Hopkinton, MA 01748
(508) 435-4077
Fax: (508) 435-6274
Small Animal
AC, BF, WH, CN, HC, HO, NU

MINNESOTA

Roger DeHaan, D.V.M.
RR 1, Box 47A
33667 Peace River Ranch Rd.
Frazee, MN 56544
(218) 846-9112 (MWF 9–12)
Fax: (218) 846-9112
Small Animal, Equine
AC(IVAS), AK, BF, CH, WH, CR
(AVCA), CN, CM, GT, HO, NU,
MT, MA PMT

William G. Winter, D.V.M.
3131 Hennepin Ave. S.
Minneapolis, MN 55408
(800) 377-6369
Holistic Veterinary Handbook
AC(IVAS), BF, CH, CN, CM, GT, H,
HC, NU, MA, WH

NEBRASKA

Diane Simmons, D.V.M.
8625'½ Q St.
Ralston, NE 68127
(402) 593-6556
Fax: (402) 593-8810
Small Animal, Equine
AC(IVAS), AK, BF, CH, WH, CR, CN,
EAV, GT, HO, NU, MT, MA, NAET

NEVADA

Joanne Stefanatos, D.V.M.
1325 Vegas Valley Drive
Las Vegas, NV 89109
(702) 735-7184
Fax: (702) 732-4266
Small Animal, Avian, Exotic
AC(IVAS), AK, BF, CH, WH,
CR(AVCA), CN, CT, CM, EAV, GT,
HC(AVH), HO Bioenergetic, IN,
NU, MT, PMT, MA, NAET, ACMOS

NEW JERSEY

Gerald Buchoff, D.V.M.
9018 Kennedy Blvd.
North Bergen, NJ 07047
(201) 868-3753
Small Animal
AC(IVAS), BF, CH, CR, CN, GT,
HC, WH

Kenneth D. Fischer, D.V.M.
Hillsdale Animal Hospital
201 Broadway
Hillsdale, NJ 07642
(201) 358-6520
Fax: (201) 358-8332
Small Animal
AC, BF, CR, CN, GT

Robert W. Mueller, D.V.M.
261 Randolph Rd.
Freehold, NJ 07728
(732) 780-2202
Fax: (732) 780-5159

Source Guide

Small Animal, Equine
WH, CR, CM, MT

Mark D. Newkirk, D.V.M.
9200 Ventnor Ave.
Margate, NJ 08402
(609) 823-3031
Fax: (609) 822-9152
Small Animal, Avian, Exotic
AK, BF, WH, CR, CN, CM, GT, H,
NU, NAET, IAT

Charles T. Schenck, D.V.M.
777 Helmetta Blvd.
East Brunswick, NJ 08816
(732) 257-8882
Fax: (732) 254-2303
AC(IVAS), BF, CH, CN, CM, IN,
NU, MT

Gloria B. Weintrub, D.V.M.
190 Rt. 70
Medford, NJ 08055
(609) 953-3502
Fax: (609) 953-5907
Small Animal
AC(IVAS), AK, BF, CH, CR(AVCA),
CN, CM, GT, HO, IN, MT, NAET

NEW MEXICO

B. Dee Blanco, D.V.M.
P.O. Box 5865
Santa Fe, NM 87502-5865
(505) 986-3434
Fax: (505) 992-8522
Small Animal
AC(IVAS), BF, WH, CN, HC(AVH)

NEW YORK

Christine E. N. Aiken, D.V.M.
400 Smith Ridge Road
South Salem, NY 10590
(914) 533-6066
Fax: (914) 533-6405
Small Animal AC(IVAS), CH, WH, CN,
CM, GT, H, NU, Immuno Augmenta-
tive Therapy for Cancer, Ozone-therapy,
Cryosurgery, Poly-Vet Therapy

Marcie Fallek, D.V.M.
247 W. 11th St.
New York, NY 10014
(212) 216-9177
Small Animal
AC(IVAS), BF, WH, GT, HC, NU

Martin Goldstein, D.V.M.
400 Smith Ridge Road
South Salem, NY 10590
(914) 533-6066
Fax: (914) 533-6405
Small Animal, Equine
AC(IVAS), BF, CH, WH, CR, CN,
H, CM, GT, HO, NU, Immuno-
Augmentative Therapy (Cancer), Ozone
Therapy, Bio Nutritional Analysis
(BNA) Poly-Vet Therapy

Douglas Kappstatter, D.V.M.
144 7th St.
Bethpage, NY 11714
(516) 932-3089
Small Animal
AC(IVAS), CH, WH, CN, GT, HC

Sue Ann Lesser, D.V.M.
20 Burgess Ave.
South Huntington, NY 11746
(631) 423-9223
Fax: (631) 549-7760
Small Animal
AC, AK, CR(AVCA), GT, NU

Pavel Mihok, D.V.M.
400 Smith Ridge Road
South Salem, NY 10590
(914) 533-6066
Fax: (914) 533-6405
Small Animal
AC, BF, CH, WH, CR, CN, CM,
EAV, GT, H, NU Bio-Nutritional
Analysis (BNA), IAT

Phillip Raclyn, D.V.M.
219 W 79th St.
New York, NY 10024
(212) 787-1993
Fax: (212) 787-1397
Small Animal
AC(IVAS), BF, CH, WH, CR, CN,
CM, GT, MT, MA, PMT

Michele A. Yasson, D.V.M.
1101 Rt. 32
Rosendale, NY 12472
(914) 658-3923
Fax: (914) 658-3884
Small Animal, Equine
Has Office hours in New York City
on Tuesdays at 47 E. 30th
AC(IVAS), BF, WH, CN, GT, HC
(AVH), NU

NORTH CAROLINA

Charles E. Loops, D.V.M.
38 Waddell Hollow Rd.
Pittsboro, NC 27312
(919) 542-0442
Fax: (919) 542-0535
Small Animal, Equine, Farm Animal,
Avian, Exotic
BF, WH, CN, GT, HC, NU

OHIO

Donn W. Griffith, D.V.M.
3859 W. Dublin-Granville Rd.
Dublin, OH 43017
(614) 889-2556
Fax: (614) 761-3623
Small Animal, Avian, Exotic
AC(IVAS), AK, BF, CH, CR(AVCA),
CN, CT, CM, EAV, GT, H, HC, HO,
NU, BI, MT, MA, WH, Dog training,
Behavior modification

OREGON

Jeffrey Judkins, D.V.M.
1431 SE 23rd
Portland, OR 97214
(503) 233-2332
Fax: (503) 233-7246
Small Animal, Exotic
AC(IVAS), BF, CH, WH, CN, HC

Richard Pitcaim, D.V.M., Ph.D.
1253 Lincoln St.
Eugene, OR 97401
(541) 342-7665
Fax: (541) 344-5356
Small Animal
HC(AVH), NU

Donna M. Starita, D.V.M.
27728 SE Haley Rd.
Boring, OR 97009
(503) 663-7277
Fax: (503) 663-4069
Small Animal, Equine
AK, BF, CH, WH, CR, CN, CT, CM,
GT, HO, NU, MT, NAET, crystal and
gom essences, Qi Gong

Bob Ulbrich, V.M.D.
1431 SE 23rd Ave.
Portland, OR 97214
(503) 233-2332
Fax: (503) 233-7246
Small Animal
BF, CH, WH, GT, HC(AVH), NU,
Pranic healing

PENNSYLVANIA

Deva Kaur Khalsa, V.M.D.
1724 Yardley-Langhorne Rd.
Yardley, PA 19067-5517
(215) 493-0621
Fax: (215) 493-1944
Small Animal
AC(IVAS), AK, BF, CH, WH, CR,
CN, CM, GT, HO, HC, IN, NU,
NAET, Reiki, Rife Machine

Louise I. Morin, V.M.D.
Delaware Valley Animal Hospital
266 Lincoln Highway
Fairless Hills, PA 19030
(215) 946-1111
Fax: (215) 946-7757
Small Animal, Avian, Exotic
AC(IVAS), AK, BF, CN, CT, CM,
NU, NAET

Susan Yatsky, V.M.D.
341 W. Butler Avenue
New Britain, PA 18901
(215) 340-0345
Small Animal
AC(IVAS), AK, BF, CH, CR, CN,
CM, GT, H, NU, NAET

TEXAS

Nancy A. Bozeman, D.V.M.
5721 SW Green Oaks Blvd.
Arlington, TX 76017
(817) 572-2400
Fax: (817) 572-2026
Small Animal, Equine
AC(IVAS), BF, CH, WH, CR(AVCA),
CN, CM, GT, HC, NU, NAET, VOM
(Vet Orthopedic Manipulation)

Madalyn Ward, D.V.M.
11608 fm 1826
Austin, TX 78737
(512) 288-0428
Fax: (512) 288-1117
Equine
AC(IVAS), CR(AVCA), HC(AVH), NU,
CN

UTAH

Kimberly Henneman, D.V.M.
150 Starview Drive
Park City, UT 84098
(435) 647-0807
Fax: (435) 647-2985
Small Animal, Equine

AC(IVAS), BF, CH, WH, CR(AVCA),
CN, CM, HC, NU, MT, MA

VERMONT

William K. Kruesl, D.V.M.
87 East Clarendon Road
Cold River Veterinary Center
North Clarendon, VT 05759
(802) 747-4076
Small Animal
AC, BF, CH, WH, CN, CM, GT, H,
NU, MA, Ozone therapy, Alternative
Cancer therapies

VIRGINIA

Cheryl A. Caputo, D.V.M.
430 Roanoke Rd.
P.O. Box 240
Daleville, VA 24083
(540) 992-4550
Fax: (540) 992-6892
Small Animal AC(IVAS), AK, BF,
WH, CR, CN, CM, GT, HC, NU

Joyce Harman, D.V.M., M.R.C.V.S.
P.O. Box 488
Washington, VA 22747-0008
(540) 675-1855
Fax: (540) 675-1447
Small Animal, Equine, Avian
AC(IVAS), BF, CH, NU, Thermagraphy

Jordan A. Kocen, D.V.M.
6136 Brandon Ave.
Springfield, VA 22150
(703) 569-0300
Fax: (703) 866-4962
Small Animal
AC(IVAS), CH, HC

Source Guide

WASHINGTON

Michael W. Lemmon, D.V.M.
P.O. Box 2085
Renton, WA 98056
(425) 226-8418
Fax: (425) 228-7065
Small Animal
AC, BF, CH, WH, CR, CN, CM, GL,
HC, NU, MT, PMT

WISCONSIN

Maria H. Glinski, D.V.M.
1405 W. Silver Spring Drive
Glendale, WI 53209
(414) 228-7655
Small Animal
AC(IVAS), BF, CH, CR, CN CM,
EAV, GT, HC, HO, LT, MT, NU, WH

Pedro Luis Rivera, D.V.M.
2555 Wisconsin St.
Sturtevant, WI 53177
(414) 886-1100
Fax: (414) 886-6460
Small Animal, Equine, Farm Animal,
Avian, Exotic
BF, CH, WH, CR(AVCA), CN, CT,
CM, GT, HC, NU, MA, Feng Shui,
Physical Therapy

Anderw Zuckerman, D.V.M.
2163 N. Farwell Ave.
Milwaukee, WI 53202
(414) 276-0701
Fax: (414) 276-7019
Small Animal
AC, BF, CH, WH, CN, CM, NU

CANADA

Edward Beltran, B.V.M., Ph.D.,
M.R.C.V.S.
Blair Animal Hospital
(613) 746-2443

Paul McCutcheon, D.V.M.

805 O'Connor Dr.
Toronto, Ontario
Canada M4B 2S7
(416) 757-3569
Fax: (416) 285-7483
Small animal
BF, CN, CM, GT, HO, NU

Section III
MANUFACTURERS

Ambrican Enterprises Ltd.
Marina Zacharias
Heel Products
P.O. Box 1436
Jacksonville, OR 97530
(541) 899-2080

Ambrican is a primary source for Heel products, as well as a multitude of glandulars, herbals, and other nutritional specialties. Ambrican also publishes the newsletter "Natural Rearing."

Arrowroot Standard Direct
83 East Lancaster Avenue
Paoli, PA 19301
(800) 234-8879

Arrow Direct is a wholesale distributor for Standard Homeopathic, Inc. (210 West 131st Street, Los Angeles, CA 90061; [800] 624-9659). Large health food stores and pharmacies order from Standard Homeopathic; doctors and veterinarians order from Arrow Direct (which accepts no retail orders). From Arrow I get our supplies of Homeopet, the line of thirteen complex homeopathic remedies for diarrhea, vomiting, skin irritations, etc. In addition, Arrow has a wide array of vitamins, herbs, and nutraceuticals.

Bayside Quality Products
315 Franklin Avenue
Valley Stream, NY 11010
(888) 724-5489

Bayside sells English flower essences for people and pets. Specifically for animals, it also sells Homeopet.

Bio-Active Nutritional, Inc.
1803 N. Wickham Road, Suite 6
Melbourne, FL 32935
(800) 288-9525

Bio-Active offers botanicals, homeopathics, and nutritionals for both people and pets, but sells only to licensed practitioners and to certain health food stores run by pharmacists (where, due to their potency, Bio-Active products must be displayed within locked cases). Bio-Active has more than fifty botanicals, extracted from herbs, which range from apizelen, a German herbal complex used to help the body fight cancer, to vermaplex, which combats parasites, including tapeworm and roundworm, and is also used for constipation and intestinal problems. It has hundreds of homeopathic combinations, as well as some pure homeopathics. Among its best-selling nutritionals are Bio-Metabolic Balancer, a source of vitamin B, and Bone Developer, for pets with fractures and calcium problems.

Bioglan Animal Products
20481 Crescent Bay Drive
Lake Forest, CA 92630
(800) 888-0171

Bioglan sells only to distributors, but readers are welcome to call its 800 number to be directed to nearby stores that carry its products. In addition to products for healthy skin and coat, Bioglan has remedies for hip and joint pain; a medicine for hot spots; digestive supplements; and various shampoos.

Biotherapies, Inc.
9 Commerce Road
Fairfield, NJ 07004
(800) 700-7325

Biotherapies offers a wide array of natural dietary supplements, for people and pets, both wholesale and retail. The product I use most often is Cartivet, a shark cartilage product that I've found to be helpful in the treatment of cancer and arthritis.

Biovet, Biotec, and Biomed
940 Royal Street, Suite 309
New Orleans, LA 70116
(888) 468-7999

Biovet has been a pioneer in the application of the age- and disease-retarding antioxidant known as superoxide dismutase (SOD), both for people and pets. My favorite is AOX/PLX, which is particularly helpful with arthritis. Biovet also has a line of combination antioxidants called "Canine Support" and "Feline Support." Its new specialty is substances that repair misshapen red blood cells in just hours or a day or two, a boon in the treatment of damaged internal organs, especially the liver.

Botanical Laboratories, Inc.
1441 West Smith Road
Ferndale, WA 98248
(800) 232-4005

Complimed is a homeopathic line of remedies both for people and pets. It's strong enough to be FDA regulated, and is sold through prescription. Along with a number of products for general pet problems—arthritis, cold and flu, trauma—I use Quietiva for stress; Thyroid for thyroid problems; Asthmica for asthma, and Gastrica for gastrointestinal problems. Botanical Laboratories also carries an over-the-counter line of homeopathics called Natra-Bio. Though not as concentrated as Complimed, it's often just as effective, and I use a lot of it, especially Bladder Irritation, Teeth and Gums, and Head Cold.

Crystal Star Herbal Nutrition
4069 Wedge Way Court
Earth City, MO 63045
(800) 736-6015

Crystal Star offers whole-herb combination remedies, as opposed to the more traditional single-herb approach. Both for people and pets, it basically has a ready-made herbal remedy for every ailment. Among my favorites are AR-Ease, for arthritis, and Tinkle Caps, for urinary problems. Both wholesale and retail orders can be placed at the above number.

Dolisos
3014 Rigel Avenue
Las Vegas, NV 89102
(800) 365-4767

Dolisos has refined and distributed homeopathic medicines since its founding in France in 1937 by a pharmacist named Jean Tetau. Still based in France, the company produces tens of millions of preparations for subsidiaries all over the world. One we use a lot is thuja. Then there's silicea, which is nutritional support and chronic suppuration. But Dolisos also manufactures many other homeopathic single remedies. Some are available only to licensed practitioners, but thuja and silicea are available over the counter.

Dr. Goodpet
P.O. Box 4547
Inglewood, CA 90309
(800) 222-9932

Dr. Goodpet carries vitamins, enzymes, homeopathics, shampoos—anything for pets' health and well-being. I use many of the products in their homeopathic line: Flea Relief, Diar-Relief, and Calm Stress. Both wholesale and retail orders may be placed at the above number.

Doctors Mutual Service, Inc.
18722 Santee Lane
Valley Center, CA 92082
(800) 952-9568

Doctors Mutual offers a wide array of glandulars, enzymes, anti-inflamatory Betathyme, and Mega-lipotropic, which contains L-carnotine and promotes weight loss. To veterinarians, it also sells a lot of Serene, a calmant; Propolis, the beehive coating that works as a natural penicillin; and Colostrex (from colostrum), which helps build immunity and is helpful for diarrhea.

Earth Animal
606 Post Road East
Westport, CT 06880
(800) 622-0260
www.earthanimal.com

Founded by my brother, Dr. Robert Goldstein, and his wife, Susan, Earth Animal offers a complete line of all-natural products for dogs and cats, including organic foods, Daily Health Nuggets, and other nutritional supplements, cookies and treats, flea and tick prevention products, and shampoos. Earth Animal's exclusive products are available at its retail store (above), as well as through mail order.

John Ewing Company
P.O. Box 188
La Salle, CO 80645
(800) 525-8601

Ewing carries nutritional supplements for horses, dogs, cats, and humans. The one I use is MSM, which is a DMSO derivative that has an aspirin-like effect for pains and inflammation, especially for the joints. Both wholesale and retail orders may be placed at the above number.

Halo, Purely for Pets®
3438 East Lake Road, #14
Palm Harbor, FL 34685
(813) 854-2214

Halo distributes Anitra's Vita-Mineral Mix, a dietary powder that helps support bones, teeth, joints, and ligaments; calms nervous pets; helps eliminate shedding, dandruff, and greasy coat syndrome; and provides all the water-soluble vitamins missing from processed foods. Mixed in with a pet's regular food, it's also a tasty supplement. Anitra's Herbal Eyewash, available through Halo, is the most useful cleanser I've found to flush out irritants and rinse reddened eyes; I've also used it medicinally, for ulcerations of the eye. Dream Coat, one of Halo's best-sellers, is a liquid blend of oils that helps stop shedding, itching, scratching, dandruff, and dry skin. All these products, along with other supplements and herbal grooming aids, may be ordered from the above number.

Heel, Inc.
11600 Cochiti SE
Albuquerque, NM 87123-3376
(800) 621-7644

In 1936, German physician Dr. Hans-Heinrich Reckeweg created the first of his Heel homeopathic complex remedies. In 1979, having moved to the U.S., he created a second line, BHI. Since his death in 1985, the Heel company has carried on his work, and is regarded as one of the most distinguished producers of homeopathic remedies today. Among the dozens of Heel products, the best-seller is Traumeel, well known as an anti-inflammatory and analgesic. BHI's products are also homeopathic combinations, designed to address the parts of the body for which they're named: Sinus, Allergy, Stomach, Headache, and so forth. Heel sells only to licensed practitioners and distributors; if you can't find their products at your local health food store, consult a holistic veterinarian.

Institute for Traditional Medicine
2017 Southeast Hawthorne
Portland, OR, 97214
(800) 544-7504

The institute sells (and in some cases formulates) Chinese herbs for both people and pets, including Seven Forests. It prefers to sell to practitioners (who can buy the herbs wholesale), especially those who are already schooled in the properties of their products. Among the products often ordered for pets by holistic veterinarians are Omphalia II, a good parasite fighter; Drynaria, for arthritis; and Akebia for kidney problems. The institute also has several herbs useful in combating cancer.

Kroeger Herbs
805 Walnut Street
Boulder, CO 80302
(303) 443-0261

Though most of its products are designed for people, Kroeger Herbs offers a number of herbal formulas meant "to create an unfriendly environment" for parasites. Rascal is for tapeworms, Wormwood Combination is for roundworms, and Spiro Kete is for spirochetes. Kroeger also provides various homeopathic remedies for pets. Though it operates only as a wholesale outlet, its products may be ordered retail through its sister operation, Hannah's Herb Shop, 5681 Valmont Road, Boulder, CO 80301; (800) 206-6722.

Lucas Meyer, Inc.
P.O. Box 3218
Decatur, IL 62524
(217) 875-3660

Lucas Meyer is a supplier of the natural, fat-like substance called Phosphatidylserine (PS), which is used in many supplements for both people and pets. PS was first extracted in the mid-1980s to combat Alzheimer's disease. Since then, it has been recognized as having broader implications in the promotion of health and the reduction of stress. Lucas Meyer's PS is actually manufactured from soybean lecithin; administered to pets as a supplement called Pet-PS, it's been observed to be an aid not only in cognitive problems (i.e., the mental confusion of advancing age) but joint problems, coat and skin conditioning, and wound healing. Though Lucas Meyer is only a raw supplier, it can advise readers how to find Pet-PS at stores in their area.

Melaleuca, Inc.
3910 South Yellowstone Highway
Idaho Falls, ID 83402
(800) 282-3000

For pets, Melaleuca offers ProCare nutritional treats, herbal shampoos, and a coat lusterizer. A number of the products Melaleuca produces for people, however, are excellent for pets. The product we use most is tea tree oil (the scientific name is . . . melaleuca!), from the Australian tea tree; it's used as an antiseptic for ringworm or fungi, but also appears in their tea tree shampoo. Both wholesale and retail orders may be placed at the above number.

Miller Pharmacal Group, Inc.
350 Randy Road, Unit 2
Carol Stream, IL 60188
(800) 323-2935

Miller, which sells mainly to doctors, is one of my principal sources of animal glandulars. A staple of my practice is Mil Adrene, a raw adrenal glandular. Miller also has glandulars for the liver, heart, kidney, and stomach, among others. For the most part, these are "straight" glandulars, which is to say that no vitamins or minerals have been mixed into them. Sometimes the vitamins and minerals can help, but in other cases, the "straight" stuff is best.

NESS
8500 Northwest River Park Drive, #233
Parkveal, MO 64152
(800) 637-7893

NESS, which distributes only to licensed practitioners, is a prime source for Smith Ridge of enzyme powders and capsules for pets. The product line is called Vetzimes: V1 is a multiple digestive enzyme for dogs, V2 is a digestive enzyme for cats, V3 is an enzyme for healthy hair, coat, and skin for both dogs and cats, V4 is an enzyme for stronger immune systems for dogs and cats, and V5 is an enzyme for the feline urinary tract. (V1, V2, V3, and V5 are powders; V4 is a capsule.)

Norfields
632³/₄ N. Doheny Drive
Los Angeles, CA 90069
(800) 344-8400

Norfields was created with the intention and commitment to provide the best and most advanced magnetic therapy available for horses. With ten years of growing experience and success, Norfields Magnetic Therapy products have been clinically tested and are equally effective on bone, soft tissue, vascular problems, and injuries. The products are extremely useful both preventatively, to soothe and relax aching joints and muscles, and post injury and/or surgery, to speed up the recovery process. Norfields products give an edge to the athletic performance of all horses. Equally effective for dogs and cats. Norfields has a strong veterinary board consisting of equine practitioners who are using and testing our products and are familiar with our application techniques. Our board includes not only veterinarians (of which Martin Goldstein is one), but physical therapists, blacksmiths, and practitioners of holistic equine health.

Nu Biologics, Inc.
30 West 100 Butterfield Road
Warrenville, IL 60555
(800) 332-3130

For the most part, Nu Biologics supplies to chiropractors. Many of its products are useful for pets, however, including its glandulars. Specifically for pets, Nu Biologics carries a product called Eco-VM (Imhotep), a topical spray from grapefruit seed extract for general irritation and first-aid needs; Eco-VM Ear Care, a cleanser; and Seed-A-Sept, another grapefruit seed extract good for soaking inflamed ears. It also carries Progressive Labs, which has a thyroid supplement called Tri-40, GSC, a glandular for stress complex, and Adrenal Chelate, for adrenal support. Both wholesale and retail orders may be placed at the above number.

Nutramax Labs, Inc.
5024 Campbell Blvd
Baltimore, MD 21236
(800) 925-5187

Nutramax has three important veterinary products, all created at its own laboratories and available only to licensed practitioners. The first is Cosequin, which stimulates the production of cartilage cells, and so is useful for stiff joints and arthritis; I think it's the best supplement available for arthritis.

Nutrition Headquarters
One Nutrition Plaza
Carbondale, IL 62901
(800) 851-3551

Mostly products for people, but a few pet products, including shampoos and nutrition tablets. We use Nutrition Headquarters as our source for the common vitamins, such as A, C, and E, though of course these vitamins are available everywhere.

Nutritional Specialties PHP
P.O. Box 5897
Pittsburgh, PA 15209
(800) 245-1313

Nutritional's Professional Health Products includes an extensive line of homeopathics. In particular, I use Renal Drops, Pancreas Drops, Thyro Drops, homeopathic and gland support. I'm also partial to several PHP nutritionals, including Collagen Complex, Immuno Complex, and Renal Complex.

The Ohio Hempery, Inc.
P.O. Box 18
Guysville, OH 45735
(800) 289-4367

Hemp seed oil. "Nature's most balanced oil," rich in omega-3 and omega-6 essential fatty acids, and GLA.

Pet Health Pharmacy
13925 West Metler CK SP Boulevard
Suite 15
Sun City West, AZ 85375
(800) 742-0516

From Pet Health, we get our natural hydrocortisone, which has the same anti-inflammatory effect as synthetic cortisone (but without the side effects), and natural estrogen for female urinary incontinence.

Pet Power, Inc.
3627 East Indian School Road
Suite 209
Phoenix, AZ 85018
(800) 875-0096 or (602) 957-0096

Pet Power makes a cartilage formula, useful for arthritis, hip dysplasia, or other joint problems. Its tranquility formula is effective without leading to drowsiness or other side effects. Its nutritional products include bee pollen and digestive enzymes, and many vitamins and minerals. It also makes a topical propolis salve with whole-herb extracts, which helps heal topical abrasions or open wounds. Retail and wholesale orders at the above numbers.

Prozyme, Inc.
2567 Greenleaf Avenue
Elk Grove, IL 60007
(800) 522-5537

Prozyme offers a proprietary blend of enzymes obtained from natural sources. Ingredients include lactobacillus, lactos, protease (to help in the digestion of protein), and lipase (for digestion of fats).

Quantum Herbal Products Ltd.
20 DeWitt Drive
Saugerties, NY 12477
(800) 348-0398 or (914) 246-1344

Most of Quantum's products are intended for people, but they help animals, too. For pets in particular, Quantum makes a very effective and utterly nontoxic spray concentrate for fleas and ticks called, logically enough, 100% Natural Flea & Tick Repellant. Its primary ingredients are oils of erigeron, cajeput, and rose geranium, but it also contains concentrates of St. John's Wort, wormwood, black walnut, neem, and rue. I order it by the caseload. Quantum also makes Pet Salve, a topical salve for hot spots and other skin irritations, which stops pets from licking. Though Quantum sells mostly wholesale to health food stores, it does do mail-order business with customers who don't live near a retail outlet that stocks its products. Orders and requests for product brochures may be made at the above number.

Similasan Homeopathic Remedies
1321 South Central, Suite D
Kent, WA 98032
(800) 426-1644

Similasan Homeopathic is the U.S. distributor for about a dozen of the hundred remedies for both people and pets produced by its Swiss parent company. Its Similasan #1 eyedrops alleviate red, dry eyes; its #2 eyedrop formula is designed for eye symptoms brought on by allergies. I'm also fond of Similasan's homeopathic nasal spray and three different homeopathic cough remedies for different cough symptoms. Though it sells directly only to practitioners, health food stores, and pharmacies, it will mail catalogs upon request and steer customers to nearby outlets that stock its products.

Smith Ridge Veterinary Center
400 Smith Ridge Road
South Salem, NY 10590
(914) 533-6066
Fax: (914) 533-6405
www.smithridge.com

The purpose of Smith Ridge is to further and expand the treatment of animals through the utilization of nontoxic therapies, and to serve as an educational example and source to the professional and general public. Therapies include Bio Nutritional Analysis™, Immuno-Augmentative Therapy, acupuncture, homeopathy, chiropractic adjustment, conventional medicine and surgery, and cryosurgery.

Spoiled, LLC
128 Davis Hill Road
Weston, CT 06883
(203) 227-0137

Susan Ellis says, "Spoil yourself and your animals with optimum health. We use magnets and Far-Infrared products. Preventative breakthrough technology with no side effects. Relief of stress, increased energy, better quality sleep."

Standard Process Labs
P.O. Box 904
1200 West Royal Lee Drive
Palmyra, WI 53156
(800) 558-8740

Standard is the company that set the standard; it is the original distributor of glandulars formulated by Dr. Royal Lee in the late 1920s. Most of Standard's products are still designed for people, but an increasing number of veterinarians are using them. I order pure glandulars from Standard such as Drenatrophin (raw adrenal concentrate), and Pancreatrophin (raw pancreas), as well as Neurotrophin for epilepsy and brain tumors. Standard also carries whole-food vitamin and mineral products that include glandulars. (Dr. Lee felt that to be effective, whole-food nutrients need vitamins, minerals, and proteins; the glandulars supply the protein.) There are specific formulations for ailments, and others for replenishing the body's nutrient storehouses. One of the most popular choices among Standard's 140 products is Immuplex, for supporting the immune system. Standard Process sells only to licensed practitioners.

Vetri-Science Laboratories
20 New England Drive
Essex Junction, VT 05453-1504
(800) 882-9993

Vetri-Science's best-selling product is Glyco-Flex, concocted from the green-lipped mussel, which contains glycosaminoglycans (including chondroitin sulfates) to help restore connective tissue. (It's similar to Cosequin.) I've used it particularly to treat arthritis and hip dysplasia, as well as torn cartilage, in dogs. Glyco-Flex also helps reduce inflammation. Vetri-Science has two other joint therapy products: Vetri-Disc (used in the treatment of spondylosis deformans); and Glucosamine (single-source and multisource), which supplies cats with needed minerals (and is essentially Cosequin at a less expensive cost). It also sells a product called Acetylator, good for treatment of inflammatory bowel disease; antioxidants; and various vitamins, chiefly Canine Plus and Nu-Cat. All of Vetri-Science's products are available only to licensed practitioners.

Washington Homeopathic Products
4914 Del Ray Avenue
Bethesda, MD 20814
(800) 336-1695

Washington Homeopathic distributes a sizable line of homeopathic products. At Smith Ridge, we use a nosode for squamous cell carcinoma, and another for feline fibrosarcoma. (The nosodes are available only to licensed practitioners; the rest of Washington Homeopathic's products are generally available.) But for pets specifically, the company also manufactures Homeopet, a line of remedies for arthritis, anxiety, and the skin; Noah's Kingdom, a line that includes Aller-Ease, Scratch Free, Arth-Ease, and Calms Pet; and Equio Pathic, a line that includes Hoof, Preperformance Stress, and Dewormer.

APPENDIX A

More hope comes almost every month now from reports of new approaches to treating cancer that show real promise. To me, one of the most intriguing comes from Dr. Merrill Garnett, a laboratory researcher at the Long Island High Technology Incubator in Stony Brook. Merrill has developed a group of products that use what he defines as a "second genetic code," which bears a bit of explaining.

There's no debate that we all have a first code of DNA containing genetic information that makes us the individuals we are and gets passed from one generation to the next. But why, Garnett asks, does a living creature's genetic code remain unchanged when it dies? What must be missing is a second code for rapid energy storage and energy retrieval that allows us to be alive. Merrill feels this second code must exist as an electronic circuit that stores the electrical charge in DNA. Perhaps the second code is contained in "junk DNA"—the 85 percent of DNA considered extraneous to the "first" genetic code.

Merrill's products are metal-organic compounds—liquid crystals that revive the second genetic code in animals sick with cancer. Because these crystals have the same electronic frequencies as DNA, they do to primitive cancer cells what the second genetic code should have done in the first place: destroy the cells' membranes with one-quarter-volt electron flows.

In this country, Merrill's products are at the investigative stage, but in other countries, they have gained registration status. I'm open to all new ideas about cancer, and so have already administered these products to many cancer patients who had not responded to other therapies. I'm excited by some of the results I've witnessed, and even more impressed by the absence of side effects. As a result, I'm working closely with Merrill's company to develop an animal-specific product for veterinary medicine that already has a name: Poly-Vet. Being open to such new approaches is more than helpful in the treatment of cancer—it's essential.

INDEX

Index

arthritis, 19, 21, 35, 69, 110, 122, 127, 131, 132, 139, 160, 167, 186–8, 235, 267; acupuncture for, 155, 156, 188; causes and treatment, 186–8; homeopathics and herbs for, 139, 144, 150, 187–8; vaccines and, 71, 90, 186

asbestos, 34, 272

ash, 52

aspirin, 14

Association of American Feed Control Officials (AAFCO), 45–7 and n., 51, 52, 54–6

asthma, 68, 148, 155, 181, 182

astragalus, 147, 235

atopy, 36–7

atropine, 236

Australia, 73, 83

autism, 73, 74

autoimmune diseases, 121, 122, 185; vaccines and, 89–90

autoimmune hemolytic anemia (AIHA), 90, 185

autoimmune thyroiditis, 227n.

Bach, Dr. Edward, 151–2

Bach's flower remedies, 151–4

bacteria, 14, 26, 29–31, 63, 82, 197, 238; antibiotics and, 29–30 and n., 39–40; infections, 14, 29–31, 39–40, 90, 148, 167, 189–91, 200–202, 241, 244–5; vaccines and, 77

bad breath, 14, 57, 193, 194, 228

balance, 10; metabolic, 107–18, 120, 125, 192, 202, 204, 225–6, 235

Banting, Frederick G., 121

barometric pressure, 35–6

beagles, 283

Beauchamp, Antoine, 30–1

behavior disorders, 53

Belfield, Dr. Wendell O., 67, 123, 126, 254, 266

Bermans, 28

Beston, Henry, *The Outer Most House,* 298

beta-carotene, 125

BHA and BHT, 52

bichon frise, 298–9

bile, 227, 230

Biological Homeopathic Industries (BHI), 137–8, 141, 144, 182, 183

Bio Nutritional Analysis (BNA),

106–18, 119, 124, 125, 126, 132, 144, 224, 245

black walnut, 223, 248

bladder, 150; cancer, 141, 151, 263, 271–2; cystitis, 188–90; infections, 36, 47, 52, 150, 151, 188–90; stones, 191 and n.

BLDR-K, 150

blindness, 85, 86, 116–17, 268

bloat, gastric, 217–18

blood, 15n., 29–30, 90, 129; analysis, 6, 106–18, 158, 167–9; anemia, 184–6; cancer and, 257–62, 265–6, 267; homeopathics for bleeding, 141, 149; internal bleeding, 285; poisoning, 228; in stool, 238, 307; sugar, 121, 123, 148, 195–6, 236; transfusions, 185, 211, 260; in urine, 191, 222

blood urea nitrogen (BUN), 108 and n., 113–14, 230

Blue Earth Dragon, 92, 148, 151

bone(s), 127, 159; broken, 286; calcium, 132–3; cancer, 94, 141, 159, 185, 239, 254, 263, 274–6; eating, 61, 194; hip dysplasia, 223–5; infections, 176–7; marrow, 115, 168, 184–5, 209, 228, 259; spinal problems, 246–7

bone meal, 51

bordetella, 78, 104, 243–4; vaccine, 78, 79, 91, 92, 97, 244

boxers, 167–70, 282

brain, 107, 112, 125, 192, 224, 239; cancer, 268–9; epilepsy, 203–5

breeding, 186, 193, 240, 241; herbs for, 149; malformations, 28, 193; vaccines and, 81, 101–2

brewer's yeast, 216

bronchitis, 30, 148, 181, 182

brown rice, 22, 23, 58

bullous pemphigoid, 90

bursitis, 35

Burton, Dr. Lawrence, 235, 251, 257–65, 272, 276–8

calceria fluorica, 140

calcium, 35, 59, 111, 132 and n.; supplements, 132–3

calendula, 140, 182

calici, 78, 79, 86, 97

Canada, 49, 145, 174

cancer, 4–5, 9, 14, 16–17, 30, 50, 54, 60, 65, 66n., 98, 114, 118, 125,

Index

A NOTE ABOUT THE AUTHOR

Dr. Martin Goldstein earned both his B.S. and D.V.M. from Cornell University. He was certified in veterinary acupuncture by the International Veterinary Acupuncture Society in 1977, and in iridology in 1981. He continues to receive advanced education credits yearly by attending the American Holistic Veterinary Medical Society's annual conferences, where he also frequently lectures. Dr. Goldstein has written numerous articles about holistic veterinary medicine and alternative therapies for many magazines, journals, and related publications. He teaches the seminar "Fundamentals of Health and Disease from an Alternative Point of View" to both veterinarians and members of the general public. The seminar, six hours long and illustrated by four hundred slides, is the culmination of over two decades of his research and work in the field of alternative veterinary medicine. He has many happy and healthy dogs and cats, all of which are living proof of the philosophy contained in this book.